Herbal
Solutions
for
Healthy Living

*A Practical Guide to Using Herbal Solutions
Safely and Effectively*

*By Richard Scalzo, Herbalist and
Dr. Michael Cronin, Naturopathic Physician*

HERBAL RESEARCH PUBLICATIONS

D1316853

HERBAL RESEARCH PUBLICATIONS
108 Island Ford Rd.
Brevard, North Carolina, 28712

Library of Congress Cataloging -in-Publication Data
Scalzo, Richard & Cronin, Michael
Herbal Solutions for Healthy Living: A Practical Guide to Using
Herbal Solutions Safely and Effectively
Includes references and index.
ISBN 0-9707936-0-X

Cover design by   Kent Constable
Formatted by   RKR Graphics

Printed in the United States of America
9 8 7 6 5 4 3 2 1

ATTENTION

The information included in this book is for informational purposes
only. It is not intended to be used as a basis for self-treatment or as
a substitute for professional medical care. The reader should consult
a qualified health professional in regard to all symptoms, treatments,
and dosage recommendations. Any reader taking prescription medication must be especially careful to seek professional medical attention before using any part of the remedies described in this book.
The dosages discussed in this book are suggested dosages for adults,
not children. The authors and publisher disclaim any responsibility
for the adverse effects related to the usage of any information presented in this book. Any application of the information contained in
this book is at the reader's own discretion and risk.

Herbal Solutions *for* Healthy Living

PREFACE ON THE USE OF
STRUCTURE/FUNCTION INFORMATION

This book provides useful information on the function of these herbs within the human body. This information comes from a wide variety of resources that we have included at the end of each chapter. Within the structure/function information that we provide, we identify the reference by a number. This is to enable the reader to make decisions about the quality and reliability of the reference source for each statement.

The information in this book is intended to represent material supported by the traditional and historical use of herbal medicine, the contemporary use of naturopathic physicians and herbalists, and the accumulated scientific knowledge from around the globe from many cultures each investigating the medicinal herbs their culture and traditions have valued. Also the scientific references made are from authoritative sources from reliable research published by authors from around the world. This authoritative scientific material represents an evolving body of investigation into the safe and effective use of herbal medicines.

Whenever a structure/function statement is made or a description of use is provided within each formula or single remedy it is followed by an asterisk (*) and is expressly understood that "This information has not been evaluated by the FDA or the FTC and is in no way intended to diagnose, treat, cure, or prevent disease." If you read and/or utilize this material, you do so with the express understanding and acceptance of the above.

DEDICATION

Dedicated to the plants, who offer so tirelessly their healing properties and vast wisdom to all of us who trod upon this great earth. May we in turn reciprocate in kindness and honor and preserve this precious relationship.

Ric Scalzo

Dedicated in profound appreciation to my wife and partner, Dr. Kyle Hawk Cronin, and our three great kids, Michael, Patrick, and Lucas. In proud recognition of the next generation of healers and Naturopathic Medicine and Health Sciences.

Mike Cronin

Information on the practice of Dr. Michael Cronin and the team of naturopathic physicians he works with in Scottsdale, Arizona is online at:

www.integrativehealthcare.com

Further information on the use and applications of quality herbs can be found at:

www.gaiaherbs.com

ACKNOWLEDGEMENTS

The authors wish to express their deep thanks to the following people who have contributed vastly to this book:

Shayne Foley for his dedicated research and writing contributions.

Dr. Eric Yarnell, *Naturopathic Physician* for his contributions on many of the descriptive formulas and research contained in Chapter 6.

Joanne Snow, *Herbalist and Botanical Researcher* for her research and writing contributions on the single herb remedies contained in Chapter 5.

Karen Hardy, *Herbalist* for her contributions in researching and writing assistance of the Cautions, Contra-Indications, and Herb/Drug Interactions contained in Chapter 9

Karen Domanski for her contributions in compiling the information on Specific Indications of Single Herbs contained in Chapter 8.

Amy Stirling for her dedicated efforts in final stage editing.

And of course the ever expanding body and mind of nature and how it manifests into the healing plants. May they continue to inspire us to learn and assist us in our healing process.

Richard Scalzo, Herbalist and Botanical Researcher

CONTENTS

———————◆◆◆◆———————

HERBAL SOLUTIONS FOR HEALTHY LIVING

FOREWORD

The object of this guide it is to provide information that enables you to identify and use Herbal Solutions safely and effectively. Your decision making process in using herbs has multiple stages that involves choosing the indicated herbs, their dosage, frequency of use, and the best manufacturer. You must decide how to use several herbal products together, possibly in addition to prescription medications that you may be taking. Each chapter is written to provide you practical information to guide your decisions toward healthy living.

Chapter one describes the vitalistic principle that empowers plants as medicine, the Vis Medicatrix Naturae. Chapter two discusses the distinctions between a therapeutic strategy that uses single herbs and compares and contrasts that to a strategy that favors multiple herbs combined together in a formula. Chapter three is essential to making cost effective decisions about purchasing herbs. It discussed the improvements in the herbal products industry and how those changes make a more potent, standardized product. We explain the process of extraction, standardization, full spectrum standardization and the properties of the different types of herbal products from teas to fluid extracts. Chapter three also explains the issues of bioavailibility, dosage and frequency of use. In Chapter four we proudly present the newest option in herbal medicine, Liquid Phyto-Caps™, a patented delivery system that has the convenience of capsules with the advantages of bioavailibility found in herbal extracts. The features of Liquid Phyto-Caps™ include being the most potent choice in herbal medicine to date and provide "Quality without Compromise."

Chapters 5-7 contains detailed and fully referenced information about the function of individual herbs and the formulas designed by the authors addressing current lifestyle and health challenges. Chapter 5 describes the use and indications of ten single herbs in the form of Liquid Phyto-Caps™. Chapter 6 details the use and indications of over 30 formulas designed by the authors. Chapter 7 details the use and indications over 50 formulas with structure/function indications. Chapter 8 has the historical descriptions of the Eclectic physicians' favorite herbs.

These specific indications are still relevant and useful references for our use of single herbs today.

The safe use of herbs and the associated risks are addressed in Chapter 9, which contains information from over 60 medical references. This chapter documents the cautions and contraindications to use in specific health conditions. It also presents an understandable description of the complex interaction of herbs and prescription medicines when used together.

Chapter 10 answers frequently asked questions about the manufacture and use of herbal solutions. It includes a quality checklist to be used when purchasing herbal products to obtain the highest quality and the most cost effective remedies in terms of dosage and bioavailibility.

A list of General References that lists the books that are the most frequently used references we use is included. Please explore this list and consider investing in some of these books for your personal health library. The time and energy that you invest in understanding your body and its function in health and disease will pay dividends to you and your family through your life.

From the Authors,
Ric Scalzo and Mike Cronin

CHAPTER 1

HERBAL SOLUTIONS FOR HEALTHY LIVING –
THE VITAL FORCE OF NATURE

The plants represented in this book are medicines that carry the healing power of nature. They work with your body's vitality. The human body is powered by a vital energy; Vis Medicatrix Naturae is the healing power of nature. It is a concept that describes the miracle of nature that life is. Human beings are living, breathing beings made up of over 100 billion cells communicating with each other. Our body is 95% water organized by our DNA. Our cellular, circulatory, digestive and neuromuscular systems operate 24 hours a day. When our bodies are diseased they are capable of self-healing though the immune and repair functions. Rest, good nutrition, clean air and water are vital components in this healing process. Removing chemical toxins and emotional stress assists our healing process.

Plants are vital medicine and effective aids to our healing. Herbs are beautifully complex organisms that have a tremendous biochemical diversity of molecules that protect, stimulate and heal. Plants contain information that somehow reminds our bodies about homeostasis. Herbal medicines have a vitality that drugs do not.

Plants have been used as medicine since prehistory. The scientific knowledge of herbal medicines has been accumulating at a rapid rate for the last one hundred years. During this time we have been integrating our scientific knowledge with the accumulated wisdom and experience of traditional healers, herbalists and physicians. As we better understand the biochemical functions of the human body we use plant medicine more skillfully than ever before. This includes learning to use herbs in conjunction with drugs as well as how to use herbs instead of drugs. Through the Internet the most recent and exciting scientific research into botanical medicine is made available to the public, conventional physicians, and natural medicine practitioners.

Our ability to grow healthy medicinal plants has greatly improved. Organic agriculture enables the scientific formulation of organic fertilizers, optimum watering schedules, seed and plant selection and Bio-dynamic gardening. While medicinal plants are growing we have the ability to test for the quantity of active ingredients and select the precise time for harvesting to maximize healing principles. By using new extraction procedures the active ingredients are preserved and concentrated with the "full spectrum" of medicinal constituents present. New extraction procedures also capture a larger quantity of the plant's active ingredients.

In order to balance this eulogy on the wonders of science and herbal technology we should recognize the shadow side of our modern culture that requires that we have stronger natural medicines available. One disadvantage of life in the 21st century is our daily exposure to chemicals in the food, air, water, building materials and household chemicals. Our children are now exposed to thousands of chemicals that never before existed. The biochemical systems of our great grandparents never experienced these pollutants. We are in new territory.

When the toxicology of a chemical is researched its effect alone is considered in determining its lethal dose and potential for human harm. But it is the combination of chemicals that have a synergistic effect that amplifies their toxicity. No studies determine our total toxic load from all possible sources. Nobody is adding up the score!

In years past an herbal tea or a dilute alcohol tincture was able to effect a significant therapeutic result. Today a cup of herb tea is not strong enough to deal with the quantity and frequency of stress in our lives. We must learn to keep our family and ourselves healthy. The Vis Medicatrix Naturae, the healing power of nature, is on our side. We must protect our bodies delicate systems through reasonable actions that limit our exposure to toxins, by assisting our body to detoxify and eliminate chemicals. We need a good multi-vitamin/mineral. We need to utilize antioxidants in our diet and supplements. We should support our immune system, enhance our liver function and engage the biochemical equipment in our cells by using high quality herbal remedies. This means is that our herbal medicines need to be stronger, more potent than in the past.

CHAPTER 2

HERBAL SOLUTIONS FOR HEALTHY LIVING - STRATEGIES FOR HERBAL USE

Herbs are used for a variety of health conditions each requiring a treatment plan that includes the dosage, the frequency and duration of use. Our goal in this book is to give you information about using herbs to create solutions that improve the quality of your life. In acute infections we use herbs for a short period of time to boost the immunity and reduce symptoms. Herbs are also used to tonify the systems of our body such as digestion, immune, liver, circulatory and nervous system. Tonification is a supportive process that should be done periodically to those functions one knows are weak. Herbs are also used to treat specific symptoms such has headaches, depression and fatigue. Many people use herbs in conjunction with prescription medication for arthritis, heart disease, autoimmune conditions and cancer.

Herbal tonics will often increase the vitality of an organ system so that when the formula is discontinued normal function continues. Herbs may have an effect that improves a particular function although it may not completely stabilize it requiring ongoing support and supplementation.

Preventive self-care is an important part of maintaining control over our health. Intelligent use of herbal products as well as nutrients and multivitamins is an important component for a healthy, happy life. In the next chapter there are some successful strategies for using herbal medicine in a self-care environment. These prescribing procedures are similar to those used by natural medicine practitioners specializing in herbal medicine.

SINGLE REMEDIES

The use of single remedies for specific conditions is the most common use of herbs. Currently all research in medicinal plants is done on single plants for a specific condition. This approach is essential for identifying the qualities, effects and specific indications for use. The research often starts by looking at the traditional herbal literature and the experience of natural medicine

specialists to identify areas of promise. Then a search of the
medical literature occurs to identify what research has already
been done. A study is then designed that will give a specific
answer regarding the herb and its therapeutic effectiveness.
When using single remedies it is easier to determine if there has
been a positive result. Determining the correct therapeutic
dosage and frequency is more accurate.

St. John's Wort is an excellent example of an herb going from
clinical experience to research to clinical acceptance. It has been
shown effective in mild to moderate depression, seasonal affective
disorder and insomnia. The use of St. John's Wort by individuals
self prescribing has been safe and effective. The few negative reactions have been mostly with individuals already taking prescribed
antidepressants.

**Please note: In discussing the use of herbs in a self-care pro-
gram the individual often has more that one condition to be
addressed. Identifying an herbal product that focuses on
each condition may require the use of several herbal products, either single herbs or formulas.**

FORMULAS

Using well designed formulas is a second strategy for self-care
using for herbal medicines. Herbal formulas incorporate multiple herbs that are known to be effective when combined for specific conditions. Herbalists, naturopathic physicians and medical
doctors experienced in the use of herbal medicine know that
using multiple herbs in a well designed formula will often create
better clinical outcomes than a single herb because of the synergistic effect of the botanical medicines. Each plant in the formula has a different sphere of activity that has complementary therapeutic results.

Because formulas have multiple ingredients the quantity of
each herb is less than in a single herb product. This produces a
therapeutic action that supports multiple organs and functions in
the body in a gentle and generalized manner. Formulas are
described a having a "tonification" effect compared to a single
ingredient herb having a more focused effect towards a specific
outcome. Some people do better with an herbal formula, others
find that the correct single herb is a better solution.

A formula for liver support may include Chinese Bupleurum, Licorice, Reishi mushroom, Maitake, Astralagus, and Chinese Skullcap. This formula provides antioxidant protection to the liver, is antiviral and decreases inflammation and addresses multiple problems that may be caused by a liver infection like Hepatitis C.

A formula designed to provide antioxidant relief to multiple body functions under chemical stress could include Bilberry for the eyes, blood vessels, and connective tissue, Hawthorne and Grape seed extract for the circulatory system, Ginkgo for the central nervous system, and Green tea for systemic protection.

COMBINING HERBAL REMEDIES

Combining a single herb in high potency with a formula often is the ideal plan for customizing an individuals herbal program. Combining a formula with a single herb often becomes necessary when there is an aggravation of symptoms. For a short time both herbal strategies may be needed. The dosage and/or frequency may need to be increased. Whenever the results of a herbal program are not being experienced a reevaluation should occur. A new formula or single herb may be needed or the illness may warrant a visit to your health professional.

Using the example of St. John's Wort for mild depression as a single herb the dosage is a 300 mg extract three times a day. If the single herb works well there may not be a need for the formula. If however there is a particular stressful time when the person feels the need for additional support, adding a formula that is a nerve tonic, supports the adrenal gland and promotes restful sleep would be helpful. When a person is planning on discontinuing the St. John's Wort gradually transitioning to a nerve tonic formula may help to stabilize the withdrawal process. If someone has used St. John's Wort, for a long time alternating onto a formula periodically may be a better strategy than staying on the St. John's Wort continually.

Another example is using only echinacea for acute infections. Using a formula that contains multiple herbs that assist the mucous membranes, immune system and has a second antiviral herb may be a better solution than echinacea alone.

CUSTOMIZED FORMULAS

Customized Formulas use herbs in a combination designed specifically for the matrix of symptoms of an individual. This customized formula may contain herbs for treating two or three conditions simultaneously. This may be two or three chronic conditions or an acute condition with 2 or 3 symptoms. A chronic respiratory problem in combination with poor digestion would require a customized herbal formula. Naturopathic physicians formulate customized formulas for many of their patients. Customized formulas often will be used in addition to both a single herb and preformulated compounds in a significant dosage for resistant health problems.

SAFETY AND MEDICAL ADVICE

When using nutritional supplements and herbal products it is important to understand some commonsense safety issues. Your investment into your supplement program is optimized by the good advice of your health care providers. Communicate with your conventional health care provider about what you are taking. Seek advice from a healthcare professional knowledgeable about herbal medicine and the treatment of your specific condition. Understand the boundaries of selfcare. Herbs are generally very safe. Even with the large numbers of people taking herbs for the first time the numbers of problems that occur annually is very few, especially if you compare it to reactions to conventional over the counter or prescribed drugs. Please refer to the chapter 9 on Herbal Medicines, Cautions, Contraindication and Drug Interactions.

Three of areas where negative reactions to herbs occur more frequently:

1. Individuals taking multiple medications for multiple health conditions. The problem medications are most often anticoagulants like coumadin (blood thinners), antidepressants, blood pressure medicine and herbs used just prior to surgery. In these cases consult with your physician, naturopathic physician or natural medicine specialist.

2. Individuals who are highly allergic to multiple environmental pollens, dust and mold may react to herbs in a negative manner and should begin any new herb at 1/4 the dosage.

3. Many negative reports regarding dietary supplements are from stimulant/recreational drugs masquerading as dietary substances including ephedrine, weight loss products, caffeine stimulants and some designer street drugs.

Taking herbs during pregnancy is not recommended unless under the direction of a health care professional. This does not include the use of herbal teas as beverages.

CHAPTER 3

UNDERSTANDING HERBAL MEDICINE QUALITY

After choosing to use herbal products a great deal of attention is given to the selection of the most indicated herb or herb formula. But an equally important understanding is the quality of the herbs and the dosage of the product. The following sections will explain the basics of herbal medicine manufacturing and production. This chapter should enable you to make informed decisions when purchasing herbal products of the highest quality and best value.

POTENCY OF HERBAL MEDICINES

There are several measures of quality and potency that consumers should be aware of when comparing herbal products.

QUALITY CONTROL OF THE PLANT MATERIAL

Strong healthy plants produce better herbal medicines.

1. Herbs can be harvested in the wild, or grown on farms. Herbs that are harvested in the wild must be done in a careful and considerate manner. Ecologically Wildcrafted Herbs describes a process for selecting plants in the plant's natural wild habitat without endangering their future from over harvesting. Plants grown on a farm can be grown Certified Organic or using non-organic commercial fertilizers and processes. Using certified organic herbs in the products you purchase is a worthy investment. It may add a small amount of cost but it insures a plant free from the residues of insecticides, herbicides and chemical fertilizers, the last thing you want in your herbal remedies.

2. Plant material should be investigated for adulterants in the form of foreign materials, dirt, metals, toxins and microbes.

3. A recent concern regarding the quality of herbs is whether the seeds or the product contain genetically modified organisms (GMO). Manufacturers currently are not required to label their product if it contains GMO material.

4. The plant should be harvested at the peak of its production of active ingredients. The ideal is to have agricultural testing carried out using high pressure liquid chromatography (HPLC) while the plants are still growing. This enables the capture of a consistent range of bioactivity in the harvested plant.

5. Once harvested, the plants should be processed as soon as possible to prevent the oxidation of the active ingredients.

STANDARDIZATION

Definition: Standardization is a chemical analytical process to make a botanical that possesses measurable, quantifiable, and replicable content of active ingredient <u>and/or biological activity.</u>[1]

No standardization methods for botanicals are available today that test <u>biological activity.</u> Currently, there are no standards established for biological testing. This should change in the future as the quality and the volume of research in botanical medicine grows. The standardization methods we have currently test for the content of "marker molecules." Plants are complex organisms composed of many compounds with one or more active medicinal ingredients. In many herbs we know what is the active ingredient, in others we are not sure. For kava we know the active ingredient is in a group of substances called kavalactones that are standardized to 30-55% total kavalactones. For St. John's Wort most extracts are standardized to contain 0.3% hypericin, although we know that hypericin is not the active antidepressant ingredient. Because there is no agreement about what is the active ingredient hypericin is used because it is easy to identify and if hypericin is present at the standardized level then so should the active ingredients.

Standardization of herbal medicines is a quality control test done on the raw plant material. It is an important step but it is essential for consumers to understand that no standardization used today indicates the bioavailability of the finished product. In fact the opposite is sometimes true, that standardization can make a low quality batch of herb look good if it passes the lab test. Many processes of standardization use methods that extract the maximum amount of marker substance out of the plant. These methods include the use of strong solvents such as hexane using high temperature and vacuum pressure. It is important to note that the amount of active ingredient that standardization identifies in the plant material does not mean that the human body can extract the same quantity (especially if the active ingredient is a purified component of the herb with the other synergistic components removed). Our bodies are not nearly as efficient as the laboratory procedures. *Standardization testing when done on the finished product, quantifies and qualifies the activity of the product.* It is the authors' belief and experience that herbal tinctures and liquid extracts are more absorbable and bioavailible than tablets or capsules made with plant material.

FULL SPECTRUM STANDARDIZATION

Through a process referred to as "Full Spectrum Standardization" the potency and consistency of an herbal product is maintained without compromising the "wholeness" characteristics of the plant. This process is accomplished through four specific procedures:

a. **Agricultural Testing**
   While the plants are still in their developmental stage, analytical testing is carried out through HPLC (High Pressure Liquid Chromatography) to determine levels of activity. Periodic sampling and testing from the field enable a determination to be made as to the peak harvest time of the plant when the constituents are highest.

b. **Extraction Methodology**
   Extraction methods are set up using only USP grade grain alcohol and pure spring water as organic solvents. Non-ingestible solvents are not used. The plants are then extracted in their entirety without any purification or isolation of inert substances. This Full Spectrum Process enables the entire chemical profile of the plant to be extracted.

c. **Concentration Technology**
   Once extracted and filtered the extract is then concentrated using low heat/low vacuum concentrators. Solvent is removed slowly so as to preserve the plants fragile constituents. As the solvents are distilled off, the extract becomes concentrated to the desired levels.

d. **Final HPLC Analysis**
   Once concentration is completed a final HPLC test is carried out to ensure the extract is concentrated

to the marker level. A marker compound is used
for each herb and this compound gives specificity
to the extract's level of full spectrum activity.

It is the author's opinion that "Full Spectrum Standardization"
is the very finest and most wholistic of all the methods used to
standardize herbal products. This method captures the chemical
"blueprint" of the plants while accomplishing the necessary concentration levels for optimum results.

HERB STRENGTH RATIO

When you shop for herbs one of the measures of quality of
the finished product is the Herb/Strength ratio. This ratio is
used on the labels of tinctures, liquid extracts, fluid extracts and
solid extracts. An herb strength ratio of 1:5 means that 1000
grams (1kilogram=2.2 pounds) of raw herbal material produced
5,000 ml (5 liters) of extract.

	Herb Strength Ratio	Raw Herbal Material	Finished Herbal Extract
Tincture	1:5	1000 grams (2.2 lbs.)	5 liters (5,000 ml)
Saturated Tincture	1:3	1000 grams	3 liters (3,000 ml)
Fluid Extract	1:1	1000 grams	1 liter (1,000 ml)
Solid Extract	2:1 (or greater)	1000 grams	1/2 liter 500 ml

CONCENTRATION

Liquid herbal extracts can be concentrated without changing
their original "fingerprint" of the plant's chemistry. This is best
done with low heat and under low pressure to vacuum off the
alcohol and water to the desired concentration. The potency of
the herbal extract is a combination of the concentration and the
bioavailability.

Alcohol Free extracts are made by using the proper alcohol
requirement when doing the extraction then utilize vacuum
extraction to remove the alcohol. Vegetable Glycerin is then
added after the extraction is complete and HPLC analysis is

done to compare the active ingredient in the alcohol extract to the alcohol free extract.

PROCEDURES USED TO PREPARE QUALITY HERBAL EXTRACTS

The following represents a check-list that should be used by manufacturers and validated by distributors of herbal extracts to ensure that correct procedures are being followed for the preparation of quality herbal extracts:

- **Selection of Plant Material** – Pre-testing of all batches of certified organic or ecologically wild-crafted plant material for microbial analysis, heavy metal contamination, and analytical/bio-activity analysis.
- **Comminution** – A process whereby the fresh or freshly dried plant material is ground into a wet slurry (if fresh) or milled into a course grind (if dry) so as to prepare the plant material for extraction.
- **Maceration** – A process whereby the ground plant material is saturated in organic solvent (USP grade grain alcohol and spring water) and agitated daily for a period of 2-4 weeks. The saturated plant material is then placed in hydraulic extractors to separate the liquid from the spent herb (marc).
- **Percolation and Battery Percolation** – A process whereby the ground plant material is saturated for a period of several days and then a slow percolation is encouraged via gravitational force to move the liquid through the plant material. Battery percolation uses the same principle however runs the solution through several tanks of herb material for greater concentration.
- **Flow Thru Extraction** – A process whereby the organic solvent (USP grain alcohol and spring water) is forced under vacuum and temperature through the ground plant material at a high rate of speed thereby extracting the components of the herb quickly and entirely.

● **Filtration** – A process whereby the sediment is removed from the liquid extract resulting in a "polished" product ready for concentration.

● **Thin Film Evaporation** – A process whereby low heat and vacuum are applied to the filtered extract to slowly remove the alcohol and water thereby enabling the extract to concentrate to desired levels.

● **Lab Analysis** – Scientific instruments such as HPLC (High Pressure Liquid Chromatography) and GC-Mass (Gas Chromatography/Mass Spectometry) and UV Spectometry are then used to analysis the finished product to assure that desired levels of "marker" compounds are present in the finished product.

FORMS OF HERBAL PRODUCTS

Herbal products are available in teas, capsules containing herbal powder or powdered extracts, tablets, soft gels, tinctures, fluid extracts, solid extracts and liquid phyto-caps. Understanding the advantages and disadvantages of each is important in comparing and using herbal remedies.

HERBAL TEAS

Herbal medicinal teas are a wonderful way to use and learn about herbal medicines, by tasting the teas, learning their names and feeling the effects. Herbal tea's can calm the nerves, assisting our digestion, promote sleep, stimulate our central nervous system, and assist with a wide variety of cold and flu symptoms. Herbal tea's make excellent beverages and a wide variety of them should be a regular part of your pantry and diet. Using herbal tea use is much healthier than coffee, black tea or soda. Their use in botanical medicine is limited because tea extracts only the water soluble, not the oil soluble, components of the herbs. Also the concentration of the herbal tea is often not strong enough to effect a therapeutic result. Finally the taste of the medicinal herbs can be difficult and after all you can only drink so much tea.

HERBAL TABLETS

Herbal tablets are made by a high-pressure tableting machine that compressing the powdered plant material into a shape that can be easily swallowed. The advantage of this method is that the herb can be taken without being tasted. Making a tablet stay together when it is made of plant material requires binding agents like magnesium stearate to keep the material together. The active ingredients in the herb are in their natural state, bound to the fiber of the plant. The human body must extract the active ingredients from the plant material. The tablet may contain dry extracts that have been extracted using either alcohol or commercial solvents. When phenol type solvents are used for extraction, quality control measures are essential to ensure that the solvents are removed as completely as possible leaving minimal residue.[1] These products are often standardized. Herbal tablets can be made in both single herb and formulas. The size of the tablet determines the quantity of plant material ingested and multiple tablets are generally needed to produce a therapeutic dose.

HERBAL CAPSULES

Herbal capsules contain the same powdered plant material that herbal tablets contain except that the powdered herb is compacted into a two-piece gelatin capsule. The advantage to a capsule is that it can be taken without being tasted. This method does not require binding agents but flow agents may be needed to smoothly inject the powder into the capsule. The active ingredients in the herb are in their natural state bound to the fiber of the plant. Herbal capsules can be made using dry extracts as described in the herbal tablet section. Capsules deliver either single herb or multiple herb formulas. The quantity of herbal material is limited by the size of the capsule. Multiple capsules are generally needed to produce a therapeutic dose. Another advantage of herbal capsules is that vitamins, nutrients and minerals may be added to create a synergistic herb/nutrient formula.

SOFT-GEL CAPSULES

Soft gel capsules contain a liquid that has powdered herb/plant material mixed with oil. Soft gel capsules have the advantage of being in a liquid yet often contain substances such as beeswax to maintain them in solution. Although soft-gels are very popular, the fact that they are made with animal gelatin capsules and carry an oil base may make them somewhat difficult to digest (except with fat soluble herbs).

TINCTURES

Tinctures are alcohol/water extracts of plant material. Tinctures are 1:4 or 1:5 liquid solutions. Tinctures contain alcohol that acts as a natural solvent that extracts out the active ingredients that are bound to the plants' fibrous material. The alcohol is also an excellent preservative for the delicate alkaloids, resins and other ingredients that make up the herbs therapeutic value. The solutions that are used for extracting may vary in the alcohol/water ratio and may include vinegar or glycerin in order to extract specific and important active ingredients. This specific process varies from plant to plant. Tinctures are considered dilute and usually are suitable for consumer use, but not for medicinal use.

LIQUID EXTRACTS OR FLUID EXTRACTS

Liquid extracts are tinctures that are concentrated. Tinctures may have a 1:5 ratio of herbal material to fluid while liquid extracts have a 1:1 herb strength ratio. The concentration method used is often a low heat/low vacuum evaporator that preserves the integrity of the plant ingredients while evaporating off the alcohol and water to make a more concentrated herbal solution. Liquid and Fluid extracts are much more concentrated than tinctures and therefore much more suitable for therapeutic use. For this reason they are preferred for use by naturopathic physicians or herbalists.

LIQUID PHYTO-CAPS™

Liquid Phyto-Caps™ are concentrated liquid extracts in a vegetarian capsule. The thin capsule contains the herbal concentrated extract. The capsules can be swallowed or bitten to release the herbal solution. Because the Liquid Phyto-Caps™ are in a fully liquid (non-oil) state, the activity and absorbability of the herbal solution is the best available. Liquid Phyto-Caps™ offer the advantages in absorbability with the convenience of taking a capsule, avoiding the taste of the tincture. The advantages of the Liquid Phyto-Caps™ are as follows:

a. Formulations for lifestyle needs
b. Full Spectrum Standerdization – The natural proportions of plants of constituents remain unchanged.
c. Each batch of herbal extract analytically verified for potency.
d. Certified Organic or Ecologically Wild-Crafted Herbs
e. 100 % Vegetarian – Vegetarian based capsule-tamper evident and leak proof
f. Phyto Caps are alcohol free and contain a non-oil base (glycerine)
g. No toxic solvents or high temperatures used in extraction or concentration

h. Stable shelf Life
i. Manufactured under current Good Manufacturing Practices (cGMP'S) following Standard Operating Procedures (SOP's)
j. Easy to Swallow #1 capsules
k. Standardized bio-active constituent/marker compound levels

Bio-Availability of Herbal Medicines

Bio-Availability of Herbal Tablets, Gelatin Capsules and Soft Gels

Herbal tablets and gelatin capsules both must go through a lengthy digestive process in order to release the active ingredients. In the stomach the herb's active ingredients are subject to the strong acid environment, they then enter the extreme alkaline environment of the duodenum. The active principles are separated from the fiber of the plant material and absorbed into the gut. They travel in the blood to the liver and its metabolic processing. The active ingredients then go through the heart and get distributed to the rest of the body. Soft Gels contains oil and powdered herbal material or dry extracts that utilized the same process of absorption as Caps and tabs other than for the presence of the oil which may help the fat soluble fractions of the herb to be absorbed. In each case the bio-availability of herbal tablets, capsules and gelatin soft-gels may take as long as 2-4 four hours once the herb has been digested. Individuals with compromised digestive functions may not benefit from the full value of the herbal product when it is ingested in these forms of herbal delivery.

Bio-Availability of Tinctures and Liquid Extracts

Tinctures and liquid extracts are already in full solution and have an increased biological activity due to efficient absorption and delivery to the blood and tissues of the body. Alcohol extracts when taken orally rapidly absorb into the mucous membranes of the mouth, tongue, throat, esophagus and stomach. These mucous membranes deliver the active principles into the lymph vessels of the mouth, neck and chest to be delivered directly by the thoracic duct into the blood as it enters the heart and is distributed to the body. The lymphatic pathway bypasses the digestive tract and liver and is a major advantage in the activity and bioavailibility of liquid preparations. This efficient mechanism is the reason that many naturopathic physicians and herbalists prefer to despense herbs in liquid solution.

The dosage of liquid preparations can be varied by the number of drops taken. The concentration or strength of a liquid can be increased by several methods. A disadvantage of liquids is that the taste of many of the herbs is not appreciated by most people. Masking the taste of liquids using grape juice or herb tea is helpful. It is clear, however, that the liquid delivery of herbal medicines will always provide the most complete and efficient form of herbal administration.

BIO-AVAILABILITY OF LIQUID PHYTO-CAPS™

Liquid Phyto-Caps™ are the most concentrated of the herbal products presented. The Liquid Phyto-Cap™ contains an herbal solution having an herb/strength ratio of at least 3:1. The herb within the vegetarian capsule remains in full solution due to the fact that the original extract is in a fully liquid state rather than a reconstituted state as in the case of soft-gels. The liquid base is pure vegetable glycerine rather than vegetable oil as in the case with soft-gels. The Liquid Phyto-Cap™ can be swallowed which presents the active ingredient to the stomach in a form that is ready to be absorbed. Because of the concentration of the active ingredient and its very absorbable state a high level of absorption occurs. The Liquid Phyto-Cap™ can also be easily bitten into releasing the active ingredients for absorption into the mouth, pharynx, esophagus and stomach. This takes advantage of the lymphatic absorption of active ingredients and is an excellent way to get the most out of one's herbal purchase. The Liquid Phyto-Cap™ delivery system represents a new advancement in herbal consumption. With a Liquid Phyto-Cap™ you have all the advantage of the liquid delivery system with all the convenience of a vegetarian capsule.

HERBAL DOSAGE AND FREQUENCY OF USE

Most fluid extracts are formulated to a recommended dose of 30 drops, 3-4 times daily. Double potency or double macerated extracts have a reduced dosage while tinctures with a 1:5 or 1:4 herb strength ratio will require an increased dose.

This recommendation would be for a 150 lb. adult. There are several methods of adjusting dosage to the individual. Two are presented here; one based on weight and the other on the age of a child. Clark's rule of dosage uses weight to adjust the dosage. It divides the weight of the person by 150 pounds to get a fraction and adjusts the recommended dose by multiplying by the fraction. A 120 pound woman (120/150) would use 4/5 of the 30 drop recommended dose or 24 drops. A 180 pound man (180/150) would take 6/5 or 36 drops. Clarks rule can also be used for children, a 60 lb. child (60/150) would take 2/5 dose or 12 drops. Young's rule is another method used for children up to age 12. It divides the child's age by their age plus 12 and multiple the fraction by the adult dose. For example a 6 year old (6/6+12) would be given 1/3 of the adult dose or 10 drops.

Common sense dictates that when starting an herb for the first time you use a 1/2 dose for 2-3 times. Individuals who are allergic or hypersensitive to their environment should start with a 1/4 dosage and increase by 1/4 increments. Elderly or those in a weakened condition should start with a 1/2 dose or less.

Herbs are best taken frequently due to rapid absorption of liquid extracts. For chronic conditions a frequency of four times per 24 hours delivers the remedy an average of every 6 hours instead of every 12 hours if it is taken twice daily. For convenience three times per day (every 8 hours) is a reasonable frequency.

For acute conditions more frequent dosing is recommended. Taking a formula for a cold every 2 hours at 10 drops is better than taking 30 drops three times per day.

As more research gets done on herbal medicine we will learn more about the half-life of specific herbs and conditions.

STRUCTURE/FUNCTION CLAIMS

Students of herbal medicine should understand the regulatory environment that herbal medicine exists within. In 1994 the US congress passed the Dietary Supplement Health and Education Act (DSHEA) that regulated how dietary supplements including botanicals can be manufactured and sold. Prior to DSHEA the FDA actively restricted information that a manufacturer could use to inform and educate consumers that created an information vacuum. There are now specific rules about the claims that a manufacturer can make about their products. These rules describe how manufacturers can use information derived from books or scientific papers to be used in connection with the sale of dietary supplements. The information must present a balanced view of the available scientific information… must not be false or misleading …and must be supported by an authoritative source.

Structure/function claims for supplements can include:[3]

1. Claims that a supplement can prevent a classical deficiency disease, Example: "Vitamin C can help prevent scurvy."
2. Claims that a supplement can affect a structure or function of the body. Example: "Calcium helps build strong bones."
3. Claims that describe documented mechanism by which an ingredient acts to maintain structure or function. Example: Antioxidants may prevent damage to cells and tissues."
4. Claims that describe a general benefit resulting from consumption of a dietary supplement. Example: St. John's Wort may promote a positive mood.
5. Permission for claims made from a traditional use of an herb as described by an appropriate reference book printed prior to 1980.
6. Section 6 requires manufacturers to label and display the disclaimer "this statement has not been evaluated by the FDA. This product is not intended to diagnose, treat, cure or prevent any disease.
7. Reference citations that support statements of "Traditional Use" and "Relevant Scientific Investigation" must be retained on file in their complete form at the manufacturer's facility.
8. All Structure/Function names and claims must be registered with the FDA.

REFERENCES

1 McKenna D. Natural dietary Supplements: a Desktop Reference; INPR, Marine on St. Croix, MN, 1998

2 Brinker f. Formula's for Healthful Living, Eclectic Medical Publications, Sandy Or, 1995,26-27.

3 McKenna D. Natural dietary Supplements: a Desktop Reference; INPR, Marine on St. Croix, MN, 1998

CHAPTER 4

WHY LIQUID HERBAL EXTRACTS?

*"The best, bioavailable form is the solution,
or suspension. It is of course,
not the dry form."*

Prof. Umberto Cornelli M.D.
Dept. of Pharmacology and Experimental Therapeutics
Loyola University Medical School in Illinois

THE LIQUID DELIVERY SYSTEM

Whether you open a textbook written for the pharmaceutical sciences or the botanical sciences you will inevitably notice that one area generally agreed upon is drug delivery, particularly as it relates to drug bio-availability. On this issue both 'sides' enthusiastically agree that superior bio-availability is obtained with drugs that are in their liquid form (solutions).

So what is drug *bio-availability?* Specifically, it is defined as 'the degree and rate at which a substance (as a drug) is absorbed into a living system or is made available at the site of physiological activity'. Simply put, it is how well and how fast you absorb a medicine.

One basic rule in this scientific field is well understood. *Before anything is absorbed across a membrane and into the body, the substance must be in solution.* The only exceptions to this are those substances that are inhaled (delivered in gaseous form).

Herbal drugs that are delivered in their liquid form have several distinct and unique advantages, including;

Superior bioavailability – Because the extract constituents are already in solution, they may be absorbed rapidly and more completely.

No need to be digested – Liquid extracts do not need to be digested. The digestive process of removing the active constituents from the plant cellulose is not required because the alcohol/water solvent extracts the active principle. Liquid extracts are **'predigested'**. They are in fact "in solution". It is important to understand that digestion is usually one of the first functions to become impaired during the disease process. Therefore, it does not make sense to deliver a medicine in a form that depends upon digestive function (i.e. dried powdered herb capsules and tablets).

Option of using fresh material – The key word here is *option*. Some plants must be extracted when fresh (including American Skullcap, Dandelion root and Kola nut). Others, on the other hand, must be extracted when dried. *Cascara sagrada* is an excellent example of a plant that must be dried (and aged) to buffer the harsh laxative effects of compounds known as anthraquinone glycosides.

Ginger is an example of a plant that may be used in *either* its fresh form or its dried form, each producing a different therapeutic effect.

Whatever the requirements of the specific herb you want to take (i.e. fresh or dried) with liquids you're able to satisfy those requirements completely, without the compromise that is associated with other deliver methods.

May by-pass the 'first pass' of the liver – Another basic rule of drug bio-availability is that whenever anything is swallowed and absorbed from the gastrointestinal tract (regardless of its form, i.e. dried crude herb, powder, liquid, etc.) it must pass via the portal vein, directly to the liver.*

Once in the liver, metabolism of the substance begins. What does not get broken down on this 'first pass' through the liver then enters systemic circulation to be delivered to its active sites (cells, tissues, etc.). When a drug bypasses this 'first pass', less is needed to effect the same results as a higher dose.

Alternatively, when a substance is absorbed sub-lingually (under the tongue), buccally (if held in the cheek of the mouth), transdermally (across the skin), or rectally, it bypasses this 'first pass' of the liver. By holding an extract in your mouth so that it may be absorbed sublingually is only possible with a liquid. This is a great advantage of liquid herbal extracts.

Having this option of enhanced absorption is very important, particularly when you need something to work quickly.

Remember, bio-availability (how well and how fast you absorb a medicine) is everything.

*The only exception to this is when fats known as triglycerides (also known as neutral fats) are absorbed directly into the lymphatic system.

Liquids can be concentrated – Liquid herbal extracts can be concentrated by removing some (or all) of their liquid, without sacrificing any of their other unique advantages.

Liquids can be standardized – By analyzing an extract and concentrating it (removing an exact amount of alcohol and water) a liquid extract may be standardized to deliver a precise number of milligrams (mg) per milliliter (ml) of a plants active constituents, without altering the original 'fingerprint' of the plants chemistry. This method of standardizing an extract is referred to as a *'Full Spectrum Standerdization'.*

The advantage of taste – The fact is that many traditional systems of medicine acknowledge the profound importance of taste. In our culture(s) almost everything we consume is either salty or sweet. This is not beneficial. What about the bitter, pungent, and astringent (also described as 'sour' by some traditions) tastes? When we taste something we set up receptivity for it throughout our body. Experiencing a range of tastes is vitally important to achieving and maintaining balanced well-being. By tasting your herbs you will achieve greater benefit from them. It may be a little difficult to get used to these other tastes at first, *but you will get used to it.* One may never actually enjoy the taste of herbal extracts (although some people do), but the health benefits one will experience make it worth it.

CHAPTER 5

LIQUID PHYTO-CAPS™ – SINGLE HERBS POTENCY AND CONVENIENCE

The following represents the features and benefits of
LIQUID PHYTO-CAPS™

Liquid Phyto-Caps™ are concentrated liquid extracts in a capsule. The thin capsule contains the herbal concentrated extract. The capsules can be swallowed or bitten to release the herbal solution. Because the Liquid Phyto-Caps™ are in a fully liquid (non-oil) state, the activity and absorbability of the herbal solution is the best available. Liquid Phyto-Caps™ offer the advantages in absorbability with the convenience of taking a capsule, avoiding the taste of the tincture. The advantages of the Liquid Phyto-Caps™ are as follows:

a. Formulations for lifestyle needs
b. Full Spectrum Standerdization – The natural proportions of plants of constituents remain unchanged.
c. Each batch of herbal extract analytically verified for potency.
d. Certified Organic or Ecologically Wild-Crafted Herbs
e. 100 % Vegetarian – Vegetarian based capsule-tamper evident and leak proof
f. Phyto Caps™ are alcohol free and contain a non-oil base (glycerine)
g. No toxic solvents or high temperatures used in extraction or concentration
h. Stable shelf Life
i. Manufactured under current Good Manufacturing Practices (cGMP'S) following Standard Operating Procedures (SOP's)
j. Easy to Swallow #1 capsules
k. Standardized bio-active constituent/marker compound levels

GINKGO LEAF
(Ginkgo biloba)
Ultimate Support to Improve Memory*

Concentration:	3:1 herb strength ratio; 24% ginkgo flavonoid glycosides (from ginkgo) 30.8 mg per 2 capsules.
Dosage:	1 Liquid Phyto-Cap, Twice Daily
Duration of use:	4-6 Months
Best taken:	Between meals, with warm water

HISTORY

Ginkgo is the oldest surviving species of tree and is often referred to as "the living fossil". Fossil records indicate that it probably originated during the Permian period about 250 million years ago.[1] The tree ranged worldwide during the Paleozoic era and went into decline before the Ice Age, eventually retreating to the mountain forests of China.

That ginkgo is the only living species of its family speaks of the tree's hardiness. The first green growth to emerge in the city of Hiroshima after the atomic blast was ginkgo. The medicinal properties of ginkgo were first recorded around 2800 BC. In Chinese folk medicine the leaf was used as an antitussive, antiasthmatic, and anodyne. [2] The modern day therapeutic effect of ginkgo is well established. In Europe it is one of the most widely prescribed medications for the treatment of cognitive deficiency. It's truly amazing that ginkgo, an ancient tree seeded millions of years ago, has survived to impart such a profound healing influence on human physiology.

SCIENTIFIC RESEARCH

Ginkgo and its constituents are the subjects of over 400 scientific publications, making it one of the most researched herbal medications. Numerous clinical trials have documented ginkgo's effects on cognitive, physiologic, and psychiatric conditions associated with neurologic and vascular diseases. Ginkgo has been shown to effect recall, recognition memory, reaction time, attention, concentration, psychomotor function, fatigue, mood, and information processing. [3]

Many clinical trials have been conducted in patients with cerebral insufficiency (dementia). Symptoms of this condition are difficulty in concentration and memory, absentmindedness, confusion, lack of energy, decreased physical performance, depressed mood, and anxiety. In one of the earliest placebo-controlled double-blind trials, patients demonstrated improvements in short term memory, concentration power, attention span, and mental flexibility. [4]

One of the first reviews of ginkgo was published in the Lancet in 1992. The authors reviewed over 40 double-blind controlled trials of ginkgo for the treatment of cerebral insufficiency. After reviewing the trials, the authors concluded that ginkgo is an effective treatment for cerebral insufficiency. [5]

A 52 week randomized, double-blind placebo-controlled, multi-center trial was conducted in 309 patients with mild to moderate dementia (primarily Alzheimer's). Subjects received either 40 mg of ginkgo extract (24% gingko flavonoids) three times a day, or a placebo. Compared to the subjects taking the placebo, those taking gingko showed either improvement or a delay in the progression of the disease. The authors concluded that ginkgo was safe and appears capable of stabilizing and improving the cognitive performance and social functioning of demented patients.[6] Recently, an intent-to-treat analysis of this study was performed to determine the efficacy of 26 weeks of treatment. After a 6 month treatment period gingko was effective in two areas of treatment: cognitive performance and daily living and social behavior. There was a significant worsening in all areas of assessment in the placebo group. There were no differences between ginkgo and placebo with regards to side effects.[7]

Randomized, double-blind placebo-controlled studies have also found ginkgo to be effective in ordinary age-related memory loss. In two trials, healthy participants demonstrated an improvement in memory and improved speed of information processing. [8,9]

MECHANISM OF ACTION

Many diverse actions contribute to the overall effectiveness of gingko. Not all of these mechanisms have been elucidated. Actions that possibly contribute to its effectiveness include direct and indirect antioxidant activity, neurotransmitter/receptor modulation, platelet activating factor antagonism, and neuroprotective actions. The combined therapeutic effects are probably greater that that of an individual mechanism and are perhaps the result of the synergistic effects of multiple constituents of the total extract.[3, 10-16]

THERAPEUTIC APPLICATIONS*

Note: The intention of the following information is to represent the traditional use of the herb and to inform the reader of any evolving inquiry relevant to the herb.

SUPPORTED BY TRADITIONAL USE

Cerebral insufficiency [4-9]

SCOPE OF RELEVANT SCIENTIFIC INVESTIGATION

Nootropic (cognitive activating) [3-7]   Antioxidant [3,11-12]

CAUTIONS, CONTRA-INDICATIONS
AND DRUG INTERACTIONS

Please reference Chapter 9. Do not use during pregnancy or lactation. Because of its antiplatelet activating factor properties, gingko should not be used without professional guidance with anticoagulant medications.

COMPLIMENTARY HERBS/FORMULAS

Anti-Oxidant Supreme, Ginkgo/Gotu Kola Supreme, Gotu Kola

REFERENCES

1. Glimn-Lacy J and Kaufman PB. *Botany Illustrated.* New York. Van Nostrand Reinhold Company; 1984: 72-73.
2. Huang KC. *The Pharmacology of Chinese Herbs.* Boca Raton.CRC Press;1993: 85-86.
3. Diamond BJ, *et al.* Ginkgo biloba extract: Mechanisms and clinical indications. *Arch Phys Med Rehabil.* 2000;81:668-678.
4. Vesper J and Hansgen KD. Efficacy of ginkgo biloba in 90 outpatients with cerebral insufficiency caused by old age. Results of a placebo-controlled double-blind trial. *Phytomedicine.* 1994; 1:9-16.
5. Kleijnen J and Knipschild P. Ginkgo biloba for cerebral insufficiency. *Br. J. Clin. Pharmaco* 1992; 34:352-358.
6. Le Bars PL, *et al.* A placeo-controlled, double blind, randomized trial of an extract of ginkgo biloba for dementia. *JAMA.* 1997; 278(16): 1327-1332.
7. Le Bars PL, *et al.* A 26-week analysis of a double-blind, placebo-controlled trial of the ginkgo biloba extract Egb 761 in dementia. *Dement Geriatr Cogn Disord.* 2000;11:230-237.
8. Rigney U, *et al.* The effects of acute doses of standardized ginkgo biloba extract on memory and psychomotor performance in volunteers. *Phytotherapy Research.* 1999: 13:408-415.

9. Mix JA and Crews WD. An examination of the efficacy of ginkgo biloba extract Egb 761 on the neuropsychologic functioning of cognitively intact older adults. *J of Alternative and Complementary Medicine.* 2000;6(3):219-229.

10. Gardès-Albert M, *et al.* Oxygen-centered free radicals and their interactions with EGb 761 or CP 202. *Advances in Ginkgo biloba Extract Research, Vol 2.* Paris. Elsevier; 1993:1-11.

11. Köse L and Do an P. Lipoperoxidation induced by hydrogen peroxide in human erythrocyte membranes. 1. Comparison of the antioxidant effect of ginkgo biloba extract (EGb 761 with those of water-soluble and lipid-soluble antioxidants. *The Journal of International Medical Research* 1995; 23: 9-18..

12. Lugasi A, *et al.* Additional information to the in vitro antioxidant activity of ginkgo biloba L. *Phytotherapy Research.* 1999; 13: 160-162.

13. Braquet P. Proofs of involvement of PAF-acether in various immune disorders using BN 52021 (ginkgolide B): a powerful PAF-acether antagonist isolated from ginkgo biloba L. *Advances in Prostaglandin, Thromboxane, and Leukotriene Research* 1986; 16: 179-198.

14. Logani S, *et al.* Actions of ginkgo biloba related to potential utility for the treatment of conditions involving cerebral hypoxia. *Life Sciences.* 2000; 67: 1389-1396.

15 Calapai G, *et al.* Neuroprotective effects of ginkgo biloba extract in brain ischemia are mediated by inhibition of nitric oxide synthesis. *Life Sciences.* 2000; 67:2673-2683.

16. Di Renzo G. Ginkgo biloba and the central nervous system. *Fitoterapia.* 2000; 71: S43-S47.

HAWTHORN SUPREME

Ultimate Support of Cardiovascular Function *
FORMULA

Hawthorn berry (Solid extract)   (*Crataegus oxycantha*)
Hawthorn flower and leaf   (*Crataegus spp.*)

Concentration:	2.5:1 Herb strength ratio
Dosage:	Liquid Extract: 40-60 drops, three times daily
Duration of use:	4-6 months or longer, for best results
Best taken:	Between meals, with warm water

DESCRIPTION OF FORMULA

A combination of the Hawthorn berry with its flower and/or leaves has traditionally been used in Europe as a highly regarded heart tonic. Its specific application includes heart weakness, particularly where nervous exhaustion is present. This highly nutritive plant, nourishes the entire cardiovascular system promoting connective and cardiovascular tissue integrity. Due to the absence of plant bioflavonoids, from foods in the American diet, simple plant compounds, such as these, will prove to become increasingly effective with many of today's chronic degenerative disorders. This compound contains two groups of active flavonoids that exert their actions upon the cardiovascular system. One group of flavonoids has been shown to enhance rhythmical activity (Positive inotropic) of the heart while the other group has been shown to reinforce the collagen tissue of the cardiovascular system.

Hawthorn berries have been used historically to tonify the heart.[G3, G5, G6, 1, 2, 3] In fact, such use for Hawthorn has been reported since the first half of the 17th century.[2] The berries have also traditionally found use as a digestive stimulant for relief of numerous gastrointestinal disturbances.[G3, G5] Primary focus, has of course fallen predominantly upon its well established cardiovascular affect. In the tradition of the American Eclectics, Hawthorn was considered to be a specific for cardiac insufficiency of virtually any kind.[G6] Today, Hawthorn is primarily recognized in the scientific literature for its influence with congestive heart disease,[G5, 7, 8] cholesterol lowering effects, antioxidant properties, and collagen stabilizing ability.[G5, 1]

Hawthorn flowers and leaves possess similar properties and chemistry to the Hawthorn berry.[3] While the berries are higher in certain constituents, the flower and leaf are higher in others.[2] They have been combined here in Hawthorn Supreme to offer the full spectrum of Hawthorn's chemistry and vast therapeutic effects. The German Commission E (Germany's equivalent of the FDA) endorses the use of the leaf and flower, of the Hawthorn for Cardiac Insufficiency, and 'the aging heart, not yet requiring digitalis'.[9] Hawthorn is considered to be one of the most gentle heart remedies in the herbal *materia medica* (materials of medicine).[3]

THERAPEUTIC APPLICATIONS*

Note: The intention of the following information is to represent the traditional use of the individual botanicals found in these formulas and to inform the reader of any evolving scientific inquiry relevant to the formula's ingredients.

SUPPORTED BY TRADITIONAL USE

Heart tonic,[G3, G5, G6, 1, 2, 3] Antisclerotic,[G3, G6] Digestive.[G3, 2]

SCOPE OF RELEVANT SCIENTIFIC INVESTIGATION

Congestive Heart Disease,[G5, 1] High Blood Pressure,[G3, G5, 1] Elevates cyclic AMP,[G5, 1, 9] Extends refractory period,[G5] Positively inotropic,[G3, G5, 1, 2, 4, 5, 9] Cholesterol lowering,[G5] Antioxidant,[G5, 1] Collagen stabalization,[G5, 1] Increased coronary and peripheral blood flow.[G3, 1, 6, 7, 8]

CAUTIONS, CONTRA-INDICATIONS AND DRUG INTERACTIONS

Please reference Chapter 9. Do not use during pregnancy or lactation.

COMPLIMENTARY HERBS/FORMULAS

Hawthorn Berry Solid Extract, Night Blooming Cereus (for MVP - Practitioners Only), Anti-Oxidant Supreme, Ginkgo Leaf

REFERENCES

1. Murray M. The healing power of herbs - The enlightened persons guide to the wonders of medicinal plants. 2nd ed. Prima publishing. Rocklin, Ca. 1995.
2. Hobbs C, Foster S. Hawthorn - A Literature Review. *Herbalgram*. 1990; 22:19-33.
3. Mitchell W. Plant Medicine. Seattle, Wa. Self-published. 2000.
4. Loew D. Phytotherapy in heart failure. *Phytomedicine*. 1997; 4(3): 267-71.
5. Popping S, *et al.* Effect of a Hawthorn Extract on Contraction and Energy Turnover of Isolated Rat Cardiomyocytes. *Arzneim.-Forsch.* 1995; 45(1): 1157-61.
6. Ammon H, Handel M. Crataegus, Toxikologie und Pharmakologie Teil II: Pharmakodynamik *Planta Med.* 1991; 43(3): 209-39.
7. Schussler M, *et al.* Functional and Antiischaemic Effects of Monoacetyl-vitexinrhamnoside in Different In Vitro Models. *Gen. Pharmac.* 1995; 26(7): 1565-70.
8. Al Makdessi S, *et al.* Myocardial Protection by Pretreatment with Crataegus oxyacantha. *Arzneim.-Forsch.* 1996; 46(1): 25-27.
9. Witchl M. (Bisset NG, Ed.) Herbal Drugs and Phytopharmaceuticals. Medpharm, CRC Press: Boca Raton. 1994.

KAVA KAVA
(Piper methysticum)
*Ultimate Support for Relaxation**

Concentration:	3:1 Herb/Strength Ratio: 55% total Kavalactones from Kava 225mg/ 3 capsules
Dosage:	1 Liquid Phyto-Cap™, Three times daily
Duration of use:	4-6 Months
Best taken:	Between meals, with warm water

HISTORY

Kava is slow growing, perennial shrub. A member of the pepper family (Piperaceae), it is native to the tropical pacific region. Islanders who use it as a ritual beverage during ceremonies have long revered it. It is traditionally used as a social beverage for chiefs and noblemen who use it for its calming, relaxing effect. The root is also used medicinally to treat a variety of ailments including headache and insomnia.[1] Kava is cultivated commercially, where it is totally dependent on human intervention for propagation.

SCIENTIFIC RESEARCH

Kava is highly regarded in Europe as an effective treatment for anxiety. Numerous clinical studies have verified its efficacy. A randomized placebo-controlled trial evaluated kava's effectiveness in 101 patients with anxiety of non-psychotic origin. Subjects were followed for 6 months. Symptoms were evaluated using the Hamilton Anxiety Scale (HAM-A). Significant improvements were seen at 8 weeks (reduction of HAM-A score from 30-17) and continued for another 16 weeks. At the end of the trial the HAM-A score was reduced to 9. In this study, long-term treatment had better efficacy than short-term treatment. [2]

Similar, but quicker results were seen in a placebo-controlled double blind study of 40 women with menopause-related symptoms of anxiety. However, unlike the previous study there was a significant decrease (measured by HAM-A) in symptoms after just 1 week of treatment. Improvement continued throughout the full 8 week study period. [3]

Several studies have been conducted comparing Kava with benzodiazepines. A double-blind study of 174 patients with anxiety compared kava with oxazepam and bromazepam. Patients were followed for 6 weeks. Similar improvements in HAM-A scores were seen in all 3 treatment groups. Statistically there was no difference in the outcome of the 3 therapies. Kava was well tolerated with none of the side effects associated with benzodiazepines. [4]

A recent meta-analysis reviewed several clinical trials to determine the efficacy of kava for the treatment of anxiety. The reviewers concluded that kava was superior to placebo as a symptomatic treatment for anxiety. The authors agreed that Kava is an herbal option for the treatment of anxiety. [5]

MECHANISM OF ACTION

The exact mechanism of kava on the central nervous system is unknown. One possible mode of action is that kava may interact with Gama-Aminobutyric acid (GABA) receptors. Early in vivo and in vitro research found that kavalactones demonstrated only weak GABA receptor binding actions.[6] However, a more recent study found that kava pyrones mediate effects in GABA-A receptors, particularly in the hippocampus and amygdala.[7] Other possible mechanisms include inhibition of noradrenaline uptake [8] and activation of mesolimbic dopaminergic neurons. [9] It is likely that there is more than one pathway responsible for kava's activity on the central nervous system.

THERAPEUTIC APPLICATIONS*

Note: The intention of the following information is to represent the traditional use of the herb and to inform the reader of any evolving inquiry relevant to the herb.

SUPPORTED BY TRADITIONAL USE

Treatment of nervous anxiety and stress. [1-5, 10,11]

SCOPE OF RELEVANT SCIENTIFIC INVESTIGATION

Anxiolytic [2-3,10,11]

CAUTIONS, CONTRA-INDICATIONS
AND DRUG INTERACTIONS

Please reference Chapter 9. Do not use during pregnancy or lactation.

COMPLIMENTARY HERBS/FORMULAS
Phyto-Proz Supreme, St. John's Wort, Valerian root

REFERENCES

1. Piscopo G. Kava Kava. Gift to the islands. *Alt Med Rev.* 1997; 2(5): 355-364.
2. Voltz HP and Kieser M. Kava Kava extract WS 1490 versus placebo in anxiety disorders- a randomized placebo-controlled 25 week outpatient trial. *Phamacopsychiat.* 1997; 30:1-5.
3. Warnecke G. [Psychosomatic dysfunctions in the female climacteric. Clinical effectiveness and tolerance of kava extract WS 1490]. *Fortschr Med.* 1991; 109 (4): 119-122. [in German]
4. Woelk H, *et al.* The treatment of patients with anxiety. A double blind study: kava extract WS 1490 vs benzodiazepine. *Zitschrift for Allgemenie Medizine.* 1993; 69: 271-277. [in German]
5. Pittler MH, *et al.* Efficacy of kava extract for treating Anxiety: Systematic review and meta-analysis. *J Clin Psychopharmacology.* 2000; 20: 84-89.
6. Davis LP, *et al.* Kava pyrones and resin: studies on GABAA, GABAB, and benzodiazepine binding sites in rodent brain. *Pharmacol Toxicol.* 1992; 71 (2): 120-126.
7. Jussofie A, *et al.* Kavapyrone enriched extract from piper methysticum as modulator of GABA biding site in different regions of rat brain. *Psychopharmacology.* 1994; 116: 469-474.
8. Seitz U, *et al.* [3H]-monoamine uptake inhibition properties of kava pyrones. *Planta Medica.* 1997; 63(6): 548-549.
9. Baum SS, *et al.* Effect of kava extract and individual kavapyrones on neurotransmitter levels in the nucleus accumbens of rats. *Prog Neuropsychopharmacol Biol Psychiatry.* 1998; 22 (7): 1105-1120.
10. Blumenthal M, *et al. The Complete German Commission E Monographs: Therapeutic Guide to Herbal Medicines.* Austin. American Botanical Council; 1998: 156 & 157.
11. Schulz V, *et al. Rational Phytotherapy.* New York; Springer-Verlag; 1998: 65-73.

MILK THISTLE SEED
(Silybum marianum)
Ultimate Support for Healthy Liver Function*

Concentration:	3:1 herb strength ratio; 80% Silymarins (from milk thistle) 240 mg per 2 capsules
Dosage:	1 Liquid Phyto-Cap, Twice Daily
Duration of use:	4-6 Months
Best taken:	Between meals, with warm water

HISTORY

Milk thistle is an herbaceous annual or biennial plant with a dense-prickly flower head with reddish-purple tubular flowers. It's native to the Mediterranean region and has been naturalized in Central Europe, North and South America, and Southern Australia. Milk thistle has an extensive history of use as an medicinal and edible plant. In the 1st century AD, Pliny the Elder reported that it improved bile flow.[1] Theophrastus (IV century BC) and Dioscorides (1st century AD) also wrote of its medicinal value.[2] The English herbalist, Nicholas Culpeper (1650) claimed it was effective for removing liver obstructions.[1] At the turn of the 20th century, Eclectic physicians used milk thistle to treat jaundice, and hepatic pain and swelling.[G6] Much of the modern day research has been conducted in Germany where it is an approved medication for the treatment of liver disease.[3]

SCIENTIFIC RESEARCH

Hundreds of scientific studies have explored milk thistle and a group of its constituents called silymarins. Numerous animal studies have found that silymarin protects the liver from several hepatotoxins including *Amanita* mushrooms, alcohol, acetaminophen, carbon tetrachloride, gamma irradiation, and benzopyrene. [2, 4-8]

Many clinical studies have also demonstrated the hepatoprotective effects of silymarin. One double-blind study was conducted in 106 patients with elevated serum liver enzymes (most induced by alcohol). Subjects received either silymarin or a placebo. The patients who received silymarin had significantly lower liver enzymes than the placebo group. Histological examination of liver biopsies also showed a significant improvement. [9]

A double-blind placebo-controlled trial followed 146 patients with cirrhosis of the liver for 3-6 years. In the silymarin group, the 4-year survival rate was 58%, compared to only 38% in the placebo group.[10] In a double-blind study of 57 patients with acute viral hepatitis, the patients who received silymarin had significantly lower liver enzymes than those in the placebo group.[11]

MECHANISM OF ACTION

The exact mechanism of milk thistle and its constituents are unknown. Many diverse actions contribute to its hepatoprotective affects. Probable mechanisms of action include antioxidation, inhibition of lipid peroxidation, liver cell membrane stabilization, increased liver cell reproduction, inhibition of leukotriene and prostaglandin synthesis, kupffer cell inhibition, and mast cell stabilization. [12-18]

THERAPEUTIC APPLICATIONS*

Note: The intention of the following information is to represent the traditional use of the herb and to inform the reader of any evolving inquiry relevant to the herb.

SUPPORTED BY TRADITIONAL USE

Supportive treatment for inflammatory liver disease and hepatic cirrhosis [1,3,9-11] Toxic liver damage [1,3,19]

SCOPE OF RELEVANT SCIENTIFIC INVESTIGATION

Hepatoprotectant [4,5,15,16] Antioxidant [2,12,15]

CAUTIONS, CONTRA-INDICATIONS AND DRUG INTERACTIONS

Please reference Chapter 9. Do not use during pregnancy or lactation.

COMPLIMENTARY HERBS/FORMULAS

Liver Health, Hep-C, Cell Wise

REFERENCES

1. Luper S. A review of plants used in the treatment of liver disease: Part 1. *Altern Med Rev.* 1998; 3(6): 410-421.

2. Morazzoni P and Bombardelli E. Silybum marianum (carduus marianus). *Fitoterapia.* 1995; 66: 3-42.

3. Blumenthal M, *et al. The Complete German Commission E Monographs: Therapeutic Guide to Herbal Medicines.* Austin. American Botanical Council; 1998: 169-170.

4. Favari L, *et al.* Comparative effects of colchicine and silymarin on CCl4-chronic liver damage in rats. *Arch Med Res.* 1997; 28(1): 11-17.

5. Kropacova K, *et al.* Protective and therapeutic effect of silymarin on the development of latent liver damage. *Radiats Biol Radioecol.* 1998; 38(3): 411-415.

6. Shear NH, *et al.* Acetaminophen- induced toxicity to human epidermoid cell line A431 and heptoblastoma cell line Hep G2, in vitro, is diminished by silymarin. *Skin Pharmacol.* 1995; 8(6): 279-291.

7. Chrungoo VJ, *et al.* Silymarin mediated differential modulation of toxicity induced by carbon tetrachloride , paracetamol, and D-galactosamine in freshly isolated rat hepatocytes. *Indian J Exp Biol.* 1997; 35(6): 611-617.

8. Parish RC and Doering PL. Treatment of amanita mushroom poisoning: a review. *Vet Hum Toxicol.* 1986; 28(4): 318-322.

9. Salmi HA and Sarna S. Effect of silymarin on chemical, functional, and morphological alterations of the liver: A double-blind controlled study. *Scan J Gastroenterol.* 1982:17(4): 517-521.

10. Ferenci P, *et al.* Randomized controlled trial of silymarin treatment in patients with cirrhosis of the liver. *J of Hepatology.* 1989; 9: 105-113.

11. Magliulo E, *et al.* [Results of a double blind study on the effect of silymarin in the treatment of acute viral hepatitis, carried out at two medical centers]. *Med Klin.*1978;73(28-29): 1060-1065. [article in German]

12. Pietrangelo A, *et al.* Antioxidant activity of silybin in vivo during long-term iron overload in rats. *Gastroenterology.* 1995; 109(6): 1941-1949.

13. Dehmlow C, *et al.* Scavenging of reactive oxygen species and inhibition of arachidonic acid metabolism by silibinin in human cells. *Life Sci.* 1996; 58(18): 1591-1600.

14. Bosisio E, *et al.* Effect of the flavanolignans of silymarin marianum L. on lipid peroxidation in rat liver microsomes and freshly isolated hepatocytes. *Pharmacol Res.* 1992: 25(2): 147-154.

15. Muzes G, *et al.* [Effect of silimarin (legalon) therapy on the antioxidant defense mechanism and lipid peroxidation in alcoholic liver disease]. *Orv Hetil.* 1990; 131(16):863-866. [article in Hungarian]

16. Dehmlow C, *et al.* Inhibition of kupffer cell functions as an explanation for the hepatoprotective properties of silibinin. *Hepatology.* 1996; 23(4): 749-54.

17. Fantozzi R, *et al.* FMLP-activated neutrophils evoke histamine release from mast cells. *Agents Actions.* 1986; 18(1-2): 155-158.

18. Hikino H, *et al.* Natural products for liver disease. In: Wagner H, *et al. Economic and Medicinal Plant Research*, vol. 2. New York. Academic Press;1988: 39-72.

19. Schulz V, *et al. Rational Phytotherapy.* New York; Springer-Verlag; 1998: 214-220.

NETTLE LEAF
(Urtica dioica)
For Ultimate Relief of Allergy Symptoms*

Concentration:	3:1 Herb strength ratio: 1% caffeic acid derevatives: 1 mg/2 capsules
Dosage:	1 Liquid Phyto-Cap, Twice Daily
Duration of use:	4-6 Months
Best taken:	Between meals, with warm water

HISTORY

Nettle is an herbaceous perennial, infamous for the stinging hairs on its leaf and stem. The genus name is from the Latin *"uro"* (to burn) in reference to the painful rash caused by its biting hairs.[1] The herb grows in fields, moist thickets and along roadsides and can be found throughout North America and Europe. Nettle has been used since ancient times as a medicinal plant. The Greek physicians Dioscorides and Galen used nettle leaf to treat asthma and pleurisy. [2] During the late 19th and early 20th centuries, Eclectic physicians used this highly nutritious herb to treat eczema and chronic cystitis. [3]

SCIENTIFIC RESEARCH

Various studies have explored the use and actions of nettle leaf, nettle roots and its constituents. A randomized, double-blind study was conducted comparing 300mg of nettle leaf with a placebo in the treatment of allergic rhinitis. In those 69 subjects that completed the study, 58% rated it effective in relieving their symptoms and 50% found it to be equally or more effective than their previous allergy medication. [4]

MECHANISM OF ACTION

The mechanism of action of nettle leaf is unknown. Several studies have investigated nettle and its constituents and their affects on the immune system. During the allergic response inflammatory substances such as histamine, leukotrienes, prostaglandins, and cytokines are released causing a variety of symptoms.[5] In vitro and ex vivo studies have found that nettle leaf extract effectively inhibited prostaglandin and leukotriene synthesis and suppressed proinflammatory cytokine production. [6-9]

These actions may possibly contribute to the effectiveness of nettle leaf in the treatment of allergies.

THERAPEUTIC APPLICATIONS*

Note: The intention of the following information is to represent the traditional use of the herb and to inform the reader of any evolving inquiry relevant to the herb.

SUPPORTED BY TRADITIONAL USE

Allergic rhinitis [4, 10-11]

SCOPE OF RELEVANT SCIENTIFIC INVESTIGATION

Anti-allergic [4] and Anti-inflammatory [6,7]

CAUTIONS, CONTRA-INDICATIONS AND DRUG INTERACTIONS

Please reference Chapter 9. Do not use during pregnancy or lactation.

COMPLIMENTARY HERBS/FORMULAS

Turmeric/Catechu Supreme, Daily C Elixir, Eyebright/Bayberry Supreme, Feverfew, Olive leaf, and Green tea.

REFERENCES

1. Hyam R and Pankhurst R. *Plants and Their Names: A Concise Dictionary.* Oxford. Oxford University Press; 1995: 513
2. Blumenthal M, *et al. Herbal Medicine: Expanded Commission E Monograph.* Austin. American Botanical Council; 2000: 367.
3. Felter HW and Lloyd JU. *King's American Dispensatory.* Portland, Oregon. Eclectic Medical Publications; 1983: 2032-2034. (originally published in 1898).
4. Mittman P. Randomized, double-blind study of freeze dried urtica dioica in the treatment of allergic rhinitis. *Planta Medica.* 1990;56:44-47.
5. Roitt I. *Essential Immunology, 8th* Edition. Oxford. Blackwell Scientific Publications; 1994.
6. Obertreis B, *et al.* Ex-vivo in vitro inhibition of lipopolysaccharide stimulated tumor necrosis factor-alpha and interleukin-1 beta secretion in human whole blood by extractum urticae dioicae foliorum. *Arzneimittelforschung.* 1996; 46(4): 389-394.
7. Obertreis B, *et al.* [Anti-inflammatory affect of urtica dioica folia extract in comparison to caffeic malic acid.] *Arzneimittelforschung.* 1996; 46(1): 52-56. [in German]
8. Riehemann K, *et al.* Plant extracts from stinging nettle (urtica dioica), an antirheumatic remedy, inhibit the proinflammatory transcription factor NF-kappaB. *FEBS Lett.* 1999; 442(1): 89-94.

9. Klingelhoefer S, *et al.* Antirheumatic effect of IDS 23, a stinging nettle leaf extract, on in vitro expression of T helper cytokines. *J. Rheumatol.* 1999; 26(12): 2517-2522.

10. Thornhill SM and Kelly AM. Natural treatment of perennial allergic rhinitis. *Altern Med Rev.* 2000; 5(5): 448-454.

11. Riva R. Naturopathic specific condition review: allergies (immediate type hypersensitivity). *Protocol J of Botanical Med.* 1995; 1(2): 60-62.

OLIVE LEAF
(Olea europaea)
Support for Healthy Immune Function *

Concentration:	3:1 herb strength ratio;
	10% oleuropein (from olive leaf)
	40 mg per two capsules
Dosage:	1 Liquid Phyto-Cap, Twice Daily
Duration of use:	4-6 Months
Best taken:	Between meals, with warm water

HISTORY

Olive is an evergreen tree that grows to 8-12 meters in height. It's native to the Mediterranean region, where it has been cultivated for over 3000 years. The Roman's called the plant Olea from *oleum* meaning oil, after the valuable oil extracted from its fruits. To both the Greeks and the Romans the olive was a symbol of peace. The ancient Egyptians used the oil to mummify their kings. The English herbalist, John Gerard (1633) reported that olive leaves and buds were useful in the treatment of shingles, carbuncles, ulcers, and wounds.[1] In the 1898 edition of *King's American Dispensatory*, it was reported that a strong decoction of olive leaves could cure the most obstinate of fevers. It was believed to be more effective than quinine. [2] Historically, Olive Leaf has been used as a folk remedy for fevers and for fever producing diseases such as malaria.[3]

SCIENTIFIC RESEARCH

Several scientific investigations have examined the constituents of olive leaves. One of the constituents that has received considerable attention is called oleuropein. First isolated in 1908, oleuropein is a bitter glycoside, the first secoiridoid to be isolated. [4]

Oleuropein has been found to exhibit antimicrobial activity against pathogenic bacteria such as *Staphylococcus aureus, Salmonella* species, *Vibrio cholerae, V. alginolyticus,* and *V. para-haemotlyticus.* Oleuropein inhibited the growth of these bacteria, some of which are responsible for intestinal or respiratory tract infections in humans. Because of the broad antimicrobial activity of some of its constituents, the authors concluded that *Olea europaea* can be considered a potential source of promising antimicrobial agents for the treatment of respiratory tract infections in humans. [5] Constituents in olive leaf have also been found to inhibit the fungi *Aspergillus flavus* and *A. parasiticus* and the bacteria *Klebsiella pneumoniae, Bascillus cereus,* and *Escherichia coli.* [6]

Oleuropein has also been found to inhibit the secretion of enterotoxin B produced by *Staphylococcus aureus.* [7]

MECHANISM OF ACTION

The exact mechanism of action of Olive leaf is unknown. In addition to its antimicrobial properties, constituents found in olive leaf have been shown to be powerful antioxidants. Constituents have also been shown to inhibit low density lipoprotein (LDL) oxidation, and to potentate the macrophage-mediated response during endotoxin challenge. [3, 8-10]

THERAPEUTIC APPLICATIONS*

Note: *The intention of the following information is to represent the traditional use of the herb and to inform the reader of any evolving inquiry relevant to the herb.*

SUPPORTED BY TRADITIONAL USE
Microbial infections [2,11]

SCOPE OF RELEVANT SCIENTIFIC INVESTIGATION
Antimicrobial [5-7]

CAUTIONS, CONTRA-INDICATIONS AND DRUG INTERACTIONS

Please reference Chapter 9. Do not use during pregnancy or lactation.

COMPLIMENTARY HERBS/FORMULAS

Echinacea Supreme, Echinacea/Goldenseal Supreme, Lomatium Supreme, Spilanthes Supreme, Hep - C

REFERENCES

1. Gerard J. *The Herbal or General History of Plants.* New York. Dover Publications; 1975: 1392-1393. [The complete 1633 edition as revised and enlarged by Thomas Johnson]

2. Felter HW and Lloyd JU. *King's American Dispensatory.* Portland, Oregon. Eclectic Medical Publications; 1983: pg 1376. (originally published in 1898).

3. Benavente-Garcia O, *et al.* Antioxidant activity of phenolics extracted from Olea europaea leaves. *Food Chemistry.* 2000; 68:457-462.

4. Budavari S, *et al.* (editors). *The Merck Index. A Encyclopedia of Chemicals, Drugs, and Biologicals.* 12th Edition. Whitehouse Station, NJ. Merck and Company; pg.1171 (6967).

5. Bisignano G, *et al.* On the in-vitro antimicrobial activity of oleuropein and hydroxytyrosol. *J Pharm Pharmacol.* 1999; 51(8): 971-974.

6. Aziz NH, *et al.* Comparative antibacterial and antifungal effects of some phenolic compounds. *Microbios.* 1998; 93(374):43-54.

7. Tranter HS, *et al.* The effect of the olive phenolic compound, oleuropein, on the growth and enterotoxin B production by staphylococcus aureus. *J Appl Bacteriol.* 1993; 74(3): 253-259.

8. Visioli F and Galli C. Oleuropein protects low density lipoprotein from oxidation. *Life Sci.* 1994; 55(24): 1965-1971.

9. Visioli F, *et al.* Oleuropein, the bitter principle of olives, enhances nitric oxide production by mouse macrophages. *Life Sci.* 1998; 62(6): 541-546.

10. Coni E, *et al.* Protective effect of oleuropein, an olive oil biophenol, on low density lipoprotein oxidizability in rabbits. *Lipids.* 2000; 35(1): 45-54.

11. Stuart M. (editor) *The Encyclopedia of Herbs and Herbalism.* New York. Orbis Publishing; 1979: 229-230.

OIL OF OREGANO
(Origanum vulgare)
Supercritical CO_2 Extract of Oregano

Concentration:	400 mg Oil of Oregano per 2 capsules
Dosage:	1 Liquid Phyto-Cap, Twice Daily
Duration of use:	4-6 Months
Best taken:	Between meals, with warm water

HISTORY

There are many different species of plants call oregano. Origanum vulgare is a hardy, aromatic, bushy perennial with rose-purple, sometimes pink to white flowers. It is a European native, where it is commonly called "wild marjoram". Oregano has been highly prized for thousands of years for its culinary, cosmetic, and medicinal uses. Ancient Greeks held the plant in such esteem that they believed that Aphrodite created it to be a symbol of happiness. The ancient Egyptians also held the plant in high regard and used it as a disinfectant and preservative.[1] The English herbalist, John Gerard (1633) wrote that oregano is good for coughs, insect bites, and itchy wounds. [2]

SCIENTIFIC RESEARCH

Oregano and its constituents have been the subject of numerous in vitro and in vivo studies. The essential oil of oregano has been shown to be antifungal against *Candida albicans*, the yeast that is responsible for candidiasis. [3,4] Oregano essential oils have also been shown to inhibit mycelial growth and aflatoxin production in *Aspergillus parasiticus* and *A. flavus*. Both fungi, which grow on stored grains, produce liver damaging aflatoxins. [5,6] Oregano is also a powerful antibacterial agent and is effective against *Staphylococcus aurens, Pseudomonas aeruginosa, Escherichia coli, Salmonella pullorum,* and other pathogenic bacteria. [7]

A recent study investigated the use of oregano oil in the treatment of enteric parasites in 14 adult patients. After 6 weeks of treatment, there was a complete disappearance of *Entamoeba hartmanni* in four cases and *Blastocystis hominis* in 8 cases. Gastrointestinal symptoms improved in 7 of the 11 patients infected with *B. hominis.* [8]

MECHANISM OF ACTION

The mechanism of action of oregano oil is unknown. In addition to its antimicrobial actions, oregano has been shown to be a powerful antioxidant.[9,10]

THERAPEUTIC APPLICATIONS*

Note: The intention of the following information is to represent the traditional use of the herb and to inform the reader of any evolving inquiry relevant to the herb.

SUPPORTED BY TRADITIONAL USE

Intestinal disorders caused by microbial pathogens [4,8]

SCOPE OF RELEVANT SCIENTIFIC INVESTIGATION

Antifungal [3-5]   Antibacterial [3,7]

CAUTIONS, CONTRA-INDICATIONS
AND DRUG INTERACTIONS

Please reference Chapter 9. Do not use during pregnancy or lactation. Do not take pure *essential* oil of oregano internally. (Oil of oregano contains essential oils, it is not a pure essential oil)

COMPLIMENTARY HERBS/FORMULAS

Candida Supreme Vital Cleanse, Black Walnut/Coptis Supreme, Artemesia/Quassia Supreme, Spilanthes Supreme.

REFERENCES

1. Bremness L. *The Complete Book of Herbs: A Practical Guide to Growing and Using Herbs.* New York. Penguin Group; 1988:104-105

2. Gerard J. *The Herbal or General History of Plants.* New York. Dover Publications; 1975: 666-667. [The complete 1633 edition as revised and enlarged by Thomas Johnson]

3. Hammer KA, *et al.* Antimicrobial activity of essential oils and other plant extracts. *J Appl Microbiol.* 1999; 86(6):985-990.

4. Birdsall TC. Gastrointestinal candidiasis: Fact or fiction? *Alt Med Rev.* 1997: 2(5):346-354.

5. Montes-Belmont R and Carvajal M. Control of Aspergillus flavus in maize with plant essential oils and their components. *J Food Prot.* 1998; 61(5): 616-619.

6. Tantaoui-Elaraki A and Beraoud L. Inhibition of growth and aflatoxin production in Aspergillus parasiticus by essential oils of selected plant materials. *J Environ Pathol Toxicol Oncol.* 1994;13(1): 67-72.

7. Dorman HJD and Deans SG. Antimicrobial agents from plants: antibacterial activity of plant volatile oils. *J of Applied Microbiology.* 2000; 88: 308-316.

8. Force M, *et al.* Inhibition of enteric parasites by emulsified oil of oregano in vivo. *Phytotherapy Research.* 2000; 14:213-214.

9. Lagouri V and Dimitrios B. Nutrient antioxidants in oregano. International J of *Food Science and Nutrition.* 1996; 47:493-497.

10. Milos M, *et al.* Chemical composition and antioxidant effect of glycosidically bound volatile compounds from oregano (Origanum vulgare L. ssp. Hirtum) *Food Chemistry.* 2000; 71:79-83.

ST. JOHN'S WORT

(Hypericum perforatum)
*Ultimate Support for Emotional Well-Being**

Concentration:	3:1: .5% total hypericins; 2.7 mg/3 capsules
Dosage:	1 Liquid Phyto-Cap, Three Times a Day
Duration of use:	4-6 Months
Best taken:	Between meals, with warm water

HISTORY

St. John's Wort is a perennial herb with bright yellow flowers. It can be found growing wild in many parts of the world. This precious herb has an extensive history of use as a medicinal plant. In the 1st century AD, Dioscorides prescribed St. John's Wort for sciatica, burns, and fevers. During the 19th and 20th centuries Eclectic physicians used the aerial parts of the herb internally for hysteria and nervous affections with depression. [1]

SCIENTIFIC RESEARCH

St. John's Wort is an established medication for the treatment of mild to moderate depression in Europe. Numerous clinical trials have confirmed its efficacy. Several placebo-controlled studies were conducted in the early 1990's. In a multi-center, double-blind study, 72 patients with moderate depression according to DSM-III criteria, were randomized into two treatment groups. One group received 300mg (.9 mg hypericins) St. John's Wort three times a day, and the other group received a placebo. Significant improvement was seen in 80% of patients after 4 weeks of study. [2]

Another multi-center, double-blind trial with 105 subjects evaluated St. John's Wort for the treatment of mild depression. Patients received either St. John's Wort or placebo. Effectiveness was judged according to the Hamilton Depression Scale. At the end of the four-week study period substantial improvements were seen in the St. John's Wort group. There were no notable side effects. [3]

A meta-analysis of 23 randomized clinical trials including a total of 1757 patients was conducted in 1996. After reviewing the trials the authors concluded that St. John's Wort was significantly more effective than placebo for the treatment of mild to moderate depression. [4]

In addition to the placebo-controlled studies, there have been several trials conducted comparing St. John's Wort with pharmaceutical antidepressants. A recent 8-week double blind trial of 263 patients, compared St. John's Wort with imipramine and a placebo.

St. John's Wort and imipramine were equally effective in relieving symptoms associated with moderate depression. The range of side effects for St. John's Wort was in the same range as the placebo group. There were considerably more side effects in the imipramine group. [5]

Further studies have compared St. John's Wort with sertraline, fluoxetine (Prozac®), and imipramine. St. John's Wort was equally effective as the pharmaceuticals in treating mild to moderate depression.[6,7,8] In the study with fluoxetine, the herb was equally effective on the HAM-D scale. However, St. John's Wort was superior to fluoxetine on the Clinical Global Impression (CGI) score. St. John's Wort's safety was substantially superior to fluoxetine in type and number of adverse events.[7] One study concluded that St. John's Wort is therapeutically equivalent to standard antidepressants and should be considered for first line treatment in mild to moderate depression, especially in the primary care setting.[8]

MECHANISM OF ACTION

The mechanism of action of St. John's Wort is unknown. As with most botanicals its effects are probably the combination of differing modes of action. Early research suggested that St. John's Wort was a monoamine oxidase (MAO) inhibitor.[9] However, later research showed that no relevant MAO inhibition could be shown. The researchers concluded that the clinically proven antidepressant effects could not be explained in terms of MAO inhibition alone.[10, 11] Possible mechanisms include inhibition of synaptosomal uptake of serotonin, norepinephrine, and dopamine[12]; L-glutamine and GABA uptake inhibition[13], and serotonin uptake inhibition by elevating free intracellular $Na+1$.[14]

THERAPEUTIC APPLICATIONS*

Note: The intention of the following information is to represent the traditional use of the herb and to inform the reader of any evolving inquiry relevant to the herb.

SUPPORTED BY TRADITIONAL USE

Mild to moderate depression [2-8; 15-16]

SCOPE OF RELEVANT SCIENTIFIC INVESTIGATION

Antidepressant [12-14, 16]

CAUTIONS, CONTRA-INDICATIONS
AND DRUG INTERACTIONS

Please reference Chapter 9. Do not use during pregnancy or lactation. St. John's Wort appears to be an inducer of the metabolic pathway cytochrome P450. Therefore it should be used with caution in any drug that is metabolized via the cytochrome P450 pathway. This includes protease inhibitors for HIV (indinavir, amprenivir), transplant rejection drugs (cyclosporine, rapamycin), heart disease (digoxin), seizure (phenobarbitol) medication, and other pharmaceuticals.[17,18] However, it is important to note that certain foods such as grapefruit inhibit the cytochrome P450 pathway. Cruciferous vegetables such as broccoli and cabbage are P450 inducers.[19] Individuals receiving medical care and medications for depression should inform their physician of the use of St. John's Wort.

COMPLIMENTARY HERBS/FORMULAS

St. John's Wort Supreme, Phyto-Proz Supreme, Kava Kava, Cell Wise

REFERENCES

1. Felter HW and Lloyd JU. *King's American Dispensatory*. Portland, Oregon. Eclectic Medical Publications; 1983: 1038-1039. (originally published in 1898).

2. Hänsgen KD, *et al.* Multi center double blind study examining the antidepressant effectiveness of the Hypericum extract LI 160. *Journal of Geriatric Psychiatry and Neurology*. 1994; 7: s15-s18.

3. Harrer G and Sommer H. Treatment of mild/moderate depressions with hypericum. *Phytomedicine*. 1994; 1:3-8.

4. Linde K, *et al.* St. John's Wort for depression- an overview and meta-analysis of randomized clinical trials. *BMJ*. 1996; 313:253-258.

5. Phillip M, *et al.* Hypericum extract versus imipramine or placebo in patients with moderate depression: randomized multicentre study of treatment for 8 weeks. *BMJ*. 1999; 319: 1534-1539.

6. Brenner R, *et al.* Comparison of an extract of hypericum (LI 160) and sertraline in the treatment of depression: a double-blind, randomized pilot study. *Clinical Therapeutics*. 2000; 22(4): 411-419.

7. Schrader E. Equivalence of St. John's Wort extract (ZE 117) and fluoxetine: a randomized, controlled study in mild to moderate depression. *Int Clin Psychopharmacol*. 2000; 15(2): 61-68.

8. Woelk H. Comparison of St. Johns's wort and imipramine for treating depression: randomized controlled trial. *BMJ*. 2000; 321: 536-539.

9. Suzuki O, *et al.* Inhibition of monoamine oxidase by hypericin. *Planta Medica*. 1984; 50: 272-274.

10. Bladt S and Wagner H. Inhibition of MAO by fractions and constituents of Hypericum extract. *Journal of Geriatric Psychiatry and Neurology*. 1994; 7: s57-s59.

11. Theide HM and Walper A. Inhibition of MAO and COMT by Hypericum extracts and hypericin. *Journal of Geriatric Psychiatry and Neurology*.1994; 7: s54-s56.

12. Muller WE, *et al.* Hyperforin represents the neurotransmitter reuptake inhibiting constituent of hypericum extract. *Pharmacopsychiatry*. 1998; 31(suppl. 1): 16-21.

13. Wonnemann M, *et al.* Inhibition of synaptosomal uptake of 3H-L-glutamate and 3H-GABA by hyperforin, a major constituent of St. John's Wort: the role of amiloride sensitive sodium conductive pathways. *Neuropsychopharmacology.* 2000; 23(2): 188-197.

14. Singer A, *et al.* Hyperforin, a major antidepressant constituent of St. John's Wort, inhibits serotonin uptake by elevating free intracellular Na +1. *J Pharmacol Exp Ther.* 1999; 290(3): 1363-1368.

15. Blumenthal M, *et al. The Complete German Commission E Monographs: Therapeutic Guide to Herbal Medicines.* Austin. American Botanical Council; 1998: 214-215.

16. Schulz V, *et al. Rational Phytotherapy.* New York; Springer-Verlag; 1998: 50-65.

17. Breidenbach TH, *et al.* Drug interaction of St. John's Wort with ciclosporin. *Lancet.* 2000;255:1912.

18. Henny JE. Risk of drug interactions with St. John's Wort. *JAMA.* 2000; 283(13): 1679.

19. McIntyre M. A review of the benefits, adverse events, drug interactions, and safety of St. John's Wort (Hypericum perforatum): The implications with regard to the regulation of herbal medicine. *Journal of Alternative and Complementary Medicine.* 2000; 6(2): 115-124.

SAW PALMETTO
SUPERCRITICAL EXTRACT
(Serenoa repens)
*Ultimate Support of Prostate Health**

Concentration:	4:1 Herb Strength Ratio: 85-90% Fatty Acids from Saw Palmetto; 270 mg/2 capsules
Dosage:	1 Liquid Phyto-Cap, Twice Daily
Duration of use:	4-6 Months
Best taken:	Between meals, with warm water

HISTORY

Saw Palmetto is a small shrub native to the Southeastern United States. The berries were used by Native Americans as both a food and a medicine. Saw palmetto was official in the National Formulary from 1926-1950. The 23rd edition of the United States Dispensatory recommended saw palmetto berries for "the enlarged prostate of old men." [1] Whereas it fell out of favor in the United States, physicians in Europe continued to utilize this invaluable herb. In Germany today, it's one of the top ten herbal medications prescribed by physicians. [2]

SCIENTIFIC RESEARCH

Saw palmetto has been the focus of numerous clinical studies that have demonstrated its effectiveness in relieving the symptoms associated with benign prostatic hyperplasia (BPH). This condition affects 50% of men over the age of 50. BPH is the slow, progressive enlargement of the prostate gland. Symptoms include frequent urination, nighttime awakening to urinate (nocturia), straining to urinate, hesitancy, weak stream, sensation of incomplete emptying, and terminal dribbling.

One of the first double-blind studies of saw palmetto in the treatment of symptoms associated with BPH involved 110 patients. A significant number of subjects showed improvement in dysuria, nocturia, flow measurement, and residual urine. The extract was well tolerated.[3] An open trial with 505 subjects with mild to moderate symptoms of BPH demonstrated similar results. After 90 days of treatment, 88% of the patients felt the therapy was effective. [4]

A large double-blind, randomized international study of 1,098 men compared saw palmetto with the pharmaceutical drug finasteride. The patients were followed for six months. Both saw palmetto and finasteride increased urinary flow rate and improved quality of life. The study showed that saw palmetto and finasteride are equally effective in the management of symptoms associated with BPH. However, 9% of the men who received finasteride experienced a decline in sexual function, while 6% of the men in the saw palmetto group felt their sexual function had improved.[5]

A recent meta-analysis of 18 randomized trials concluded that saw palmetto improves urinary tract symptoms and urinary tract flow measures. Compared with finasteride, saw palmetto produces similar responses in urologic symptoms and has a much lower rate of erectile dysfunction. [6]

MECHANISM OF ACTION

The mechanism of action of saw palmetto is not yet fully understood. As with most herbal medicines, saw palmetto's effectiveness is probably the result of several differing actions. Possible explanations include inhibition of 5-alpha reductase, antiestrogenic activity in prostate tissue, prostate volume reduction, $alpha_1$- adrenergic receptor antagonism, and anti-inflammatory effects. [7-11]

THERAPEUTIC APPLICATIONS*

Note: The intention of the following information is to represent the traditional use of the herb and to inform the reader of any evolving inquiry relevant to the herb.

SUPPORTED BY TRADITIONAL USE

Reduction of symptoms associated with <u>benign prostatic hyperplasia</u> [3-6, 12]

SCOPE OF RELEVANT SCIENTIFIC INVESTIGATION

<u>Antiandrogenic</u> [12,13,14]   <u>Antiestrogenic</u> [8]

CAUTIONS, CONTRA-INDICATIONS AND DRUG INTERACTIONS

Please reference Chapter 9. Do not use during pregnancy or lactation.

COMPLIMENTARY HERBS/FORMULAS

Nettle root, Saw Palmetto Supreme

REFERENCES

1.Wood HC and Osol A. *United States Dispensatory*, 23rd Edition. Philadelphia. JP Lippincott; 1943:971-972.

2. Schulz V, *et al. Rational Phytotherapy*. New York; Springer-Verlag; 1998: 288.

3. Champault G, *et al.* A double-blind trail of an extract of the plant serona repens in benign prostatic hyperplasia. *British Journal of Clinical Pharmac.* 1984;18:461-462.

4. Braeckman J. The extract of serenoa repens in the treatment of benign prostatic hyperplasia: A multicenter open study. *Current Therapeutic Research.* 1994; 55(7): 776-784.

5. Carraro JC, *et al.* Comparison of phytotherapy (permixon) with finasteride in the treatment of benign prostatic hyperplasia: a randomized international study of 1,098 patients. *Prostate.* 1996; 29 (4): 231-240.

6. Wilt TJ, *et al.* Saw palmetto extracts for the treatment of benign prostatic hyperplasia: A systematic review. *JAMA.* 1998; 280 (18): 1604-1609.

7. Niederprüm HJ, *et al.* Testosterone 5_-reductase inhibition by fatty acids from sabal serrulata fruits. *Phytomedicine.* 1994;1: 127-133.

8. DiSilverio F, *et al.* Evidence that serenoa repens extract displays an antiestrogenic activity in prostatic tissue of benign prostatic hypertrophy patients. *European Urology* 1992; 21: 309-314.

9. Goepel M, *et al.* Saw palmetto extracts potently and noncompetively inhibit human a 1- adrenoceptors in vitro. *Prostate.* 1999; 38:208-215.

10. Gerber GS, *et al.* Saw palmetto (serenoa repens) in men with lower urinary tract symptoms: effects on urodynamic parameters and voiding symptoms. *Urology.* 1998; 51: 1003-1007.

11. Plosker GL and Brogden RN. Serenoa repens (permixon). A review of its pharmacology and therapeutic efficacy in benign prostatic hyperplasia. *Drugs Aging*. 1996; 9(5): 379-395.

12. Blumenthal M, *et al. The Complete German Commission E Monographs: Therapeutic Guide to Herbal Medicines*. Austin. American Botanical Council; 1998. Page 201.

13. Carilla E, *et al*. Binding of permixon, a new treatment for prostatic benign hyperplasia, to the cytosolic androgen receptor in rat prostate. *Journal Steroid Biochem*. 1984; 20: 521-523.

14. Sultan C, *et al*. Inhibition of androgen metabolism and binding by a liposterolic extract of Serenoa repen B in human foreskin fibroblasts. *Journal of Steroid Biochem*. 1984; 20: 515-519.

SIBERIAN GINSENG

(Eleutherococcus senticosus)
An Herb for Energy and Stamina *

Concentration:	3:1 herb strength ratio; 3.2 mg of Eleutheroside B & E per 2 capsules.
Dosage:	1 Liquid Phyto-Cap, Twice Daily
Duration of use:	4-6 Months
Best taken:	Between meals, with warm water

HISTORY

Siberian ginseng is a thorny shrub native to East Russia, Northeast China, Korea, and Japan. It is often confused with Panax ginseng, which is in the same family (Araliaceae) as Siberian (Eleutherococcus) ginseng. However, both are distinctly different plants. To help avoid this confusion, Europeans refer to Siberian ginseng as "eleuthero root".

During the 1950's and 1960's Russian scientists began to extensively study the constituents and activities of this plant. A new terminology was about to be born, as scientists studied substances that were able to bring about an "increased non-specific resistance" to an organism. These substances and the plants that contained them were called "adaptogens".

An adaptogen is a substance that helps the body adapt to stresses of various kinds. It must be absolutely harmless. It must have a "non-specific" broad therapeutic spectrum of action. It must also have a normalizing action that brings an organism back to homeostasis. Through Russian research, Siberian ginseng became the model of an adaptogen. [1]

SCIENTIFIC RESEARCH

Numerous clinical studies performed in Russia have documented the efficacy of Siberian Ginseng as an adaptogen. In the late 1960's and 1970's studies were conducted in over 2,100 healthy people. These studies showed the Siberian ginseng increased the ability of the subjects to withstand stresses such as heat, noise, motion, exercise, and increase in workload. Subjects also experienced increases in mental alertness and work output. [2]

One study was conducted with 100 children with acute diarrhea. Children were treated with either an antibiotic (monomycin) and Siberian ginseng, or the antibiotic alone. The children who received the Siberian ginseng recovered much earlier than those that received just the antibiotic. [3]

MECHANISM OF ACTION

The mechanism of action of Siberian ginseng is unknown. It is certain however, that many diverse actions contribute to the overall effectiveness of the herb. Constituents of Siberian ginseng have been shown to exhibit antioxidant, anti-cancer, hypocholesterolemic, immunomodulatory, immunostimulatory, radioprotectant, anti-pyretic, and anti-inflammatory activities. It is not known how these actions contribute to the adaptogenic affect of Siberian ginseng. [1-2, 4-6]

THERAPEUTIC APPLICATIONS*

Note: The intention of the following information is to represent the traditional use of the herb and to inform the reader of any evolving inquiry relevant to the herb.

SUPPORTED BY TRADITIONAL USE

Tonic for invigoration and fortification in times of fatigue and debility or declining capacity for work and concentration [7]

SCOPE OF RELEVANT SCIENTIFIC INVESTIGATION

Adaptogen [2-4]

CAUTIONS, CONTRA-INDICATIONS AND DRUG INTERACTIONS

Please reference Chapter 9. Do not use during pregnancy or lactation. The Commission E states that Siberian Ginseng is contraindicated in high blood pressure [7] However, some constituents may actually lower blood pressure. [G8]

COMPLIMENTARY HERBS/FORMULAS

Ginseng/Schizandra Supreme, Siberian Ginseng Tonic, Energy/Vitality Phyto-Caps

REFERENCES

1. Davydov M and Krikorian AD. Eleutherococcus senticosus (rupr. & Maxim.) Maxim. (Araliaceae) as an adaptogen: a closer look. *J of Ethnopharmacol.* 2000; 72:345-393.

2. Farnsworth NR, *et al.* Siberian Ginseng (eleutherococcus senticosis): current status as an adaptogen. In: Wagner H, *et al. Economic and Medicinal Plant Research*, vol. 1. New York. Academic Press;1985: 155-215.

3. Vereshchagin IA. [Treatment of dysentery in children with a combination of monomycin and eleutherococcus.] *Antibiotiki.* 1978;23(7):633-636. [in Russian]

4. Brekhman II and Dardymov IV. New substances of plant origin which increase non-specific resistance. *Annual Review of Pharmacology.* 1969; 9: 419-430.

5. Monakhov BV. [The effect of Eleutherococcus senticosus maxim on the therapeutic activity of cyclophosphamide, ethymide or benzotepa.] *Vopr Onkol.* 1967; 13(8): 94-97. [in Russian]

6. Bohn B, *et al.* Flow-cytometric studies with Eleutherococcus senticosus extract as an immunomodulatory agent. *Arzneimittelforschung.* 1987; 37:1193-1196.

7. Blumenthal M, *et al. The Complete German Commission E Monographs: Therapeutic Guide to Herbal Medicines.* Austin. American Botanical Council; 1998: 124-125.

VALERIAN ROOT

(Valeriana officinalis)
*Ultimate Support of Restful Sleep *

Concentration:	3:1 Herb Strength Ratio: .9% Valerenic Acid from Valerian 1.8 mg/2 capsules
Dosage:	2 liquid Phyto-Caps 1 hour before bedtime
Duration of use:	4-6 Months
Best taken:	1 hour before bedtime, with warm water

INTRODUCTION

Valerian is a perennial herb with a lengthy tradition of use in the treatment of insomnia. The root (rhizome) was official in the United States Pharmacopeia from 1820-1936 and in the

National Formulary from 1888-1946. [1] It is an approved over the counter sleep aid in Germany, France, Belgium, and Switzerland. [G4, 2, 3]

SCIENTIFIC RESEARCH

Numerous clinical studies have substantiated the efficacy of Valerian root in the treatment of insomnia. Insomnia is the inability to sleep under normal conditions. People with insomnia experience one or more of the following: inability to fall asleep (> 30 minutes) upon retiring; intermittent waking after falling asleep; or early morning awakenings.

One of the earliest studies was a placebo-controlled double-blind trial of 128 subjects. Participants received 400 mg of valerian extract, a valerian combination, or a placebo, 1 hour before bedtime. Subjects felt that they had a significant improvement in sleep quality and in time to fall asleep. Valerian had no detectable "hangover" effect the next morning. However, subjects who took the valerian formula reported morning sleepiness. [4]

A recent randomized, double-blind, placebo controlled study was conducted with 16 patients with established psychophysiological insomnia. Those persons taking the valerian extract had improvements in sleep structure and sleep perception. An interesting finding was that there were less side effects experienced with valerian (3 vs. 18) than with the placebo. [5]

There have been several studies comparing valerian or a valerian combination formula with pharmaceutical drugs used to treat insomnia. A randomized, double-blind study compared valerian with oxazepam. Sleep quality improved significantly in both groups. There was no statistical difference between the efficacy of valerian compared to oxazepam. This study was important because oxazepam has far more adverse effects and potential risks than valerian. [6]

MECHANISM OF ACTION

The exact mechanism of action by valerian is not yet known. We do know that a range of constituents and various modes of action contribute to its pharmacological activity. The mechanism is likely to be associated with increase levels of Gama-Aminobutyric Acid (GABA) in the brain. Studies suggest that sedation may partly result from an interaction of valerian with GABA receptors. [7] Constituents have also been shown to inhibit enzyme-induced breakdown of GABA in the brain. [8,9] Some studies have found GABA itself in valerian roots, however it is questionable if the body can assimilate it. [10]

THERAPEUTIC APPLICATIONS*

Note: *The intention of the following information is to represent the traditional use of the herb and to inform the reader of any evolving inquiry relevant to the herb.*

SUPPORTED BY TRADITIONAL USE

Insomnia [G4, G10, 2,4,5]

SCOPE OF RELEVANT SCIENTIFIC INVESTIGATION

Sedative, Hypnotic (produces sleep) [4,5,6,7]

CAUTIONS, CONTRA-INDICATIONS AND DRUG INTERACTIONS

Please reference Chapter 9. Do not use during pregnancy or lactation.

COMPLIMENTARY HERBS/FORMULAS

Valerian/ Poppy Supreme, Skullcap/ St. John's Wort Supreme, Sound Sleep, Serenity with Kava Kava

REFERENCES

1. Hobbs C. Valerian: a literature review. *Herbalgram.* 1989; 21:19-34.
2. Blumenthal M, *et al. The Complete German Commission E Monographs: Therapeutic Guide to Herbal Medicines.* Austin. American Botanical Council; 1998. Pg. 226, 227.
3. Upton R, editor. *Valerian Root, Valeriana officinalis: Analytical, Quality Control, and Therapeutic Monograph.* Santa Cruz, CA. American Herbal Pharmacopeia; 1999.
4. Leathwood PD, *et al.* Aqueous extract of valerian root (Valeriana officinalis L.) Improves sleep quality in man. *Pharmacology Biochemistry and Behavior.* 1982; 17: 65-71.
5. Donath F, *et al.* Critical evaluation of the effect of valerian extract on sleep structure and sleep quality. *Pharmacopsychiatry.* 2000; 33 (2): 47-53.
6. Dorn M. [Efficacy and tolerability of baldrian versus oxazepam in non-organic and non-psychiatric insomnia]. *Forsch Komplementarmed Klass Naturheilkd* 2000; 7(2) 79-84. [article in German]
7. Houghton PJ. The scientific basis for the reputed activity of valerian. *J. Pharm. Pharmacol.* 1999; 51: 519-526.

8. Wagner J, *et al.* Beyond benzodiazepines: Alternative pharmacologic agents for the treatment of insomnia. *The Annals of Phamacotherapy.* 1998; 32: 680-691.

9. Ortiz JG, *et al.* Effects of Valeriana officinalis extracts on [3H] flunitrazepam binding, synaptosomal [3H] GABA uptake , and hippocampal [3H] GABA release. *Neurochemical Research.* 1999; 24 (11): 1373-1378.

10. Santus MS, *et al.* The amount of GABA present in aqueous extracts of valerian is sufficient to account for [3H] GABA release in synaptosomes. *Planta Medica* 1994; 60: 475-476.

CHAPTER 6
Liquid Phyto-Caps™ – Formulas
Potency and Convenience

The following chapter represents Liquid Phyto-Cap™ formulations. This chapter is formatted somewhat differently than Chapter 5 in that each ingredient in the formula is discussed separately. Based on the supportive material present, "Traditional Use" and "Relevant Scientific Investigation" statements are then made suggesting the use(s) of the formula.

ANTI-OXIDANT SUPREME

*Whole Body Plant Anti-Oxidant**
FORMULA

Bilberry	(*Vaccinium myrtillus*)
Hawthorn berry	(*Crataegus oxyacantha*)
Ginkgo leaf	(*Ginkgo biloba*)
Green Tea	(*Camellia sinensis*)
Rosemary leaf	(*Rosmarinus officinalis*)
Prickly Ash bark	(*Xanthoxylum clava-herculis*)
Astaxanthin	

Concentration:	3:1
Dosage:	1 Liquid Phyto-Cap two times daily
Duration of use:	4-6 months or longer
Best taken:	Between meals with warm water

DESCRIPTION OF FORMULA

Free radicals, which are atoms that have an unpaired electron, are both essential to life and harmful. The body produces oxygen free radicals as a natural part of making energy (in the form of ATP) in most cells. Because making energy and thus free radicals cannot be avoided, the body has evolved a variety of defenses against free radicals known as antioxidants. These quench or neutralize the free radicals after they are produced, allowing cells to make ATP energy without building up toxic levels of free radicals. Natural antioxidants include such familiar substances as vitamin C, vitamin E, coenzyme Q10, superoxide dismutase, and catalase. The problem arises when the body comes under free radical assault above and beyond the burden from normal metabolic processes. When the air, water, and food all contain significant sources of free radicals, the body now has to quench these or face cellular damage and disease. Chronic inflammation causes a great increase in free radicals because immune cells produce free radicals to damage and kill infectious organisms and cancer cells. Additionally, white blood cells are very active, thus they require and produce a lot of energy and free radicals. Medicinal plants contain numerous types of vitamin and non-vitamin antioxidants that can bolster the body's defenses against free radicals.

Bilberry contains proanthocyanidin (PCO) molecules that are well-established as strong antioxidants.[1 2] Bilberry has shown the strongest affinity for the eyes, blood vessels, heart, and connective tissue (collagen).[3] It also protects the digestive tract and the skin. Bilberry can protect the blood-brain barrier and other blood vessels from becoming disrupted, as can happen when blood pressure is elevated.[4 5] Bilberry and its close cousin blueberry are used in traditional herbal medicine for ulcers, diarrhea, constipation, and diabetes.[6 7]

Hawthorn berry has a long history of use in traditional medicine for supporting normal heart function and structure.[8] The usefulness of hawthorn for heart concerns has been confirmed in research.[9] Modern research has also proven that hawthorn has potent antioxidant activity, in particular protecting collagen and the cardiovascular system.[10] Hawthorn is recommended by experienced clinicians for long term intake to obtain optimal benefits.[11]

Ginkgo leaf is a modern antioxidant phenomenon. The nuts were used traditionally but the leaves only rarely.[12] A great wealthy of studies in the past 50 years have thoroughly documented the antioxidant activity of this versatile herb.[13 14] Ginkgo's antioxidant effects appear to be most pronounced in the brain, nerves, and cardiovascular system.[15][16] In addition to quenching the common oxygen free radicals, ginkgo is also able to eliminate excessive nitric oxide, another type of free radical.[17]

Green Tea contains polyphenols and flavonoids that give it strong antioxidant activity according to most research.[18][19] Green tea is considered to be partly responsible for the low incidence of free radical-related conditions in Japan, China, and other places where green tea is widely consumed.[20]

Rosemary leaf has been demonstrated in numerous studies to be a powerful antioxidant.[21] Traditional reports of the benefits of rosemary include improving dementia and poor memory ("weakness of the brain"), preventing and eliminating infections, headaches, digestive upset, flatulence, colic, dandruff, edema, palpitations, and many other problems.[22]

Prickly Ash bark is considered a circulatory stimulant and nerve tonic in traditional herbal medicine.[23] It may accomplish some of its actions by being antioxidant, and it may theoretically help distribute other antioxidants throughout the body by increasing circulation.

Astaxanthin is the pink carotenoid that gives salmon, crabs, shrimp, and flamingos their color because these animals eat microorganisms that contain large quantities of it. Like other carotenoids, astaxanthin has proven to be a remarkably effective fat-soluble antioxidant.[24] This may be important in protecting cell membranes, that have a high fat content, against free radicals.[25]

THERAPEUTIC APPLICATIONS*

Note: The intention of this following information is to represent the traditional use of the individual botanicals found in these formulas and to inform the reader of any evolving scientific inquiry relevant to the formula's ingredients.

SUPPORTED BY TRADITIONAL USE

Ulcers, Diarrhea,[26] Constipation, Diabetes,[27] Atherosclerosis,[28] Dementia and memory loss,[29] Infections, Headache, Indigestion, Flatulence, Dandruff, Liver disease, Arthritis, Rheumatism, Venous insufficiency, Eczema

SCOPE OF RELEVANT SCIENTIFIC INVESTIGATION

Quenching free radicals,[30] antioxidant,[31] blocking induction of cancer in cells,[32] inhibiting formation of atherosclerosis,[33] chronic venous insufficiency,[34] varicose veins, prevention of free radical-related damage to nerves,[35] dementia, Alzheimer's disease,[36] arthritis, autoimmune diseases, diabetes mellitus, macular degeneration[37], congestive heart failure,[38] limiting free radical damage due to radiation exposure,[39] limiting blood vessel damage due to hypertension[40]

CAUTIONS, CONTRA-INDICATIONS AND DRUG INTERACTIONS

Please reference Chapter 9. Do not use during pregnancy or lactation. Anti-Oxidant Supreme should be used with caution in combining it with aspirin, non-steroidal anti-inflammatory drugs (NSAIDs) such as ibuprofen, warfarin (Coumadin), heparin, or any other drug that affects blood clotting.

Use of this formula should be discussed with a physician knowledgeable in herbal medicine before combining it with cancer chemotherapy or radiation therapy.

COMPLIMENTARY HERBS/FORMULAS

Whenever free radical overload is due to excessive inflammation, Anti-Oxidant Supreme should be combined with Infla-Profen, Migra-Profen, or Cell Wise. If macular degeneration is a problem, or to help prevent this condition, use Vision Enhancement together with Anti-Oxidant Supreme.

REFERENCES

1 Cunio L. *Vaccinium myrtillus. Australian J Med Herbalism* 1993;5:81-85.

2 Murray M. Bilberry (*Vaccinium myrtillus*). *Am J Nat Med* 1997;4:18-22.

3 Cunio L. *Vaccinium myrtillus. Australian J Med Herbalism* 1993;5:81-85.

4 Detre A, Jellinke H, Miskulin M, Robert AM. Studies on vascular permeability in hypertension: Action of anthocyanosides. *Clin Physiol Biochem* 1986;4:143-9.

5 Robert AM, Godeau G, Moati F, Miskulin M. Action of the anthocyanosides of *Vaccinium myrtillis* [sic] on the permeability of the blood brain barrier. *J Med* 1977;8:321-32.

6 Weiss RF. *Herbal Medicine.* Gothenberg, Sweden: Ab Arcanum and Beaconsfield: Beaconsfield Publishers Ltd, trans. Meuss AR, 1985:101-2.

7 Leung AY, Foster S. *Encyclopedia of Common Natural Ingredients Used in Food, Drugs and Cosmetics* 2nd ed. New York: John Wiley & Sons Inc, 1996:84-85.

8 Felter HW. *Eclectic Materia Medica, Pharmacology and Therapeutics.* Sandy, OR: Eclectic Medical Publications, 1922:325-6.

9 Reuter HD. *Crataegus* (hawthorn): A botanical cardiac agent. *Z Phytother* 1994;15:73-81. Reprinted in Q *Rev Nat Med* 1995;summer:107-17.

10 Murray MT, Pizzorno JE Jr. *Crataegus oxyacantha* (hawthorn). In: Pizzorno JE Jr, Murray MT (eds) *Textbook of Natural Medicine* vol 1. Edinburgh: Churchill Livingstone, 1990:683-7.

11 Weiss RF. *Herbal Medicine.* Gothenberg, Sweden: Ab Arcanum and Beaconsfield: Beaconsfield Publishers Ltd, trans. Meuss AR, 1985:162-9.

12 Squires R. *Ginkgo biloba.* ATOMS (*Austral Trad Med Soc*) 1995;autumn:9-14.

13 Yan LJ, Droy-Lefaix MT, Packer L. *Ginkgo biloba* extract (EGb 761) protects human low density lipoproteins against oxidative modification mediated by copper. *Biochem Biophys Res Comm* 1995;212:360-6.

14 Haramaki N, Aggarwal S, Kawabata T, *et al.* Effects of natural antioxidant *Ginkgo biloba* extract (EGB 761) on myocardial ischemia-reperfusion injury. *Free Rad Biol Med* 1994;16:780-94.

15 Oken BS, Storzbach DM, Kaye JA. The efficacy of *Ginkgo biloba* on cognitive function in Alzheimer disease. *Arch Neurol* 1998;55:1409-15.

16 Peters H, Kieser M, Hölscher U. Demonstration of the efficacy of *Ginkgo biloba* special extract EGb 761" on intermittent claudication--a placebo controlled, double-blind multicenter trial. *Vasa* 1998;27:106-10 [in German].

17 Marcocci L, Maguire JJ, Droy-Lefaix MT, *et al.* The nitric oxide-scavenging properties of *Ginkgo biloba* extract EGb 761. *Biochem Biophys Res Commun* 1994;201:748-55.

18 Brown MD. Review of green tea's role in cancer prevention. *Alt Med Rev* 1999;4(5):360-70.

19 Katiyar SK, Agarwal R, Mukhtar H. Inhibition of spontaneous and photo-enhanced lipid peroxidation in mouse epidermal microsomes by epicatechin derivatives from green tea. *Cancer Lett* 1994;79:61-66.

20 Imai K, Nakachi K. Cross sectional study of effects of drinking green tea on cardiovascular and liver diseases. *BMJ* 1995;310:693-6.

21 Ho CT, Ferraro T, Chen QY, *et al.* Phytochemicals in teas and rosemary and their cancer-preventive properties. In: Ho CT, Osawa T, Huang MT, Rosen RT (eds) *Food Phytochemicals for Cancer Prevention II: Teas, Spices and Herbs.* Washington, DC: American Chemical Society, 1994:2-19.

22 Grieve M. *A Modern Herbal* vol 2. New York: Dover, 1931, 1971:681-3.

23 Ellingwood F. *American Materia Medica, Pharmacognosy and Therapeutics* 11th ed. Sandy, OR: Eclectic Medical Publications, 1919:165-6.

24 Maher TJ. Astaxanthin continuing education module. Boulder, CO: New Hope Institute of Retailing, 2000.

25 Kurashige M, Okimasu M, Utsumi K. Inhibition of oxidative injury of biological membranes by astaxanthin. *Physiol Chem Phys Med NMR* 1990;22:27-38.

26 Weiss RF. *Herbal Medicine.* Gothenberg, Sweden: Ab Arcanum and Beaconsfield: Beaconsfield Publishers Ltd, trans. Meuss AR, 1985:101-2.

27 Leung AY, Foster S. *Encyclopedia of Common Natural Ingredients Used in Food, Drugs and Cosmetics* 2nd ed. New York: John Wiley & Sons Inc, 1996:84-85.

28 Hoffmann D. *The Complete Illustrated Herbal.* New York: Barnes & Noble Books, 1996:82.

29 Grieve M. *A Modern Herbal* vol 2. New York: Dover, 1931, 1971:681-3.

30 Naguib Y. Antioxidants: A technical overview. *Nutraceuticals World* 1999;March/April:40-42, 44.

31 Murray MT. Flavonoids: Tissue-specific antioxidants. Gaia Symposium Proceedings on Naturopathic Herbal Wisdom, 1994:107-10.

32 Brown MD. Review of green tea's role in cancer prevention. *Alt Med Rev* 1999;4(5):360-70.

33 Imai K, Nakachi K. Cross sectional study of effects of drinking green tea on cardiovascular and liver diseases. *BMJ* 1995;310:693-6.

34 Bombardelli E, Morazzoni P. *Vitis vinifera* L. *Fitoterapia* 1995;66:291-317.

35 Oyama Y, Fuchs PA, Katayama N, Noda K. Myricetin and quercetin, the flavonoid constituents of *Ginkgo biloba* extract, greatly reduced oxidative metabolism in both resting and Ca^{2+}-loaded brain neurons. Brain Res 1994;635:125-9.

36 Oken BS, Storzbach DM, Kaye JA. The efficacy of *Ginkgo biloba* on cognitive function in Alzheimer disease. *Arch Neurol* 1998;55:1409-15.

37 Age-Related Macular Degeneration Study Group. Multicenter ophthalmic and nutritional age-related macular degeneration study--part 2: Antioxidant intervention and conclusions. *J Am Optometric Assoc* 1996;67:30-49.

38 Reuter HD. *Crataegus* (hawthorn): A botanical cardiac agent. *Z Phytother* 1994;15:73-81. Reprinted in Q Rev Nat Med 1995;summer:107-17.

39 Emerit I, Oganesian N, Sarkisian T, *et al*. Clastogenic factors in the plasma of Chernobyl accident recovery workers: Anticlastogenic effect of *Ginkgo biloba* extract. *Rad Res* 1995;144:198-205.

40 Detre A, Jellinke H, Miskulin M, Robert AM. Studies on vascular permeability in hypertension: Action of anthocyanosides. *Clin Physiol Biochem* 1986;4:143-9.

CELL WISE

For Optimum Intra-Cellular Communication *
FORMULA

Coleus Forskohlii	(*Coleus forskohlii*)
Bupleurum root	(*Bupleurum falcatum*)
Feverfew herb	(*Tanacetum parthenium*)
Chinese Skullcap root	(*Scutellaria baicalensis*)
Jujube dates	(*Ziziphus jujuba*)
Licorice root	(*Glycyrrhiza glabra*)
Ginger rhizome	(*Zingiber officinale*)

Concentration:	3:1 Herb strength ratio
Dosage:	1 Liquid Phyto-Cap, Twice Daily
Duration of use:	4-6 Months
Best taken:	Between meals, with warm water

DESCRIPTION OF FORMULA

This unique formula addresses cellular dysfunction by restoring the integrity of cellular *memory*, where it has been lost. In effect, this formula helps a cell to *remember* the correct response to the body's water-soluble hormones.

The primary pharmacodynamic focus of this formula is to increase intra-cellular levels of the cyclic nucleotide adenosine monophosphate (cyclic AMP). It has been well established in the literature that low levels of this important secondary messenger are directly associated with immune and inflammatory processes in many Chronic Inflammatory Disease (CID) states. From mast cell degranulation in asthma and immediate-type hypersensitive reactions, to its role in the oxidative-stress induced hyperproliferative state of fibroblasts in psoriasis, it is clear that low cyclic AMP levels are associated with many deleterious processes. This formula serves to elevate cyclic AMP levels via those receptor-dependent and independent mechanisms associated with the diterpenoid molecule, forskolin (from *Coleus forskohlii*), as well as via the inhibition of the phosphodiesterase regulated hydrolysis of the cyclic AMP nucleotide to its ester group.

Coleus Forskohlii is by far one of the world's most researched medicinal plants. The majority of research has focused on forskolin, which is believed to be the plants most active constituent. It is well know to activate an enzyme that forms cyclic AMP within cells.[2, 14] Cyclic AMP, which is perhaps the most important cell regulating molecule, carries out the message of water soluble hormones within the cell. The plants traditional uses include; cardiovascular disease, eczema, abdominal colic, disorders of the respiratory system, insomnia, convulsions and painful urination.[1]

Bupleurum root has also been shown to increase cAMP.[2] This 'liver herb' is said to be anti-inflammatory and an immune stimulant that regulates and restores liver and gastrointestinal function. Its reported 'protective' properties encompass liver and kidney function.[3]

Feverfew herb is known to stimulate the formation of cyclic AMP.[2] As its name suggests it was traditionally used to reduce fever. It is also well known as an anti-inflammatory, used primarily for the relief and prevention of migraine headaches, arthritis, and menstrual disorders. [G10, 4,]

Chinese Skullcap root possesses cyclic AMP stimulating activity.[2] It is anti-inflammatory, and as such has been noted for its use with allergies, [G8] specifically asthma. [G7] Antibacterial, antiviral, and antioxidant properties have also been reported. [G16]

Jujube dates are reported to possess liver protective, anti-allergic and sedative properties (with particular mention for asthma). [G1, G3] Cyclic AMP is also increased by this invigorating and nutritive plant. [G1, 2]

Licorice root is included in this formula as an excellent anti-inflammatory and antispasmodic. It is well known to be anti-allergic, immunostimulating, and soothing the mucosal lining of the respiratory tract. [G1, G4]

Ginger root is known in the Ayurvedic tradition as vishwabhesaj, meaning the universal medicine.[6] It is a powerful anti-inflammatory which is known for its pronounced effect upon gastrointestinal function. [G1, 6] It is also known to increase cyclic AMP.[2] The value that this botanical brings to this formula is simply too vast to sum up here.

THERAPEUTIC APPLICATIONS*
Note: The intention of the following information is to represent the traditional use of the individual botanicals found in these formulas and to inform the reader of any evolving scientific inquiry relevant to the formula's ingredients.

SUPPORTED BY TRADITIONAL USE
Allergies, [G1, G3, G8] Inflammation, [G10, 4, 5] (where liver/digestive influence is evident), Asthma, [G1, G3, G7], Spasmodic cramping, Cardiovascular disease (where positive inotropic action is of benefit), Eczema, Hypothyroidism, Psoriasis, Abdominal colic, Respiratory disorders, Insomnia, Convulsions, Painful urination, and Liver toxicity.[3]

SCOPE OF RELEVANT SCIENTIFIC INVESTIGATION
Activates the formation of cyclic AMP (cyclic adenosine monophosphate) via activation of adenylate cyclase and inhibition of phosphodiesterase, [G1, 1, 14] antiallergic, [1, 13] mast cell stabalization, [1, 13] inhibits histamine release, [1, 13] inhibits tumor cell growth, [11, 12] cancer metastases, [1, 12] weight loss, [1, 10] glaucoma.[9]

CAUTIONS, CONTRA-INDICATIONS AND DRUG INTERACTIONS
Please reference Chapter 9. Do not use during pregnancy or lactation.

COMPLIMENTARY HERBS/FORMULAS

May be used to accompany any formula or therapeutic approach that works to restore correct cellular function. Such situations include; allergies of all types (combined with Turmeric/Catechu Supreme), asthma (combined with Grindela/Camelia Supreme), autoimmune conditions, weight loss (when used with small doses of *Corynanthe yohimbe* - under the supervision of a qualified holistic practitioner), abnormal cell growth (combined with Daily Detox and Hep C), and endocrine disorders too numerous to mention. The breadth of the use of this formula cannot be overstated.

REFERENCES

1. Pizzorno J, Murray M. Textbook of Natural Medicine. New York: Churchill Livingstone; 1999.
2. NAPRALERT Search results. Program for Collaborative Research in the Pharmaceutical Sciences College of Pharmacy, University of Illinois at Chicago. October 1994.
3. Bone K. Bupleurum: A natural steroid effect. *Canadian Journal of Herbalism.* 1996; Early Winter: 22-41.
4. Anonymous. Feverfew. *The Lawrence Review of Natural products.* 1994;September: 1-3.
5. Heptinstall S. Parthenolide content and bioactivity of Feverfew (*Tanacetum parthenium* (L.) Schultz-Bip.). Estimation of commercial and authenticated Feverfew Products. *J. Pharm. Pharmacol.* 1992; 44:391-395.
6. Newmark T, Schulick P. Beyond aspirin. Prescott. Hohm Press; 2000.
7. Brown D. Common Drugs and Their Potential Interactions with Herbs or Nutrients. *HNR.* 1999; 6(3): 209-22.
8. Brown D. Common Drugs and Their Potential Interactions with Herbs or Nutrients. *HNR.* 1999; 6(2): 124-141.
9. Snow JM. *Coleus forskohlii* Wild. (Lamiaceae). *PJBM.* 1995 Autumn; 1(2): 39-42.
10. Arner P, *et al.* Importance of the cyclic AMP concentration for the rate of lipolysis in human adipose tissue. *Clin Sci.* 1980; 59(3): 199-201.
11. Verma AK, *et al.* Croton oil and benzo(a)pyrene induced changes in cyclic adenosine 3'5'-monophosphate and cyclic guanosine 3'5' monophosphate phosphodiesterase activities in mouse epidermis. *Canc Res.* 1976; 36:81-7.
12. Agarwal KC, *et al.* Forskolin: A potent antimetastatic agent. Int J Cancer. 1983; 32(6): 801-804.
13. Marone G, *et al.* Inhibition of IgE mediated release of histamine and peptide leukotriene from human basophils and mast cells by forskolin. Biochem Pharmacol. 1987; 36(1): 13-20.
14. Snow JM. *Coleus forskohlii* Wild. (Lamiaceae). *The Protocol Journal of Botanical Medicine.* 1995; 1(2): 39-42.

DAILY DETOX
Ultimate Support of Internal Cleansing *
FORMULA

Corydalis tubers	(*Dicentra canadensis*)
Black alder bark	(*Alnus serrulata*)
Mayapple root	(*Podophyllum peltatum*)
Figwort	(*Scrophularia nodosa*)
Yellowdock root	(*Rumex crispus*)

Concentration:	3:1 Herb strength ratio
Dosage:	Liquid Phyto-Cap™: 1 Twice daily
Duration of use:	2 months
Best taken:	Between meals, with warm water

DESCRIPTION OF FORMULA

Originally compounded by Dr. John Scudder, MD, this alterative formula has long been known as Scudder's Alterative. Alteratives improve the removal of cellular wastes and promote correct nutrition. When this balance of basic cellular operation is normalized, we remove the 'obstacles to cure', and allow the healing force within the body to overcome disorder. This type of formula represents the most profound, yet basic, principle underlying Naturopathic Botanical Medicine. This Daily Detox formula is of value where the use of 'blood cleansers' are required.

Corydalis tubers were held in high regard by the physiomedicalists and the Eclectic physicians of the last century. [G15, 1, 3] It is said that "all the excretive avenues of the body are more or less emptied of injurious and impure contents"[1] and that "its efficacy is not equaled by any other agent as an alterative tonic". [G12] It is also of value in this formula for its ability to improve digestion. [G15]

Black Alder bark has a long history of use as a pain-relieving alterative. [G12] Dr. John Scudder, the medical doctor who created this formula, said that the Black Alder is simply the ideal alterative - due to the fact that "it exerts a specific influence upon the processes of waste and nutrition, increasing one and stimulating the other". [2] It is reported to have particular affect where indigestion, [G12, G15] or lymphatic congestion is present. [G12] Dr. Scudder also noted its use with conditions of the skin and mucous membranes. [2]

Mayapple root is another example of a highly respected alterative. [G12, 1, 3] Dr. Scudder discovered that if Mayapple is extracted in hot water, that the alterative compounds within the plant are extracted and the laxative compounds in the plant are left behind. The hot water extracted Mayapple is used here. Its reported affinity for improving weakened digestion, [G12] along with its established use with liver disorders, [G12, 3] make it of particular benefit in this formula.

Figwort joins this formula of noted alteratives. It has been described as a "mild and gently stimulating alterative", [1] "probably as certain in its action as any of the vegetable alteratives". [2] It is particularly respected for its influence with conditions of the skin. [1, 2]

Yellow Dock root is considered a tonic alterative with mild laxative action. [G12, 3] It is interesting that Native Americans and the Eclectic physicians of the last century used the Yellow Dock for its mild laxative quality, and for the treatment of skin conditions. [G12, 4] The Eclectic physicians noted that it was particularly useful where lymphatic congestion was present. [G12] Yellow Dock is also noted to improve digestion and reduce liver congestion, [3] making it of particularly useful here.

THERAPEUTIC APPLICATIONS*

Note: The intention of the following information is to represent the traditional use of the individual botanicals found in these formulas and to inform the reader of any evolving scientific inquiry relevant to the formula's ingredients.

SUPPORTED BY TRADITIONAL USE

<u>Alterative</u>, [G12, G15, 1, 2, 3] Improves digestion, [G12, G15, 3] <u>Lymphatic congestion</u>, [G12] Skin conditions, [G12, 1, 2, 4] Liver disorders, [G12, 3]

SCOPE OF RELEVANT SCIENTIFIC INVESTIGATION

None relevant

CAUTIONS, CONTRA-INDICATIONS AND DRUG INTERACTIONS

Please reference Chapter 9. Do not use during pregnancy or lactation.

COMPLIMENTARY HERBS/FORMULAS
Cell Wise, Supreme Cleanse

REFERENCES
1. Lyle TJ. Physiomedical Therapeutics, Materia Medica and Pharmacy. London. National Association of Medical Herbalists; 1897.
2. Scudder JM. Specific Medication. Eclectic Medical Publications. 1985.
3. Culbreth D. A manual of materia medica and pharmacology. Philadelphia. Lea & Febiger; 1927.
4. Willard T. Wild Rose Scientific Herbal. Wild rose College of Natural Healing; Alberta; 1991.

DIET-SLIM
*Ultimate Support for Weight Loss**
FORMULA

Green Tea	(*Camellia sinensis*)
Garcinia-Malabar Tamarind	(*Garcinia cambogia*)
Coleus Forskohlii	(*Coleus forskohlii*)
Elderberry	(*Sambucus canadensis*)
Gymnema leaf	(*Gymnema sylvestre*)
Bladderwrack fronds	(*Fucus veisiculosus*)
Turmeric root	(*Curcuma longa*)
Ginger root	(*Zingiber officinale*)
Yohimbe bark	(*Corynanthe yohimbe*)
Bitter Orange Peel	(*Citrus aurantium*)

Concentration:	3:1 Average Herb Strength Ratio
Dosage:	1 Liquid Phyto-Cap, Three times daily
Duration of use:	3-4 months
Best taken:	Between meals, with a small amount of warm water

DESCRIPTION OF FORMULA

This formula helps to correct fat cell metabolism by promoting a state of utilization rather than storage. It is particularly useful for what is known as the classic 'Venus' body type, where fat storage is concentrated around the hips, thighs and buttocks. Likewise, for individuals who lose weight - only to have it return - this formula is of particular benefit.

The primary pharmacodynamic focus of this formula is to establish a metabolic environment where adrenergic-receptor mediated lipolysis is enhanced. Two primary adrenergic receptors control lipolysis (beta-1 and alpha-2 type). The beta-1 receptor is coupled positively to adenylate cyclase, whereas the alpha-2 sites are negatively coupled the enzyme. It has been well established in the literature that lipolysis is co-related to the intra-lipocyte formation of the cyclic nucleotide adenosine monophosphate (cyclic AMP).

As one might expect, the underlying strategy of this botanical formula is three-fold:

> To block the negatively coupled alpha-2 adrenergic sites - thereby reducing their impact of decreasing cyclic AMP
> Activate positively coupled beta-1 sites to encourage the formation of cyclic AMP
> Prevent the breakdown of cyclic AMP via phosphodiesterase inhibition

In summary, this compound serves to elevate intra-cellular cyclic AMP levels via those receptor-dependent and independent mechanisms associated with the diterpenoid molecule, forskolin (from *Coleus forskohlii*), as well as via the inhibition of the phosphodiesterase regulated hydrolysis of the cyclic AMP nucleotide to its ester group. This strategy results in a net increase of cyclic AMP and an associated increase in the conversion of triglycerides into fatty acids and glycerols (lipolysis).

Other strategies of this important formula are to

> enhance thermogenisis thereby promoting fat metabolism
> balance sugar metabolism thereby correcting food cravings

> ➤ promote healthy liver metabolism thereby correcting detoxification and elimination patterns.

Note: Dietary and lifestyle adjustments must be made in conjunction with this formulas use. The 3 Season Diet by Dr. John Douillard, D.C., Ph.D. is recommended reading.

Green Tea has traditionally been used to enhance mental function, promote digestion, reduce flatulence, and to regulate body temperature.[1] It is used here for the established affect of several of its components to stimulate lipolysis (utilization of fat), by preventing the breakdown of cyclic AMP. Cyclic AMP is a molecule that affects hormonal messages within a fat cell. This 'message' helps to amplify the response of a fat cell to adrenaline; the hormone that tells it to *burn fat.*[2] Coleus is also valuable here as an established antioxidant[1] and as a moderate stimulant, further assisting the underlying function of the formula.[G3]

Garcinia-Malabar Tamarind is a natural source of hydroxycitric acid (HCA). HCA is known to cause an increase in fat metabolism; possibly via its influence over liver function.[2]

Coleus Forskohlii is perhaps Green Tea's best friend when it comes to weight-loss. As mentioned above, utilization of fat is in part controlled by the hormone adrenaline; along with its capacity to form cyclic AMP inside a fat cell.[4] Green Tea and Coleus both modify the fat *burning* affect of adrenaline (via modification of beta-1 adrenergic-receptor cAMP expression).[1, 2] Forskolin, one of the main active molecules in Coleus, is also antidepressive,[4] and has the ability to increase thyroid hormone production, making it particularly well suited for weight management.[4]

Elderberries bring a number of desirable qualities to this formula. They are recognized as being diuretic, laxative[G2, G12, 5] and liver protective.[5] Via these actions, the Elderberry promotes the removal of cellular wastes and helps to correct metabolism. [G12]

Gymnema leaf is a digestive or stomach tonic with well-known diuretic properties.[6] It has been reported to "neutralize the excess sugar present in the body in diabetes".[6] Gymnema is also known as *gur-mur* (which literally means, sugar destroying) because of its noted ability to abolish the taste of sugar.[6]

Bladderwrack fronds have been widely used, medicinally, for weight management.[G1, G2, G4] Such benefit quite possibly results from its stimulating effect on thyroid function.[G4] Bladderwrack fronds must be harvested however from pristine water, as they are known to absorb toxic waste metals from polluted waters.[G1, G12]

Turmeric root serves this formula through its outstanding antioxidant,[9] anti-inflammatory, and liver protective effects.[9, G1, G3] Normalizing liver function during weight management is highly desirable, as the liver is actively involved in regulating blood sugar availability, and metabolism of the 3-ketosteroids, which is a group of hormones which in part affect fat metabolism.

Ginger root addresses indigestion, and works as an antioxidant,[G3] anti-inflammatory, and as a carminative (reduces intestinal gas).[G3, G4] In addition to these benefits, Ginger is useful here as a circulatory stimulant,[G3, G4] helping to deliver the entire formula throughout the body.

Yohimbe has been included in this formula specifically for its ability to redirect adrenaline toward the receptors on a fat cell that burn fat (Beta-1), by blocking those which result in fat storage (Alpha-2).[10]

THERAPEUTIC APPLICATIONS*

Note: The intention of the following information is to represent the traditional use of the individual botanicals found in these formulas and to inform the reader of any evolving scientific inquiry relevant to the formula's ingredients.

SUPPORTED BY TRADITIONAL USE

Diuretic,[6, G2, G12, 5] Sugar taste reducer,[6] Digestive tonic[6]

SCOPE OF RELEVANT SCIENTIFIC INVESTIGATION

Weight loss,[G2, G4, 1, 2, 3, 10] Antioxidant,[1, 9] Anti-inflammatory, [G1, G3, G4, 7, 9] Cyclic AMP formation,[1, 2, 4, 10]

CAUTIONS, CONTRA-INDICATIONS
AND DRUG INTERACTIONS

Please reference Chapter 9. Do not use during pregnancy or lactation.

COMPLIMENTARY HERBS/FORMULAS

Cell Wise, Daily Detox, Supreme Cleanse

REFERENCES

1. Snow JM. *Camellia sinensis* (L.) Kuntze (Theaceae). *The Protocol Journal of Botanical Medicine.* 1995;1(2):47-51.

2. Fredholm BB, Lindgren E. The effect of alkylxanthines and other phosphodiesterase inhibitors on adenosine-receptor mediated decrease in lipolysis and cyclic AMP accumulation in rat fat cells. *Acta Pharmacol Toxicol* (Copenh).1984; 54(1):64-71.

3. McCarty MF, Gustin JC. Pyruvate and hydroxycitrate/carnitine may synergize to promote reverse electron transport in hepatocyte mitochondria, effectively 'uncoupling' the oxidation of fatty acids. *Med Hypothese.* 1999;52(5):407-16

4. Murray M. The unique pharmacology of Coleus Forskohlii. *The American Journal of Natural Medicine.* 1994; 1(3):10-13.

5. Anonymous. Elderberry. *The Lawrence Review of Natural Products.*1992; Jul.

6. Kapoor LD. Handbook of Ayurvedic Medicinal Plants. Florida. CRC Press; 1990.

7. Snow JM. *Curcuma longa* L. (Zingiberaceae). *The Protocol Journal of Botanical Medicine.* 1995;1(2):43-46.

8. Mitchell W. Foundations of Natural Therapeutics – Biochemical Apologetics of Naturopathic Medicine. Tempe, Arizona. Southwest College Press. 1997.

ECHINACEA SUPREME

Ultimate Support for Healthy Immune Function *

FORMULA

Fresh Echinacea root   (*Echinacea angustifolia*)

Fresh Echinacea root,   (*Echinacea purpurea*)

flower & ripe seed

Concentration:	3:1 Herb strength ratio (Standardized to 1.5% Tetranoic Isobutylamide using Full Spectrum Process™)
Dosage:	Liquid Phyto-Cap: 2 capsules every 2 hours at the onset of symptoms of cold or flu.
Duration of use:	5-10 days
Best taken:	Between meals, with warm water

DESCRIPTION OF FORMULA

Echinacea Supreme is an alterative formula that may be of assistance when immune stimulation is necessary. The many actions of this formula make it an appropriate choice for invasive and inflammatory conditions; specifically congestive disorders of the respiratory system.

In 1997, *Echinacea spp.* were the focus of over 350 studies. Madaus led some of the first pharmacological studies on Echinacea in the early 1950s, using the fresh expressed juice of *E. purpurea.*

Several activities have been documented for *Echinacea spp.*, including;

> ➤ Anti-inflammatory activity (cyclooxygenase and 5-lipoxygenase inhibition has been shown)
> ➤ Hyaluronidase inhibition and hyaluronic stabalization (established by Busing in the early 1950s)
> ➤ Non-specific immune stimulation
> ➤ Increased numbers of granulocytes in the blood
> ➤ Increases phagocytes
> ➤ Increased phagocytic performance by granulocytes and macrophages
> ➤ Inhibition of virus productivity
> ➤ Activation of cytokines
> ➤ Promotes a shift in the T4/T8-cell ratio in the direction of T4 cells
> ➤ Activation of macrophages cytotoxicity against tumor cells
> ➤ Macrophage produced tumor necrosis factor
> ➤ Increases macrophage production of interleukin-1, interferon-beta2 and oxygen radicals
> ➤ Increases B-lymphocyte proliferation

Echinacea has also been reported to be active against *Candida albicans, Streptococci, E. coli, Pseudomonas aeruginosa, S. aureus,* and *Listeria* monocytogenes

Note: In the context of this formula, *Echinacea angustifolia* and *Echinacea purpurea* will be discussed together. While there are certainly several distinct differences between the two species, exploration of such differences will only cloud the issue unnecessarily with semantics. Simply, *E. angustifolia* has a much longer documented history of traditional use, while *E. purpurea* has been the focus of more scientific research. Clinically (in practice), their actions are similar. Both species have been included in this formula to offer the full benefit of their collective chemistry, and individual subtleties.

Echinacea - It has been said that Native Americans used Echinacea to treat more conditions than any other remedy. It is an immune-stimulant, anti-inflammatory, antibacterial, antiviral, and has wound healing properties. [G1, G4] Traditionally, Echinacea has been used by Native Americans to treat colds, coughs, sore throats, and snakebite.[1] The Eclectic medical doctors, from the first half of the last century, also praised Echinacea for its benefits with various chronic catarrhal (congestive) conditions of the respiratory tract. [G12] Today, modern science is beginning to support much of its established traditional use, by showing that extracts of Echinacea spp. have the ability to increase antibody production, along with resistance to various infections.[3] Research has further shown that alcohol/water extracts of Echinacea significantly enhance natural killer cell function, [4] and have phagocytic, metabolic and bactericidal influence on macrophages.[5]

THERAPEUTIC APPLICATIONS*

Note: The intention of the following information is to represent the traditional use of the individual botanicals found in these formulas and to inform the reader of any evolving scientific inquiry relevant to the formula's ingredients.

SUPPORTED BY TRADITIONAL USE

Immune-stimulant, [G1, G4, 4, 5, 6] Anti-inflammatory, [G1, G4] Antibacterial, [G1, G4] Antiviral, [G1, G4] Wound healing, [G1, G4] respiratory catarrh, [G12] alterative, [G1] blood purifier. [G6]

SCOPE OF RELEVANT SCIENTIFIC INVESTIGATION

Immunostimulant, [G1, G4, G10, 2, 3] anti-inflammatory, antibacterial, antiviral, [G1, G4, G10, 2] wound healing, antitumor activity. [G1, G4, G10]

CAUTIONS, CONTRA-INDICATIONS AND DRUG INTERACTIONS

Please reference Chapter 9. Do not use during pregnancy or lactation.

COMPLIMENTARY HERBS/FORMULAS

Diaphoretics (promote perspiration): Yarrow, Elder flowers, Peppermint, Ginger, Sage, and Boneset. Composition Essence.

REFERENCES

1. Snow JM. *Echinacea* (Moench) Spp. Asteraceae. *The Protocol Journal of Botanical Medicine.* 1997; 2 (2): 18-24.

2. Bauer R, Wagner H. *Echinacea* species as potential immunostimulatory drugs. Economic and Medicinal Plant Research. San Diego: Academic press Ltd.; 1991.

3. Schranner I, Wurdinger M, *et al.* Modification of avian humeral immunoreactions by Influx and *Echinacea angustifolia* extract. *Zentralbl Veterinarmed* (B) 1989; 36.

4. Broumand N, Sahl L, Tilles JG. The in vitro effects of *Echinacea* and ginseng on natural killer and antibody-dependent cell cytotoxicity in healthy subjects and chronic fatigue syndrome or acquired immune-deficiency syndrome patients. *Immunopharmacology.* 1997; 35.

5. Bukovsky M, Kostalova D, Magnusova R, Vaverkova S. Testing for immunomodulating effects of ethanol-water extracts of the above ground parts of the plants *Echinaceae* and *Rudbeckia*. *Cesk Farm.* 1993; 42.

6. Witchl M. (Bisset NG, Ed.) Herbal Drugs and Phytopharmaceuticals. Medpharm, CRC Press: Boca Raton. 1994.

ECHINACEA/GOLDENSEAL

*Ultimate Support for Healthy Immune Function**
FORMULA

Echinacea root	(*Echinacea angustifolia*)
Echinacea root, flower, & seed	(*Echinacea purpurea*)
Goldenseal rhizome and root	(*Hydrastis canadensis*)
Oregon grape root	(*Berberis aquifolium*)
Barberry root	(*Berberis vulgaris*)
St. John's Wort flower buds	(*Hypericum perforatum*)

Concentration:	3:1 Herb strength ratio
Dosage:	Liquid Phyto-Caps™:
	2 capsules every 2 hours at the onset of symptoms of cold or flu.
Duration of use:	5-10 days*
Best taken:	Between meals, with warm wate

DESCRIPTION OF FORMULA

This formula activates immunity at times of invasion or infection or threatened infection. It is particularly useful with acute conditions when they are accompanied by inflammation of the mucous membranes. As you can see from the traditional use of this compound's ingredients (described below), it has been formulated to be broad acting in such situations.

In addition to the pharmacodynamic merits of Echinacea this formula employs the broad antmicrobial effects of the berberine containing botanicals.

Berberine has been shown to be active against the following organisms:

Candida albicans, Candida tropicalis, Trichophyton mentagrophytes, Microsporum gympseum, Cryptococcus neoformans, Sporotrichum schenkii, and *Entomoeba histolytica* (moderate activity), *Bacillus* spp., *Staph. aureus, Strep. pyogenes, Vibrio cholerae, Mycobacterium tuberculosis* var. *hominis, Xanthomonas* spp., some strains of *E. coli,* and *Shigella boydii.*

Echinacea is an immuno-stimulant, [G1, G4, G10, 1, 2, 3] whose anti-inflammatory, antibacterial, antiviral, and wound healing properties have been widely reported. [G1, G4] Almost any alterative formula that focuses on enhancing immunity could well benefit from this powerful botanical. (For additional information, please see the Echinacea Supreme description on the proceeding pages)

Goldenseal root is native to North America. It has traditionally been used with allergic/inflammatory[G1, 1] or infectious conditions that require soothing of the mucous membranes.[1] Like several other ingredients of this formula (i.e. Oregon grape root and Barberry root), Goldenseal contains the antibiotic[G4, 1] and immunostimulatory[1] alkaloid, Berberine. Along with one other key alkaloid (hydrastine), berberine has also been shown to be antispasmodic. [G4]

Oregon grape root has a history of traditional use closely resembling that of Goldenseal.[1] Oregon grape has distinguished itself, however, by its therapeutic effect with skin conditions, such as psoriasis, eczema, and acne.[1]

Barberry root is a bitter tonic[1] which, pharmacologically, shares many properties with Goldenseal and Oregon grape root. [G3, 1] And, as one may expect of plants with closely related chemistry, the traditional use of Barberry is also similar to other Berberine containing plants.[1] Fever-reducing activity has also traditionally been associated with Barberry, making it particularly valuable here.[G3]

St. John's Wort flower buds have been used as a medicine for more than 2000 years. Beyond its widely reported antidepressant[G3, 1] effect, it is utilized here for its affect with anxiety,[G1, G3] as well as to act as a valuable antiinflammatory[G1, G3] and an antiviral agent. [G3]

Propolis extract has been reported to be an immune stimulant[4, 5] with antiinflammatory[4, 5] effects (particularly when the mucous membranes are involved).[4]

THERAPEUTIC APPLICATIONS*

Note: The intention of the following information is to represent the traditional use of the individual botanicals found in these formulas and to inform the reader of any evolving scientific inquiry relevant to the formula's ingredients.

SUPPORTED BY TRADITIONAL USE

Immune enhancement,[G1, G4, G10, 1, 2, 3] antiinflammatory,[G1, G4, 1]

SCOPE OF RELEVANT SCIENTIFIC INVESTIGATION

Immune enhancement,[G1, G3, G4, G10, 1, 2, 3, 4, 5] antimicrobial [G1, G3, G4, 5, 6]

CAUTIONS, CONTRA-INDICATIONS
AND DRUG INTERACTIONS

Please reference Chapter 9. Do not use during pregnancy or lactation. *Note: Although there are conflicting beliefs surrounding the negative impact of using berberine-containing plants, it is suggested that you follow the use of this formula with probiotic treatment (L. acidophilus, L. bifidus, etc.). If Crohn's disease is present, please consult a licensed health-care professional before commencing probiotic use.

COMPLIMENTARY HERBS/FORMULAS

Warming remedies may also be used, as needed (Composition Essence, Ginger, & Boneset,).

REFERENCES

1. Murray M. The Healing Power of Herbs - The enlightened persons guide to the wonders of medicinal plants. Rocklin, Ca. Prima publishing; 1995.

2. Bauer R, Wagner H. *Echinacea* species as potential immunostimulatory drugs. Economic and Medicinal Plant Research. San Diego: Academic press Ltd.; 1991.

3. Schranner I, Wurdinger M, *et al.* Modification of avian humoral immunoreactions by Influx and *Echinacea angustifolia* extract. *Zentralbl Veterinarmed* (B) 1989; 36.

4. Balch JF, Balch PA. Prescription for Nutritional Healing. New York; Avery Publishing

5. Anonymous. Propolis. *The Lawrence Review of Natural Products.*1986; FEB: 1-2.

6. Tosi B, Donini A, *et al.* Antimicrobial Activity of Some Commercial Extracts of Propolis Prepared with Different Solvents. *Phytotherapy Research.* 1996; 10:335-336.

ENERGY & VITALITY

Ultimate Enhancement of Mental and Physical Stamina *

FORMULA

Korean Ginseng	(*Panax ginseng*)
Green Tea	(*Camellia sinensis*)
Nettle seed	(*Urtica dioica*)
Siberian Ginseng root	(*Eleutherococcus senticosis*)
Chinese Schizandra berry	(*Schisandra chinensis*)
Cola nut	(*Cola nitida*)
Licorice root	(*Glycyrrhiza glabra*)
Gingko leaf	(*Gingko biloba*)
Prickly Ash bark	(*Xanthoxylum clava-herculis*)

Concentration:	3:1 Herb strength ratio
Dosage:	1 Liquid Phyto-Cap, Three times daily
Duration of use:	4-6 months
Best taken:	Between meals, with warm water

DESCRIPTION OF FORMULA

This formula is useful for anyone who suffers from fading vitality and depleted energy, particularly those individuals who are constantly exposed to overwork, stressful environments or situations, and excess strain to mind or body. This formula efficiently combines herbs which are well known for their energy restoring influence, with those that address adrenal response, circulatory insufficiencies, and non-specific resistance to stress (including oxidative / free radical stress).

There is some evidence to suggest that Ginseng influences the Hypothalamus-Pituitary-Adrenal (HPA) axis, resulting in a net increase in ACTH and corticosterone production from the adrenal cortex. Central neuroendocrine changes have been noted with Ginseng use, as have changes in carbohydrate metabolism and increased synthesis of glycogen.

Korean Ginseng belongs to a genus (a sub-group of a family) named Panax - which is derived from the word *panacea* - meaning 'cure-all'.[2] The common name also honors this highly useful herb, for Ginseng means 'wonder of the world'.[1] It has traditionally been used to restore energy (both mental and physical) in the most debilitated of conditions.[G3, G5, 2] Interestingly, modern research convincingly supports this restorative/adaptogenic affect.[G5, 2, 3] As an adaptogen it builds resistance to stressors of both biological and physical origin.[G5, 3] This plant is the energy tonic *par excellence*.

Green Tea has a long history of use, dating back to around 2700 B.C. It is a stimulant and a powerful antioxidant[4, 5, 11, 12, 13] having been shown to effect liver detoxification in a manner that reduces free-radical damage to the liver tissue.[4] Free-radical damage has been linked to syndromes that result in low energy and chronic fatigue.[5, 6, 7] As oxidative (free-radical) damage is also associated with decreasing intracellular levels of cyclic AMP, it is beneficial that Green Tea increases levels of this important secondary messenger.[8, 9, 10] This cyclic AMP supporting effect, coupled with its mild stimulant influence, is highly desirable in a formula that aims to restore vital energy, particularly where it has been lost due to Chronic Inflammatory Disease (CID).

Nettle seed has been included here solely on the basis of empirical use with mental exhaustion. The authors have, on many occasions, used an extract of the Nettle seed to allay drowsiness. Its effect is not as a noticeable stimulant, but as what might be termed a mental adaptogen (enhances resistance to stress).

Siberian Ginseng, unlike the Nettle seed discussed above, is well known and well researched as an adaptogen. Traditionally it has been regarded as a treatment for fatigue, stress,[G5] and chronic illness due to deficiency.[14, 15] Modern research has shown it to be a stimulant with powerful antioxidant and stress-resistant qualities. It is widely reported to build resistance to the affect of both physical and mental stressors.[G5, 16, 17, 18, 19]

Chinese Schizandra berry has historically been used to treat physical exhaustion.[G3, G8] Modern research has highlighted its strong antioxidant and liver protective properties, along with its capacity to improve work performance and endurance.[G3, G8] Use of Schizandra has been shown to result in modification of the physiological response to stress.[20]

Cola nut is a caffeine containing plant that is used medicinally with nervous depression and debility.[G1] Although many individuals may initially think of Cola nut as a stimulant, it is well respected for use during convalescence by practitioners of the physiomedical system of medicine. In fact, it is said that Cola counters fatigue and restores nervous integrity; making it a valuable addition to this formula.[21]

Licorice root is often used with physical fatigue that is related to adrenal insufficiency.[G1, 22, 23] Whereas Siberian Ginseng reduces the adrenal gland's hormonal response to stress, Licorice prevents the breakdown of such hormones,[G3, 23] resulting in an overall reduction of the load that is placed on this important glandular function. Compounds isolated from licorice have also been shown to be immune-stimulating and potentially antidepressant.[G1, 23]

Gingko leaf has been shown to maintain energy levels in cells that might otherwise be adversely affected.[24] As with a number of this formulas ingredients, Ginkgo is recognized as a powerful antioxidant.[24, 25, 26] Its influence of increasing circulation[24, 25, 26] is also of benefit here.

Prickly Ash bark has traditionally been used for circulatory insufficiency.[G1, G3, G4, G20] Its use here is to help deliver the entire formula throughout the body. Traditionally, it was said that Prickly Ash has the ability to 'increase tonicity and functional activity' and to 'sustain the vital force through any crisis that occurs'.[G6]

THERAPEUTIC APPLICATIONS*

Note: The intention of the following information is to represent the traditional use of the individual botanicals found in these formulas and to inform the reader of any evolving scientific inquiry relevant to the formula's ingredients.

SUPPORTED BY TRADITIONAL USE

Energy restorative,[G3, G5, 2] Fatigue,[G1, G3, G5, G8, 2, 21, 23]

SCOPE OF RELEVANT SCIENTIFIC INVESTIGATION

Adaptogen (non-specifically enhances resistance to stress),[G5, 2, 3, 16, 17, 18, 19] Cyclic AMP elevation,[8, 9, 10, 23] Antioxidant,[4, 5, 11, 12, 13]

CAUTIONS, CONTRA-INDICATIONS AND DRUG INTERACTIONS

Please reference Chapter 9. Do not use during pregnancy or lactation.

COMPLIMENTARY HERBS/FORMULAS

Ginseng/Schizandra Supreme, Siberian Ginseng Tonic

REFERENCES

1. Coon N. Using plants for healing. Philadelphia, Pa. Rodale Press. 1979.

2. Sonnenborn U, Proppert Y. Ginseng (Panax ginseng C.A. Meyer). *British Journal of Phytotherapy.* 1991; 2(1) 3-14.

3. Bahrke MS, Morgan WP. Evaluation of the Ergonomic Properties of Ginseng. *Sports Med.* 1994; 18(4): 229-248.

4. Snow JM. Camellia sinensis (L.) Kuntze (Theaceae). *The Protocol Journal of Botanical Medicine.* 1995; Autumn: 47-51.

5. Pizzorno J, Murray M. Textbook of Natural medicine. New York. Churchill Livingstone; 1999.

6. Richards RS, *et al.* Free radicals in chronic fatigue syndrome: cause or effect? *Redox Rep.* 2000; 5(2-3): 146-7.

7. Richards RS, *et al.* Blood parameters indicative of oxidative stress are associated with symptom expression in chronic fatigue syndrome. *Redox Rep.*2000; 5(1): 35-41

8. Mahomed AG, *et al.* Anti-oxidative effects of theophylline on human neutrophils involve cyclic nucleotides and protein kinase A. *Inflammation* 1998; 22(6): 545-57.

9. Pizurki L, Polla BS. cAMP modulates stress protein synthesis in human monocytes-macrophages. *J Cell Physiol* 1994; 161(1): 169-77.

10. Yamamoto M, *et al.* Induction of human thioredoxin in cultured human retinal pigment epithelial cells through cyclic AMP-dependent pathway; involvement in the cytoprotective activity of prostaglandin E1. *Exp Eye Res* 1997; 65(5): 645-52.

11. Katiyar, SK, *et al.* Inhibition of spontaneous and photo-enhanced lipid peroxidation in mouse epidermal microsomes by epicatechin derivatives from green tea. *Cancer Let.* 1994; 79: 61-66.

12. Kahn SG, *et al.* Enhancement of Antioxidant and Phase II Enzymes by Oral

Feeding of Green Tea Polyphenols in Drinking Water to SKH-1 Hairless Mice: Possible Role in Cancer Chemoprevention. *Cancer Res.* 1992; 52: 4050-2.

13. Tanizawa H, *et al.* Natural Antioxidants. I. Antioxidative Components of Tea Leaf (*Thea sinensis* L.) *Chem Pharm Bull.* 1984; 32(5): 2011-14.

14. Bensky D, Gamble A. *Chinese Herbal Medicine: Materia Medica.* Seattle: Eastland, 1986.

15. Tierra M. *Planetary Herbology.* WI: Lotus Press, 1988.

16. Brekhman II, Dardymov IV. New Substances of Plant Origin Which Increase Nonspecific Resistance. *Ann Rev Pharmacol.*1969; 9:419-430.

17. Werbach M, Murray M. Botanical Influences on Illness: A sourcebook of clinical research. CA: Third Line Press, 1994.

18. Kamen B. Siberian Ginseng: latest research on the fabled oriental tonic herb. CT: Keats, 1988.

19. Fulder SJ. Ginseng and the hypothalamic-pituitary control of stress. *Am J Chin Med.*1981; 9(2): 112-8.

20. Panossian AG, *et al.* Effects of heavy physical exercise and adaptogens on nitric oxide content in human saliva. *Phytomedicine* 1999;6(1):17-26.

21. Priest AW, Priest LR. Herbal medication. A clinical dispensary handbook. 1982.

22. Baschetti R. Letter: Chronic Fatigue Syndrome and Liquorice. New Zealand Med Journ. 1995; Apr:156-157.

23. Snow JM. *Glycyrrhiza glabra* L. (Leguminaceae). *The Protocol Journal of Botanical Medicine.* 1996; Winter:9-14.

24. Willard T. Wild Rose Scientific Herbal. Wild rose College of Natural Healing; Alberta; 1991.

25. Squires R. Ginkgo biloba. *Journal of the Australian Traditional Medicine Society.* 1995; Autumn:9-14.

26. Snow JM. *Ginkgo biloba* L. (Ginkgoaceae). *The Protocol Journal of Botanical Medicine.* 1996; 2(1):9-15

GINKGO/GOTU KOLA
*Ultimate Support to Improve Memory**
FORMULA

Gotu Kola leaf & root	(*Centella asiatica*)
Siberian Ginseng root	(*Eleutherococcus senticosus*)
Ginkgo leaf	(*Ginkgo biloba*)
Wild Oats Milky seed	(*Avena sativa*)
Chinese Fo-Ti root	(*Polygonum multiflorum*)
Peppermint leaf	(*Mentha piperita*)
Rosemary leaf	(*Rosmarinus officinalis*)

Concentration:	3:1 Herb strength ratio
Dosage:	Liquid Phyto-Caps™: 1 capsule, Two times daily
Duration of use:	3-4 months for best results
Best taken:	Between meals, with warm water

DESCRIPTION OF FORMULA

This formula specifically focuses on enhancing mental function and circulation, particularly where such processes have become enfeebled due to stress and nervous exhaustion. This formula is adaptogenic; it promotes overall health and stamina, along with the ability to deal with stress, both physical and emotional.

Ingredients of this formula have been shown to improve peripheral circulation and oxygen transport, increase cerebral and memory function, exhibit neuroprotective influence, act as anti-oxidants, inhibit lipid peroxidation, protect against the effects of radiation, and reduce platelet aggregation (with implications in allergy, inflammation, bronchoconstriction, tachycardia, arrhythmias, and coronary flow - to name a few). Reports on the formula's ingredients also bring to light the ability to increase skin tissue integrity, improve connective tissue maintenance, increase formation of connective tissue structural components, and increase keratization of the epidermis. Improvement in capillary permeability and microcirculation have also been noted, making it potentially well suited to aid in the treatment of varicosities, or wherever structural weakness in also evident.

Gotu Kola leaf & root is considered to be one of the so-called 'elixirs of life'.[1, 2] It has long been used in India to improve intelligence and mental function.[G3] Several studies suggest that Gotu Kola may be useful with improving memory, reducing fatigue and stress, increasing general mental ability, and increasing I.Q. in developmentally disabled children.[G3, 2]

Siberian Ginseng root has been in use in China for over 4000 years. Used regularly, it is said to increase longevity, improve general health, improve the appetite, and restore memory.[2] Today, as an adaptogen, it is known to produce improvement in overall metabolic efficiency, as well as to increase resistance to disease and stressful influences.[G3, G4]

Ginkgo leaf is a plant that derives the majority of its medicinal support from modern science, not from established traditional use. Ginkgo leaf has been shown to reduce symptoms related to Cerebral Vascular Insufficiency (CVI), including impaired mental performance, dizziness, headache, depression, ringing in the ears, and short-term memory loss.[2, 3] Many studies today focus on its influence with repairing short-term memory loss.[3]

Wild Oat milky seed has a reputation as a trophorestorative (rejuvenating tonic).[5] It is useful in states of nervous debility, exhaustion, depression, sleeplessness and wherever convalescence is required.[G1, 4]

Chinese Fo-Ti root is traditionally said to replenish the vital essence of the kidneys and the liver.[G8] It is an excellent tonic to include in any formula that endeavors to support those functions whose loss is associated with aging and an overall loss of vitality.

Peppermint has traditionally been used as a digestive stimulant, and to provide relief from intestinal flatulence.[G3, G4, G5, 6] The oil from the plant is also reported to be antispasmodic, via its ability to relax smooth muscle.[G3, G4] Peppermint improves the taste of the formula.

Rosemary leaf is a natural antioxidant[G3] and anti-inflammatory.[G1] It has been proposed that natural antioxidants, such as Rosemary, may be useful to help reduce the free-radical damage that occurs with Alzheimer's disease.[7] Rosemary has been used for centuries as a tonic and stimulant, and as remedy for intestinal flatulence, indigestion, and nervous disorders.[G3] Known as the 'herb of remembrance', Rosemary has a long history as a memory-enhancing medicine.[7]

THERAPEUTIC APPLICATIONS*

Note: The intention of the following information is to represent the traditional use of the individual botanicals found in these formulas and to inform the reader of any evolving scientific inquiry relevant to the formula's ingredients.

SUPPORTED BY TRADITIONAL USE

Improve mental function,[G3, 2, 7] Tonic[G1, G3, G4, 1, 2, 4, 5]

SCOPE OF RELEVANT SCIENTIFIC INVESTIGATION

Improve mental function,[G3, G4, 2, 3] Reduce fatigue and stress,[G3, G4]

CAUTIONS, CONTRA-INDICATIONS AND DRUG INTERACTIONS

Please reference Chapter 9. Do not use during pregnancy or lactation.

COMPLIMENTARY HERBS/FORMULAS

Siberian Ginseng Tonic Elixir, Daily Nutrition Elixir with Elderberry, Vitality Herbal Elixir, Hawthorn Supreme, Ginkgo Liquid Phyto-Cap.

REFERENCES

1. Duke J. CRC Handbook of Medicinal Herbs. Boca Raton. CRC Press. 1985.
2. Murray M. The Healing Power of Herbs - The enlightened persons guide to the wonders of medicinal plants. 2nd ed. Prima publishing. Rocklin, Ca. 1995.
3. Snow JM. *Ginkgo biloba* L. (Ginkgoaceae). *The Protocol Journal Of Botanical Medicine.* 1996; 2(1): 9-15.
4. Witchl M. Herb drugs and phytopharmaceuticals. CRC Press.1994
5. Priest AW, Priest LR. Herbal medication. A clinical dispensary handbook. 1982.
6. Hutchens AR. A handbook of Native American herbs. Shambhalla publications. 1992.
7. Duke J. The Green pharmacy. Emmaus, Pa. Rodale Press. 1997.

HEP C
DEEP LIVER SUPPORT

*For Optimum Liver Function**
FORMULA

Chinese Bupleurum root	(*Bupleurum falcatum*)
Licorice root	(*Glycyrrhiza glabra*)
Reishi mushroom	(*Ganoderma lucidum*)
Maitake mushroom	(*Grifola frondosa*)
Astragalus root	(*Astragalus membranaceus*)
Chinese Skullcap root	(*Scutellaria baicalensis*)

Concentration:	3:1
Dosage:	1 Liquid Phyto-Cap two times daily
Duration of use:	6-12 months or longer
Best taken:	Between meals with warm water

DESCRIPTION OF FORMULA

The liver is the most important organ for carrying out many detoxification and metabolic functions. It helps the elimination of environmental toxins from the body and transforms food into the nutrients needed by the body. When the liver is disrupted by infection with the hepatitis C virus, its various functions become compromised. The immune system becomes overactive in an attempt to rid the body of the virus. Unfortunately, this is usually impossible and the result is that the immune system begins to damage healthy tissue throughout the body as well as attacking the virus. A large portion of this damage is due to generation of free radicals by immune cells. Free radicals normally kill microbes of all kinds, but they can also kill healthy cells. Hep C Deep Liver Support addresses these multiple problems caused by hepatitis C. It helps restore normal liver function and it helps calm the immune system. The formula also provides antioxidant defenses against free radicals.

Chinese Bupleurum root has primarily been researched as part of a traditional Chinese formula known as sho-saiko-to (which contains about 20% bupleurum). Sho-saiko-to has been shown to foster normal liver function in people with hepatitis C, hepatitis B, and other situations in which the liver is compromised.[1, 2, 3] Chinese bupleurum appears to protect the liver by decreasing inflammation, calming the immune system, and possibly by directly supporting protein synthesis in the liver.[4, 5, 6] Preliminary research also suggests that bupleurum may help to block fibrosis of the liver.[7] Bupleurum is highly regarded in traditional Chinese herbal medicine where it is considered helpful for infections, fever, liver problems, chest pain, and hemorrhoids.[8]

Licorice root is one of the most widely researched herbs. In particular it has been shown to support normal liver function in people with hepatitis C as well as other forms of viral hepatitis.[9, 10] It has been shown to prevent long-term problems in people with hepatitis C.[11] Licorice root blocks the breakdown of the body's own cortisol,[12] thus acting as an indirect anti-inflammatory throughout the body. The presence of higher amounts of natural cortisol would also tend to act as a break on excessive immune reactions. Studies suggest that in fact part of the benefit of licorice in people with hepatitis is mediated by the effects of this herb on the immune system.[13] Licorice has been used in traditional Western herbalism as a demulcent and expectorant for coughs,[14] to heal stomach ulcers,[15] to relieve Addison's disease (low adrenal function),[16] and for people with asthma, diabetes, urinary tract infections, tumors, and pain.[17] In traditional Chinese herbalism, licorice was widely used, including liver problems, asthma, coughs, abdominal problems including ulcers, and to make other herbs work together well in a formula.[18]

Reishi mushroom helps modulate the immune system, eliminate free radicals, and protect normal liver function.[19, 20] Numerous studies have confirmed its uses in traditional Chinese medicine for cancer, hypertension, heart disease, infections, diabetes, and liver disease.[21]

Maitake mushroom is one of many mushrooms used in traditional Asian and European herbal medicine that, like reishi, helps maintain normal immune function.[22]

Astragalus root restores normal function to the immune system and protects the liver from harm.[23, 24] Astragalus has a long history of use in traditional Chinese medicine for fatigue, loss of appetite, edema, debility, weakness, chronic ulcers, and wasting.[25]

Chinese Skullcap root provides potent antioxidant and anti-inflammatory defenses.[26] It is considered useful for people with viral hepatitis in China.[27] In traditional Chinese medicine it was recommended for all manner of "hot" (inflammatory) conditions and infections including dysentery, hepatitis, meningitis, jaundice, allergies, and hypertension.[28]

THERAPEUTIC APPLICATIONS*
Note: The intention of this following information is to represent the traditional use of the individual botanicals found in these formulas and to inform the reader of any evolving scientific inquiry relevant to the formula's ingredients.

SUPPORTED BY TRADITIONAL USE

Viral hepatitis,[29, 30] Jaundice,[31] Hypertension,[32] Infections,[33] Fatigue[34]

SCOPE OF RELEVANT SCIENTIFIC INVESTIGATION

Supports normal liver function despite viral infection of the liver,[35, 36] Hepatitis B,[37] Hepatitis C,[38] Immune Deficiency,[39, 40] Prevention of liver cancer[41]

CAUTIONS, CONTRA-INDICATIONS AND DRUG INTERACTIONS

Please reference Chapter 9. Do not use during pregnancy or lactation. Used in the recommended amount, adverse effects are not anticipated. If edema, high blood pressure, headache, or great thirst occur while taking this formula, consult with your physician. The risk of this unlikely situation can be further reducing by eating a diet high in fruits and vegetables and/or consumption of potassium in a multivitamin while taking Hep C Deep Liver Support.

Use with caution when combining this formula with aspirin, warfarin (Coumadin), heparin, or any other medication that blocks platelets or otherwise increases bleeding. Also use caution when combining this formula with digitalis or related heart medications.

There are reports that bupleurum combined with interferon can very rarely lead to serious inflammation of the lungs. Do not combine bupleurum with interferon without first consulting a physician knowledgeable in herbal medicine.

COMPLIMENTARY HERBS/FORMULAS

Anti-Oxidant Supreme is a useful combination with Hep C Deep Liver Support, as most people with chronic hepatitis have excessive free radical production and require additional antioxidant support. The Liver Health formula may provide additional nourishment to the liver. Milk thistle seed should be combined with this formula as it has been repeatedly shown to be beneficial for people with hepatitis C. If fatigue is a particularly strong symptom, Energy and Vitality may be useful to bring relief. If autoimmune complications occur, Infla-Profen may be useful in addition to Hep C Deep Liver Support.

REFERENCES

1 Gibo Y, Nakamura Y, Takahashi N, *et al.* Clinical study of sho-saiko-to therapy for Japanese patients with chronic hepatitis C (CH-C). *Prog Med* 1994;14:217-9.

2 Oka H, Yamamoto S, Kuroki T, *et al.* Prospective study of chemoprevention of hepatocellular carcinoma with sho-saiko-to (TJ-9). *Cancer* 1995;76:743-9.

3 Reichert R. Phytotherapeutic alternatives for chronic active hepatitis. Q *Rev Natural Med* 1997;summer:103-8.

4 Werbach M, Murray M. *Botanical Influences on Illness.* Tarzana, CA: Third Line Press, 1994:176-83

5 Mizoguchi Y, Sakagami Y, Okura Y, *et al.* Effects of sho-saiko-to (TJ-9) in hepatitis patients and on the metabolism of arachidonic acid. In: Hoyosa E, Yamamura Y (eds) *Recent Advances in the Pharmacology of Kampo (Japanese Herbal) Medicines.* Amsterdam: Excerpta Medica, 1988:396-404.

6 Yamamoto M, Kumagai A, Yamamura Y. Structure and actions of saikosaponins isolated from *Bupleurum falcatum* L. I. Anti-inflammatory action of saikosaponins. *Arzneim Forsch* 1975;25:1021-3.

7 Shimizu I, Ma YR, Mizobuchi Y, *et al.* Effects of sho-saiko-to, a Japanese herbal medicine, on hepatic fibrosis in rats. *Hepatology* 1999;29:149-60.

8 Bensky D, Gamble A, Kaptchuk T. *Chinese Herbal Medicine Materia Medica*, Revised Edition. Seattle: Eastland Press, 1993: 49-50.

9 Van Rossum TGJ, Vulto AG, Hop WCJ, *et al.* Intravenous glycyrrhizin for the treatment of chronic hepatitis C: A double-blind, randomized, placebo-controlled phase I/II trial. *J Gastroenterol Hepatol* 1999;14:1093-9.

10 Suzuki H, Ohta Y, Takino T, *et al.* Effects of glycyrrhizin on biochemical tests in patients with chronic hepatitis. Double blind trial. *Asian Med J* 1983;26:423-38.

11 Arase Y, Ikeda K, Murashima N. The long term efficacy of glycyrrhizin in chronic hepatitis C patients. *Cancer* 1997;79:1494-500.

12 Tamura Y, Nishikawa T, Yamada K, *et al.* Effects of glycyrrhetinic acid and its derivatives on 4-sulpha- and 5-beta-reductase in rat liver. *Arzneim Forsch* 1979;29:647-9.

13 Yoshikawa M, Matsui Y, Kawamoto H, *et al.* Effects of glycyrrhizin on immune-mediated cytotoxicity. *J Gastroenterol Hepatol* 1997;12:243-8.

14 Felter HW. *Eclectic Materia Medica, Pharmacology and Therapeutics.* Sandy, OR: Eclectic Medical Publications, 1922:395.

15 Weiss RF. *Herbal Medicine.* Gothenberg, Sweden: Ab Arcanum and

Beaconsfield: Beaconsfield Publishers Ltd, trans. Meuss AR, 1985:59-61.

16 Hoffmann D. *The Complete Illustrated Herbal*. New York: Barnes & Noble Books, 1996;:99.

17 Davis EA, Morris DJ. Medicinal uses of licorice through the millennia: The good and plenty of it. *Mol Cell Endocrinol* 1991;78:1-6.

18 Foster S, Yue CX. *Herbal Emissaries: Bringing Chinese Herbs to the West*. Rochester VT: Healing Arts Press, 1992:112-121.

19 Shiao MS, Lee KR, Lin LJ, Wang CT. Natural products and biological activities of the Chinese medicinal fungus *Ganoderma lucidum*. In: Ho CT, Osawa T, Huang MT, Rosen RT (eds) *Food Phytochemicals for Cancer Prevention II: Teas, Spices and Herbs*. Washington, DC: American Chemical Society, 1994: 342-54.

20 Lin JM, Lin CC, Chen MF, *et al*. Radical scavenger and antihepatotoxic activity of *Ganoderma formosanum, Ganoderma lucidum* and *Ganoderma neo-japonicum*. *J Ethnopharmacol* 1995;47:33-41.

21 Jones K. Reishi mushroom: Ancient medicine in modern times. *Alt Compl Ther* 1998;4(4):256-67.

22 Schar D. *Grifola frondosa*: A "new" immunostimulant? *Br J Phytother* 1997;4:168-75.

23 Zhang ZL, Wen QZ, Liu CX. Hepatoprotective effects of astragalus root. *J Ethnopharmacol* 1990;30:145-9.

24 Murray M, Pizzorno P. *An Encyclopedia of Natural Medicine*. Rocklin, CA: Prima Publishing, 1991:230.

25 Bensky D, Gamble A, Kaptchuk T. *Chinese Herbal Medicine Materia Medica*, Revised Edition. Seattle: Eastland Press, 1993:318-20.

26 van Loon IM. The golden root: Clinical applications of *Scutellaria baicalensis* Georgi flavonoids as modulators of the inflammatory response. *Alt Med Rev* 1997;2:472-80.

27 Huang CK. *The Pharmacology of Chinese Herbs*. 290-1.

28 van Loon IM. The golden root: Clinical applications of *Scutellaria baicalensis* Georgi flavonoids as modulators of the inflammatory response. *Alt Med Rev* 1997;2:472-80.

29 Salmond S. Herbs and hepatitis C. *Int J Alt Compl Med* 1997;15:17-19.

30 Foster S, Yue CX. *Herbal Emissaries: Bringing Chinese Herbs to the West*. Rochester VT: Healing Arts Press, 1992.

31 Bensky D, Gamble A, Kaptchuk T. *Chinese Herbal Medicine Materia Medica*, Revised Edition. Seattle: Eastland Press, 1993.

32 Willard T, Jones K. *Reishi Mushroom: herb of spiritual potency and medical wonder*. Issaquah, WA: Sylvan Press, 1990.

33 Foster S, Yue CX. *Herbal Emissaries: Bringing Chinese Herbs to the West*. Rochester VT: Healing Arts Press, 1992.

34 Foster S, Yue CX. *Herbal Emissaries: Bringing Chinese Herbs to the West*. Rochester VT: Healing Arts Press, 1992.

35 Gibo Y, Nakamura Y, Takahashi N, *et al*. Clinical study of sho-saiko-to therapy for Japanese patients with chronic hepatitis C (CH-C). *Prog Med* 1994;14:217-9.

36 Arase Y, Ikeda K, Murashima N. The long term efficacy of glycyrrhizin in chronic hepatitis C patients. *Cancer* 1997;79:1494-500.

37 Suzuki H, Ohta Y, Takino T, *et al*. Effects of glycyrrhizin on biochemical tests in patients with chronic hepatitis. Double blind trial. *Asian Med J* 1983;26:423-38.

38 Van Rossum TGJ, Vulto AG, Hop WCJ, *et al*. Intravenous glycyrrhizin for the treatment of chronic hepatitis C: A double-blind, randomized, placebo-controlled phase I/II trial. *J Gastroenterol Hepatol* 1999;14:1093-9.

39 Jones K. Reishi mushroom: Ancient medicine in modern times. *Alt Compl Ther* 1998;4(4):256-67.

40 Schar D. *Grifola frondosa*: A "new" immunostimulant? *Br J Phytother* 1997;4:168-75.

41 Arase Y, Ikeda K, Murashima N. The long term efficacy of glycyrrhizin in chronic hepatitis C patients. *Cancer* 1997;79:1494-500.

42 Ishizaki T, Saski F, Ameshima S, *et al*. Pneumonitis during interferon and/or herbal drug therapy in patients with chronic active hepatitis. 1996;9:2691-6.

INFLA-PROFEN

*Ultimate Relief of Inflammation and Back Pain**

FORMULA

Devil's Claw tuber	(*Harpagophytum procumbens*)
Feverfew leaf	(*Tanacetum parthenium*)
Yucca root	(*Yucca spp*)
Jamaican Dogwood bark	(*Piscidia erythrina*)
Nettle leaf & seed	(*Urtica dioica*)
Burdock root & seed	(*Arctium lappa*)
Celery seed	(*Apium graveolens*)
Ginger rhizome	(*Zingiber officinale*)
Turmeric root	(*Curcuma longa*)

Concentration:	3:1
Dosage:	1 Liquid Phyto-Cap, Twice Daily
Duration of use:	4-6 Months
Best taken:	Between meals, with warm water

DESCRIPTION OF FORMULA

The Infla-Profen formula provides multiple herbs that help regulate the immune system and its signaling compounds, particularly cytokines and prostaglandins. These compounds are essential for maintaining normal function in most parts of the body such as the joints and the musculoskeletal system, particularly when they are stressed. The body normally responds to trauma by activating what is known as the inflammatory cascade. This is another way of saying the immune system's cells send out signals telling the damaged area to protect and repair itself. Scientific research has demonstrated, however, that this reaction can become abnormal and establish counterproductive, chronic inflammation in the joints, muscles, and most other parts of the body. Arthritis and chronic low back pain are two common examples of this problem. This formula helps normalize abnormal inflammatory processes and relieve the many problems they can cause by interfering with abnormal communication and promoting healthy communication between the immune system and damaged cells.

Devil's Claw tuber is a plant from southern Africa long valued by the native peoples there as an anti-inflammatory, for migraines, wounds, labor pains, and as a digestive tonic.[1] It is still not known how devil's claw works, though it does not work like non-steroidal anti-inflammatory drugs (NSAIDs like ibuprofen).[2] Thus it does not damage the stomach like these drugs do. In fact, it may even help maintain healthy digestion.[3] Regardless of how it works, devil's claw is well established to maintain normal joint function and back mobility.[4][5]

Feverfew leaf is perhaps best known for its ability to offset inflammation in the head.[6] Extensive study has shown that feverfew acts on immune cells to normalize theirs signals to other cells, including by blocking release of precursors to prostaglandin production, inhibiting production of inflammation-promoting prostaglandins, and interfering with serotonin's pro-inflammatory effects.[7] Feverfew also seems to act to prevent platelets from releasing chemical messengers that provoke inflammation.[8] This may be particularly important for preventing problems in the blood vessels of the brain. Not all studies have confirmed the efficacy of this plant for inflammatory conditions.[9] Feverfew was traditionally used for headaches, migraines, arthritis, dizziness, tinnitus, and painful periods (dysmenorrhea).[10,11]

Yucca root is a common desert plant in the southwestern United States. Saponins in yucca root have been shown to help counter chronic joint inflammation, though the mechanisms of action are unknown.[12] Yucca root was and is widely used for dandruff, arthritis, and prostatitis by traditional herbalists in the desert Southwest.[13]

Jamaican Dogwood bark has not been well researched but has shown muscle relaxing properties.[14] Its mechanism of action is unknown. Jamaican dogwood was valued in traditional herbal medicine for relief of pain, muscle cramps, rheumatism, spasmodic coughs, insomnia, and neuralgia (nerve pain).[15, 16]

Nettle leaf & seed are able to exert numerous effects on the signals sent by the immune system that provoke chronic inflammation. Studies have shown that nettle can block formation of pro-inflammatory cytokines[17] and prostaglandins.[18] It may even be able to convert some T cells, cells that control the rest of the immune system, into forms that inhibit rather than promote inflammatory reactions.[19] Nettle has been shown to help maintain a healthy urine flow.[20] Nettle leaf and seed were widely used in traditional medicine to relieve arthritis pain, help fight bladder infections, and for gout, chronic skin diseases such as eczema, autoimmune diseases such as lupus and rheumatoid arthritis, bleeding, diarrhea, kidney inflammations, wounds, and sciatica.[21]

Burdock root & seed have long been used in traditional herbalism for inflammatory conditions including rheumatism and arthritis, gout, and inflammatory skin problems like eczema and psoriasis.[22, 23] Burdock root acts as an antioxidant and interferes with a messenger chemical known as platelet-activating factor that strongly promotes excessive inflammation.[24, 25]

Celery seed has traditionally been used as a remedy for arthritis, gout, rheumatism, bladder infections, congestive heart failure, anxiety, gas, and loss of appetite.[26] It is included because of its anti-inflammatory properties.

Ginger rhizome is one of the most powerful botanical inhibitors of 5-lipoxygenase,[27, 28, 29] an enzyme responsible for excessive production of pro-inflammatory prostaglandins and thromboxanes. Ginger is used in many traditional Ayurvedic formulas that were traditionally employed in people with arthritis and other inflammatory disorders.[30] Ginger is also valued in traditional Western herbalism for arthritis, rheumatism, muscle aches, migraine, and flatulence.[31] It is also highly regarded for its effect on gastrointestinal function.[32]

Turmeric root is similar to ginger in that it is one of the most powerful inhibitors of formation of prostaglandins and thromboxanes that promote excessively inflammation.[33, 34] Turmeric has also been shown to specifically not interfere with beneficial prostaglandins, such as those that protect the stomach, unlike aspirin.[35] Turmeric is traditionally used in Ayurvedic medicine for rheumatoid arthritis and a wide variety of other inflammatory diseases as well for wounds, upset stomach, liver problems, and eczema.[36, 37]

THERAPEUTIC APPLICATIONS*

Note: The intention of this following information is to represent the traditional use of the individual botanicals found in these formulas and to inform the reader of any evolving scientific inquiry relevant to the formula's ingredients.

SUPPORTED BY TRADITIONAL USE

Osteoarthritis,[38, 39] Rheumatoid arthritis,[40, 41] Rheumatism, [42, 43] Low back pain, Lumbago, Muscle aches,[44, 45, 46] Headaches where muscle tension is involved,[47] Dysmenorrhea (menstrual cramps), Gout, Prostatitis, Neuralgia, and Lupus.

SCOPE OF RELEVANT SCIENTIFIC INVESTIGATION

Inhibits formation and secretion of pro-inflammatory cytokines, prostaglandins and cytokines,[48] inhibits 5-lipoxygenase,[49] anti-inflammatory,[50, 51, 52] anti-spasmodic,[53] osteoarthritis,[54] rheumatoid arthritis,[55, 56] low back pain,[57] and interfering with serotonin's pro-inflammatory effects.[58]

CAUTIONS, CONTRA-INDICATIONS AND DRUG INTERACTIONS

Please reference Chapter 9. Do not use during pregnancy or lactation. Excessively high doses may cause intestinal upset or loose stools. Do not exceed the recommended dose. This formula should not be used during pregnancy or lactation. Nettle leaf has been shown to make NSAIDs such as diclofenac work more effectively in people with arthritis.[59]

COMPLIMENTARY HERBS/FORMULAS

Infla-Profen would work well combined with Migra-Profen for migraine, headaches, and menstrual cramps. Infla-Profen could also be combined with Cell Wise formula for chronic inflammatory disorders of any kind including arthritis, low back pain, and autoimmune diseases like lupus.

REFERENCES

1 Mills S, Bone K. *Principles and Practice of Phytotherapy: Modern Herbal Medicine*. Edinburgh: Churchill Livingstone, 2000:345-9.

2 Moussard C, Alber D, Toubin MM, *et al.* A drug used in traditional medicine, *Harpagophytum procumbens*: No evidence for NSAID-like effect on whole blood eicosanoid production in human. *Prostagland Leukotr Essential Fatty Acids* 1992;46:283-6.

3 Blumenthal M, Busse WR, Goldberg A, *et al.* (eds). *The Complete German Commission E Monographs: Therapeutic Guide to Herbal Medicines*. Austin: American Botanical Council and Boston: Integrative Medicine Communications, 1998:120-1.

4 Chantre P, Cappelaere A, Leblan D, *et al.* Efficacy and tolerance of *Harpagophytum procumbens* versus diacerhein in the treatment of osteoarthritis. *Phytomedicine* 2000;7:177-83

5 Chrubasik S, Junck H, Breitschwerdt H, *et al.* Effectiveness of *Harpagophytum* extract WS 1531 in the treatment of exacerbation of low back pain: A randomized placebo-controlled double-blind study. *Eur J Anaesthesiol* 1999;16:118-29.

6 Vogler BK, Pittler MH, Ernst E. Feverfew as a preventive treatment for migraine: A systematic review. *Cephalalgia* 1998;18:704-8.

7 Mills S, Bone K. *Principles and Practice of Phytotherapy: Modern Herbal Medicine*. Edinburgh: Churchill Livingstone, 2000:385-93.

8 Heptinstall S, White A, Williamson L, *et al.* Extracts of feverfew inhibit granule secretion in blood platelets and polymorphonuclear leucocytes. *Lancet* 1985;i:1071-4.

9 Pattrick M, Heptinstall S, Doherty M. Feverfew in rheumatoid arthritis: a double blind, placebo controlled study. *Ann Rheum Dis* 1989;48:547-9.

10 Hoffmann D. *The Complete Illustrated Herbal*. New York: Barnes & Noble Books, 1996:150.

11 Hobbs C. Feverfew: *Tanacetum parthenium*. *HerbalGram* 1989;20:26-35, 47.

12 Bingham R, Bellew BA, Bellew JG. Yucca plant saponin in the management of arthritis. *J Appl Nutr* 1975;27:45-50.

13 Moore M. *Medicinal Plants of the Desert and Canyon West*. Santa Fe: Museum of New Mexico Press, 1989:134-5.

14 Della Loggia R, Zilli C, Del Negro P, *et al.* Isoflavones as spasmolytic principles of *Piscidia erythrina*. *Prog Clin Biol Res* 1988;280:365-8.

15 Ellingwood F. *American Materia Medica, Pharmacognosy and Therapeutics* 11th ed. Sandy, OR: Eclectic Medical Publications, 1919:110-12.

16 Felter HW. *Eclectic Materia Medica, Pharmacology and Therapeutics*. Sandy, OR: Eclectic Medical Publications, 1922:548-9.

17 Obertreis B, Ruttkowski T, Teucher T, *et al.* Ex-vivo in-vitro inhibition of lipopolysaccharide stimulated tumor necrosis factor-_ and interleukin-1_ secretion in human whole blood by extractum Urticae dioicae foliorum. *Arzneim Forsch* 1996;46:389-94.

18 Obertreis B, Giller K, *et al.* (1996) Antiphlogistic effects of *Urtica dioica* folia extract in comparison to caffeic malic acid. *Arzneim Forsch* 1996;46:52-6 [in German].

19 Klingelhoefer S, Obertreis B, Quast S, Behnke B. Antirheumatic effect of IDS 23, a stinging nettle leaf extract, on in vitro expression of T helper cytokines. *J Rheumatol* 1999;26:2517-22.

20 Kirchhoff HW. Urtica juice as a diuretic. *Z Phytother* 1983;4:621-6 [in German].

21 Yarnell E. Stinging nettle: A modern view of an ancient healing plant. *Altern Complem Ther* 1998;4:180-6.

22 Newall CA, Anderson LA, Phillipson JD. *Herbal Medicines: A Guide for Health-Care Professionals*. London: Pharmaceutical Press, 1996:52-3.

23 Ellingwood F. *American Materia Medica, Pharmacognosy and Therapeutics* 11th ed. Sandy, OR: Eclectic Medical Publications, 1919:378.

24 Lin CC, Lu JM, Yang JJ, et al. Anti-inflammatory and radical scavenge effects of *Arctium lappa*. *Am J Chin Med* 1996;24:127-37.

25 Iwakami S, Wu J, Ebizuka Y, Sankawa U. Platelet activating factor (PAF) antagonists contained in medicinal plants: Lignans and sesquiterpenes. *Chem Pharm Bull (Tokyo)* 1992;40:1196-8.

26 Leung AY, Foster S. *Encyclopedia of Common Natural Ingredients Used in Food, Drugs and Cosmetics* 2nd ed. New York: John Wiley & Sons Inc, 1996:141-3.

27 Srivastava KC. Isolation and effects of some ginger components on platelet aggregation and eicosanoid biosynthesis. *Prostaglandins Leukotrienes Med* 1986;25:187-98.

28 Kawakishi S, Morimitsu Y, Osawa T. Chemistry of ginger components and inhibitory factors of the arachidonic acid cascade. In: Ho CT, Osawa T, Huang MT, Rosen RT (eds) *Food Phytochemicals for Cancer Prevention vol 2: Tea, Spices and Herbs*. Washington, DC: American Chemical Society, 1994:244-50.

29 Kiuchi F, Iwakami S, Shibuya M, et al. Inhibition of prostaglandin and leukotriene biosynthesis by gingerols and diarylheptanoids. *Chem Pharm Bull* 1992;40:387-91.

30 Chopra A, Lavin P, Patwardhan B, Chitre D. Randomized double blind trial of an Ayurvedic plant derived formulation for treatment of rheumatoid arthritis. *J Rheumatol* 2000;27:1365-72.

31 Srivastava CK, Mustafa T. Ginger (*Zingiber officinale*) in rheumatism and musculoskeletal disroders. *Medical Hypoth* 1992;39:342-48.

32 Bone ME, Wilkinson DJ, Young JR, et al. Ginger root--a new antiemetic: The effect of ginger root on postoperative nausea and vomiting after major gynaecological surgery. *Anaesthesia* 1990;45:669-71.

33 Srivastava R, Dikshit M, Srimal RC, Dhawan BN. Anti-thrombotic effect of curcumin. *Thromb Res* 1985;404:413-7.

34 Shah BH, Nawaz Z, Pertani SA, et al. Inhibitory effect of curcumin, a food spice from turmeric, on platelet-activating factor- and arachidonic acid-mediated platelet aggregation through inhibition of thromboxane formation and Ca2+ signaling. *Biochem Pharmacol* 1999;58:1167-72.

35 Srivastava R, Puri V, Srimal RC, Dhawan BN. Effect of curcumin on platelet aggregation and vascular prostacyclin synthesis. *Arzneim Forsch* 1986;36:715-7.

36 Deodhar SD, Sethi R, Srimal RC. Preliminary study on antirheumatic activity of curcumin (diferuloyl methane). *Indian J Med Res* 1980;71:632-4.

37 Nadkarni AK, Nadkarni KM. *Indian Materia Medica vol 2*. Bombay: Popular Prakashan. 1976:414-18.

38 Mills S, Bone K. *Principles and Practice of Phytotherapy: Modern Herbal Medicine*. Edinburgh: Churchill Livingstone, 2000.

39 Moore M. *Medicinal Plants of the Desert and Canyon West*. Santa Fe: Museum of New Mexico Press, 1989.

40 Mills S, Bone K. *Principles and Practice of Phytotherapy: Modern Herbal Medicine*. Edinburgh: Churchill Livingstone, 2000.

41 Hoffmann D. *The Complete Illustrated Herbal*. New York: Barnes & Noble Books, 1996.

42 Ellingwood F. *American Materia Medica, Pharmacognosy and Therapeutics* 11th ed. Sandy, OR: Eclectic Medical Publications, 1919.

43 Felter HW. *Eclectic Materia Medica, Pharmacology and Therapeutics.* Sandy, OR: Eclectic Medical Publications, 1922.

44 Mills S, Bone K. *Principles and Practice of Phytotherapy: Modern Herbal Medicine.* Edinburgh: Churchill Livingstone, 2000.

45 Hoffmann D. *The Complete Illustrated Herbal.* New York: Barnes & Noble Books, 1996.

46 Ellingwood F. *American Materia Medica, Pharmacognosy and Therapeutics* 11th ed. Sandy, OR: Eclectic Medical Publications, 1919.

47 Hoffmann D. *The Complete Illustrated Herbal.* New York: Barnes & Noble Books, 1996.

48 Ronzio B. Polyphenols as anti-inflammatory agents. *J Naturopathic Med* 2000;9:44-50.

49 Ronzio B. Polyphenols as anti-inflammatory agents. *J Naturopathic Med* 2000;9:44-50.

50 Handa SS, Chawla AS, Sharma AK. Plants with antiinflammatory activity. *Fitoterapia* 1992;63:3-31.

51 Werbach M, Murray M. *Botanical Influences on Illness.* Tarzana, CA: Third Line Press, 1994.

52 Mills S, Bone K. *Principles and Practice of Phytotherapy: Modern Herbal Medicine.* Edinburgh: Churchill Livingstone, 2000.

53 Della Loggia R, Zilli C, Del Negro P, *et al.* Isoflavones as spasmolytic principles of *Piscidia erythrina. Prog Clin Biol Res* 1988;280:365-8.

54 Werbach M, Murray M. *Botanical Influences on Illness.* Tarzana, CA: Third Line Press, 1994.

55 Chopra A, Lavin P, Patwardhan B, Chitre D. Randomized double blind trial of an Ayurvedic plant derived formulation for treatment of rheumatoid arthitis. *J Rheumatoli* 2000;27:1365-72.

56 Weiss RF. *Herbal Medicine.* Gothenberg, Sweden: Ab Arcanum and Beaconsfield: Beaconsfield Publishers Ltd, trans. Meuss AR, 1985.

57 Chrubasik S, Junck H, Breitschwerdt H, *et al.* Effectiveness of *Harpagophytum* extract WS 1531 in the treatment of exacerbation of low back pain: A randomized placebo-controlled double-blind study. *Eur J Anaesthesiol* 1999;16:118-29.

58 Mills S, Bone K. *Principles and Practice of Phytotherapy: Modern Herbal Medicine.* Edinburgh: Churchill Livingstone, 2000:385-93.

59 Chrubasik S, Enderlein W, Bauer R, Grabner W. Evidence for the antirheumatic effectiveness of herba *Urticae dioicae* in acute arthritis: A pilot study. *Phytomedicine* 4:105-8.

LIVER HEALTH
Ulimate Support of Healthy Liver Function *
FORMULA

Milk Thistle seed	(*Silybum marianum*)
Turmeric root	(*Curcuma longa*)
Schizandra berry	(*Schisandra chinensis*)
Licorice root	(*Glycyrrhiza glabra*)
Chinese Skullcap	(*Scutellaria baicalensis*)
MSM	(*Methylsulfonylmethane*)

Concentration:	3:1 Herb strength ratio
Dosage:	Liquid Phyto-Caps™:1 capsule, Two Times Daily
Duration of use:	4-6 Months
Best taken:	Take 2 capsules in the evening hours daily

DESCRIPTION OF FORMULA

This powerful liver-protective formula helps to prevent the free-radical damage to liver tissue that is generated at times of stress. There is an understanding in modern Naturopathic medicine, that "it's not the 'toxin' that does the damage, but your body's response to it". When a substance is metabolized in the liver, free-radicals are generated, this is a simple fact of Nature. What this formula endeavors to achieve, is a reduction in the damage that might occur as a consequence of the generation of these highly active free radical molecules. By direct antioxidant action, as well as by restoring levels of the livers own antioxidants, this formula exerts a powerful influence in this regard. Tissue regenerative properties are also relevant for a number of herbs in this formula.

The pharmacodynamic goals of this formula include mediating phase 1 mixed-function oxidase enzyme activity by supporting phase 2 hepatic biotransformation of hydrophilic dietary substances, endogenous metabolites, xenobiotics and drugs. Phase 1 oxidation, reduction or hydrolysis pathways are well known to generate reactive oxygen species (ROS). Under normal conditions phase 1 pathways, and therefore their oxidative damage, are kept to a minimum by the glutathione (GSH) dependant conjugation reactions of phase 2. When phase 2 pathways are compromised, due to metabolic overload or GSH depletion, phase 1 responds and consequently generates ROS, in addition to other highly reactive intermediary metabolites.

Botanicals in this formula directly
➤ reduce oxidative-stress induced lipid peroxidation
➤ increase hepatic cyclic AMP, stabilize hepatocyte membranes
➤ increase GSH levels in hepatocytes
➤ promote the safe regeneration of hepatic tissue by stimulating DNA dependant ribosomal RNA polymerase 1.

Milk Thistle seed has a long history of traditional use, having been used primarily for disorders of liver congestion.[G12] In modern times, however, it is used more for its ability to protect liver tissue from the free-radical stress generated during liver metabolism.[1,2] Such stress on the liver may be the result of enhanced detoxification requirements placed on its function by so-called 'toxins' from either within the body itself (hormones, by-products of inflammation and stress, etc), or those which have been introduced from the environment (alcohol, caffeine, pharmaceutical drugs, bacterial poisons, etc.).[1,3]

Simply stated, Milk Thistle seed has the following effects on the liver: [G5, 1, 2]

A. It is a powerful antioxidant with anti-inflammatory effects
B. It increases the livers natural antioxidant levels
C. It protects against damage from dangerous chemicals and drugs
D. It regenerates liver tissue, without producing the negative effects associated with this influence.

Turmeric root has traditionally been recognized as a medicine for the treatment of numerous disorders, including those related to digestive [G3, G5, 4, 5, 6] and liver dysfunction.[G3, G5, 4, 6] It is interesting to note that the powerful medicinal benefits of a number of 'spice cabinet' herbs (such as Black Pepper, Ginger, Cayenne, Garlic, Turmeric, etc.) are being brought more fully to light by modern science. As a cousin of Ginger, Turmeric is a powerful antioxidant [G3, G5, 4, 6] and anti-inflammatory.[G1, G3, G5, 4, 5] In fact, curcumin - a constituent of Turmeric - has been shown to be as effective an anti-inflammatory as phenylbutazone (and almost as effective as cortisone for acute inflammation), without the well known gastric side-effects associated with these drugs.[G5, 5] It has also been shown to possess liver-protective,[G1, G3, 4, 5] antiplatelet, antitumor, anticancer, antiviral, and cholesterol lowering effects.[G5, 4, 5] Like the Milk Thistle, Turmeric aids liver function primarily by reducing the damage caused by the free-radicals that are generated during metabolism. Reducing this stress allows a return to normalized function of the liver.

Schizandra berry is a valued kidney and male tonic of the Traditional Chinese system of medicine.[G3] Within this system it is often referred to as a 'king' or 'harmonizing' remedy, alluding to the broad-reaching influence of this small 'five flavored' berry.[G17] It is also deserving of great respect as an adaptogen (increases non-specific resistance). In fact, the power of its adaptogenic influence has been compared Siberian Ginseng.[G3] It has been shown, specifically, to promote liver detoxification,[G3, 7] as well as to protect the liver during chronic hepatitis and acute intoxication from poisons of various origin[3], including the deadly carbon tetrachloride, [G3, 7, 8] acetaminophen,[G3, 7] digitoxin, and indomethacin.[G3] In China, compounds derived from Schizandra are being used to treat viral hepatitis with greater effect than the silymarins from the Milk Thistle.[G3] In a similar manner as the Milk Thistle, Schizandra increases the livers antioxidant levels, and in addition promotes the regeneration of liver tissue, apparently without the related concern of tumor-promoting side-effects.[G3, 8] Schizandra has also been shown to increase liver cyclic AMP (see cAMP - Coleus Forskohlii Supreme).[G3]

Licorice root has found use as a medicine for more than 3,000 years.[9, 10, 11] Interestingly, its use for asthma during this early period is now being 'rediscovered' by modern scientific research.[9] Among a long list of reported effects, research on licorice has confirmed it as an anti-inflammatory, with antiviral, antiulcer,[9, 11] antiarthritic, and hormone balancing properties.[9] Like Schizandra, it also increases cyclic AMP.[1, 9] Perhaps most relevant to this formula, however, is the ability of Licorice to protect against the damage caused by free-radicals to liver cells.[1, 9, 11] Research with chronic active hepatitis has also shown that compounds from Licorice may protect against the body's self-inflicted liver damage which is associated with this condition.[9] In addition, Licorice is able to enhance the ability of the liver to safely detoxify, in a manner that does not cause the excessive generation of damaging free-radicals.

Chinese Skullcap has a long list of traditional applications to its credit, including use as a detoxifying herb[G3] and as an anti-inflammatory of noted importance.[G10] Modern science confirms its anti-inflammatory influence.[G3, G8] In fact, Chinese Skullcap is now recognized as one of many highly revered medicinal plants that selectively inhibit the enzyme known as COX-2.[12] This COX-2 inhibitory action means that it is able to reduce inflammation, without the highly destructive gastric side-effects of the class of pharmaceutical drugs known as Non-Steroidal Anti-inflammatory Drugs (NSAID's)[12] (many also inhibit the gastric-protective COX-1). Its value here is as an anti-inflammatory and a powerful antioxidant.[G10] Similar to the other ingredients of this formula, Chinese Skullcap provides further support for the reduction of the inflammation-induced free-radical stress that is well-known to be generated at times of enhanced detoxification or challenge from a powerful external 'toxin'.

THERAPEUTIC APPLICATIONS*

Note: The intention of the following information is to represent the traditional use of the individual botanicals found in these formulas and to inform the reader of any evolving scientific inquiry relevant to the formula's ingredients.

SUPPORTED BY TRADITIONAL USE

Liver disorders, [G3, G5, G12, 4, 6] Digestive disorders, [G3, G5, 4, 5, 6]

SCOPE OF RELEVANT SCIENTIFIC INVESTIGATION

Hepato-protective,[G1, G3, G5, 1, 2, 4, 5, 7, 8] Antioxidant,[G3, G5, 1, 2, 4, 6, 8] Hepatic-tissue regenerative, [G5, 1, 2] Antiinflammatory,[G1, G3, G5, G8, 1, 4, 5, 9, 11] Cholesterol lowering, [G5, 4, 5] Antiviral, [G3, G5, 4, 5, 9, 11] Anticancer, [G5, 4, 5] Antitumor, [G5, 4, 5] Hepatic CP450 biotransformation enhancer,[G3, 7] Increases cyclic AMP, [G3, 9, 11]

CAUTIONS, CONTRA-INDICATIONS AND DRUG INTERACTIONS

Please reference Chapter 9. Do not use during pregnancy or lactation.

COMPLIMENTARY HERBS/FORMULAS

Sweetish Bitters Elixir, Cell Wise, Hep C

REFERENCES

1. Pizzorno J, Murray M. Textbook of Natural medicine. New York. Churchill Livingstone; 1999.

2. Legalon. Madaus Education Monograph. Madaus. Germany. 1/2/10.94

3. Detoxification Profile. GSDL Education Monograph. Great Smokies Diagnostic Lab (GSDL). Asheville, NC. 1998.

4. Snow JM. *Curcuma longa* L. (Zingiberaceae). *The Protocol Journal of Botanical Medicine.* 1995; Autumn: 43-46.

5. Srimal RC. Turmeric: A brief review of medicinal properties. *Fitoterapia*; 1997; 68(6):483-493.

6. Selvam R. The antioxidant activity of turmeric (Curcuma longa). *Journal of Ethnopharmacology.* 1995; 47:59-67.

7. Gengtao L. Hepato-pharmacology of Fructus Schizandrae. Advances in Chinese Medicinal Materials Research. 1985.

8. Ko KM, *et al.* Effect of a lignan-enriched Fructus Schizandrae extract on hepatic glutathione status in rats: Protection against carbon tetrachloride toxicity. *Planta Medica.* 1995; 61: 134-137.

9. Kent C. Licorice - More than just candy. *Journal of the Australian Traditional Medicine Society.* 1994; Autumn: 9-14.

10. Davis E, Morris DJ. Medicinal uses of Licorice through the millennia: The good and plenty of it. *Molecular and Cellular Endocrinology.* 1991; 78:1-6.

11. Snow JM. Glycyrhizza glabra L. (Leguminaceae). *The Protocol Journal of Botanical Medicine.* 1996; Winter: 9-14

12. Newmark TM, Schulick P. Beyond Aspirin. Prescott, Az. HOHM Press. 2000.

LOMATIUM/OSHA SUPREME

*Ultimate Support for Healthy Upper Respiratory Function**

FORMULA

Lomatium root	(*Lomatium dissectum*)
Oshá root	(*Ligusticum porteri*)
Echinacea/Goldenseal Supreme	
Garlic bulb	(*Allium sativum*)
Mullein leaf	(*Verbascum olympicum*)
Grindelia buds	(*Grindelia robusta*)
Hyssop herb	(*Hyssopus officinalis*)
Irish Moss	(*Chondrus crispus*)
Lobelia herb & seed	(*Lobelia inflata*)

Concentration:	3:1
Dosage:	Acute problems: 2 caps every three to four hours
	Chronic problems: 1-2 caps two to three times per day
Duration of use:	Acute problems: until three days after all symptoms are gone (5-14 days)
Best taken:	Between meals, with warm water

DESCRIPTION OF FORMULA

Humans are constantly exposed to viruses and bacteria. Despite our best efforts it is almost impossible to avoid contact with at least some of these, and many people end up with what is known as the common cold. The winter months are generally the worst season for such exposures, in part because people spend much more time indoors and in contact with another. Despite the name, the common cold is not caused by or related to cold weather except for the crowding factor mentioned above. However, many people who are exposed to viruses and bacteria do not develop a common cold. This is likely due to the fact that the various components of their immune systems defend them against infection. Lomatium/Oshá Supreme combines several healing herbs together to both support healthy immune function and to maintain a healthy respiratory tract, particularly in the winter when the greatest threats exist.

Lomatium root is a classic herb for supporting the immune system and respiratory tract, originally known to the Native Americans and then spread to Europeans.[1] It is said that one Nevada researcher found that people who used lomatium during the influenza epidemic of 1920-22 did far better than people who did not.[2] In test tubes lomatium is able to kill a wide range of bacteria.[3] Lomatium is also traditionally used for skin infections, gingivitis, candida infections, and pneumonia.[4]

Oshá root and a similar plant in China have been used in traditional medicine for centuries as a remedy for viral infections including influenza and the common cold, rheumatism, bruises, headache, diarrhea, menstrual cramps, ringworm, and scabies.[5, 6, 7] It has not been researched in modern times but it included for its renown in traditional herbalism.

This formula contains the **Echinacea/Goldenseal Supreme formula**. More information is available about this formula in its own section.

Garlic bulb is mentioned in some of the oldest written records that exist, dating back to 2600 BC in the Middle East. It is repeatedly mentioned in traditional medicine as a remedy for coughs, the common cold, lung infections, diarrhea, worm infestations, and a large number of other problems.[8] Garlic and its various constituents have repeatedly been shown to be antibacterial and antiviral in the test tube.[9] Garlic can also stimulate immune cells in laboratory tests.[10] It doesn't hurt that garlic also helps support a healthy cardiovascular system.[11]

Mullein leaf as well as the very similar flower are officially approved in Germany for use in supporting a healthy respiratory tract.[12] In traditional herbalism it is respected for relieving the common cold, coughs, chronic bronchitis, and ear infections.[13, 14] It has shown antiviral, specifically anti-influenza, activity in test tube studies.[15]

Grindelia buds contain an aromatic resin and in traditional medicine is considered to be an important tonic for the lungs and to help relieve asthma, cough, the common cold and other respiratory infections.[16, 17]

Hyssop herb has long been utilized in traditional herbalism as a remedy for the common cold and spasmodic coughs of any kind and is considered mildly relaxing.[18] Test tube studies suggest it may be antiviral.[19]

Irish Moss is used traditionally for coughs in European herbalism.[20]

Lobelia herb & seed were considered by the Eclectic physicians in the late nineteenth century to be one of the most important medicinal plants. They utilized it to strengthen people with any type of respiratory weakness including infections, to help make coughing more effective in clearing mucus, cardiovascular weakness, angina, spasms, and anxiety.[21] It is surprising given the high regard and widespread use of lobelia that there is so little investigation of its properties in modern research. This is likely due to the fact that in overdose it can cause nausea, and apparently researchers have not thought to go back to the traditional method of giving small amounts of lobelia in combination with other herbs more frequently to avoid the side effects while maximizing its benefits.

THERAPEUTIC APPLICATIONS*

Note: The intention of this following information is to represent the traditional use of the individual botanicals found in these formulas and to inform the reader of any evolving scientific inquiry relevant to the formula's ingredients.

SUPPORTED BY TRADITIONAL USE

Common cold,[22, 23, 24] Bronchitis,[25, 26] Cough,[27] Pneumonia,[28] Respiratory infections[29]

SCOPE OF RELEVANT SCIENTIFIC INVESTIGATION

Support of immune function particularly in mucous membranes of the upper respiratory tract,[30] antiviral,[31, 32, 33] antibacterial,[34] expectorant, antitussive, spasmolytic

CAUTIONS, CONTRA-INDICATIONS AND DRUG INTERACTIONS

Please reference Chapter 9. Do not use during pregnancy or lactation. If a skin rash appears while taking the formula, its used should be discontinued and a physician knowledgeable in herbal medicine consulted.

If nausea occurs then the formula should be taken with food. If nausea persists the amount being taken should be decreased by half. If vomiting occurs, the formula should be discontinued and a physician or herbalist knowledgeable in herbal medicine should be consulted.

COMPLIMENTARY HERBS/FORMULAS

In acute situations, Echinacea Supreme might be combined with Lomatium/Oshá Supreme for optimum immune system support. For chronic or recurrent problems, Anti-Oxidant Supreme and Energy and Vitality formulas may increase the benefits of Lomatium/Oshá Supreme.

REFERENCES

1 Moore M. *Medicinal Plants of the Pacific West.* Santa Fe: Red Crane Books, 1993:167-71.

2 Moore M. *Medicinal Plants of the Pacific West.* Santa Fe: Red Crane Books, 1993:167-71.

3 Carlson JH, Douglas HG. Antibiotic agents separated from the root of lace-leaved leptotaenia. *J Bacteriol* 1948;55:615-21.

4 Moore M. *Medicinal Plants of the Pacific West.* Santa Fe: Red Crane Books, 1993:167-71.

5 Moore M. *Medicinal Plants of the Mountain West.* Santa Fe: Museum of New Mexico Press, 1979:119-21.

6 Curtin LSM; Moore M (ed). *Healing Herbs of the Upper Rio Grande: Traditional Medicine of the Southwest.* Santa Fe: Western Edge Press, 1947, reprinted 1997:121-4.

7 Leung AY, Foster S. *Encyclopedia of Common Natural Ingredients Used in Food, Drugs and Cosmetics* 2nd ed. New York: John Wiley & Sons Inc., 1996:552-3.

8 Koch HP, Lawson LD (eds). *Garlic: The Science and Therapeutic Application of Allium sativum L and Related Species,* 2nd ed. Baltimore: Williams & Wilkins, 1996:1-24.

9 Reuter HD. *Allium sativum and Allium ursinum:* part 2. Pharmacology and medicinal application. *Phytomedicine* 1995;2:73-91.

10 Salman H, Bergman M, Bessler H, *et al.* Effect of a garlic derivative (alliin) on peripheral blood cell immune responses. *Int J Immunopharmacol* 1999;21:589-97.

11 Warshafsky S, Kamer RS, Sivak SL. Effect of garlic on total serum cholesterol: A meta-analysis. *Ann Intern Med* 1993;119:599-605.

12 Blumenthal M, Busse WR, Goldberg A, *et al.* (eds). *The Complete German Commission E Monographs: Therapeutic Guide to Herbal Medicines.* Austin: American Botanical Council and Boston: Integrative Medicine Communications, 1998:173.

13 Felter HW. *Eclectic Materia Medica, Pharmacology and Therapeutics.* Sandy, OR: Eclectic Medical Publications, 1922, reprinted 1998:693.

14 Weiss RF. *Herbal Medicine.* Gothenberg, Sweden: Ab Arcanum and Beaconsfield: Beaconsfield Publishers Ltd, trans. Meuss AR, 1985, 197-8.

15 Zgórniak-Nowosielska I, Grzybek J, Manolova N, *et al.* Antiviral activity of flos verbasci infusion against influenza and herpes simplex viruses. *Arch Immunol Ther Exp* 1991;39:103-8.

16 Felter HW. *Eclectic Materia Medica, Pharmacology and Therapeutics.* Sandy, OR: Eclectic Medical Publications, 1922, reprinted 1998:397-8.

17 Hoffmann D. *The Complete Illustrated Herbal.* New York: Barnes & Noble Books, 1996:100.

18 Hoffmann D. *The Complete Illustrated Herbal.* New York: Barnes & Noble Books, 1996:104.

19 Leung AY, Foster S. *Encyclopedia of Common Natural Ingredients Used in Food, Drugs and Cosmetics* 2nd ed. New York: John Wiley & Sons Inc., 1996:312-4.

20 Weiss RF. *Herbal Medicine.* Gothenberg, Sweden: Ab Arcanum and Beaconsfield: Beaconsfield Publishers Ltd, trans. Meuss AR, 1985, 199.

21 Ellingwood F. *American Materia Medica, Pharmacognosy and Therapeutics* 11th ed. Sandy, OR: Eclectic Medical Publications, 1919, reprinted 1998:235-42.

22 Felter HW. *Eclectic Materia Medica, Pharmacology and Therapeutics.* Sandy, OR: Eclectic Medical Publications, 1922, reprinted 1998.

23 Weiss RF. *Herbal Medicine.* Gothenberg, Sweden: Ab Arcanum and Beaconsfield: Beaconsfield Publishers Ltd, trans. Meuss AR, 1985.

24 Hoffmann D. *The Complete Illustrated Herbal.* New York: Barnes & Noble Books, 1996.

25 Felter HW. *Eclectic Materia Medica, Pharmacology and Therapeutics.* Sandy, OR: Eclectic Medical Publications, 1922, reprinted 1998.

26 Weiss RF. *Herbal Medicine.* Gothenberg, Sweden: Ab Arcanum and Beaconsfield: Beaconsfield Publishers Ltd, trans. Meuss AR, 1985.

27 Ellingwood F. *American Materia Medica, Pharmacognosy and Therapeutics* 11th ed. Sandy, OR: Eclectic Medical Publications, 1919, reprinted 1998.

28 Felter HW. *Eclectic Materia Medica, Pharmacology and Therapeutics.* Sandy, OR: Eclectic Medical Publications, 1922, reprinted 1998.

29 Hoffmann D. *The Complete Illustrated Herbal.* New York: Barnes & Noble Books, 1996.

30 Barrett B. Echinacea for upper respiratory infection: An assessment of randomized trials. *HealthNotes Review of Complementary and Integrative Medicine* 2000;7:211-8.

31 Koch HP, Lawson LD (eds). *Garlic: The Science and Therapeutic Application of Allium sativum L and Related Species,* 2nd ed. Baltimore: Williams & Wilkins, 1996:172-3.

32 Zgórniak-Nowosielska I, Grzybek J, Manolova N, *et al.* Antiviral activity of flos verbasci infusion against influenza and herpes simplex viruses. *Arch Immunol Ther Exp* 1991;39:103-8.

33 Leung AY, Foster S. *Encyclopedia of Common Natural Ingredients Used in Food, Drugs and Cosmetics* 2nd ed. New York: John Wiley & Sons Inc., 1996.

34 Amin AH, Subbaiah TV, Abbasi KM. Berberine sulfate: Antimicrobial activity, bioassay, and mode of action. *Can J Microbiol* 1969:15:1067-76.

MALE LIBIDO
*Ultimate Enhancement of Male Stamina & Performance**
FORMULA

Maca	(*Lepidium meyenii*)
Tribulus	(*Tribulus terrestris*)
Horney Goat Weed	(*Epimedium grandiflorum*)
Saw Palmetto berry	(*Serenoa repens*)
Sarsaparilla root	(*Smilax officinalis*)
Muira puama	(*Ptychopetalum olacoides*)
Chinese Fo-Ti	(*Polygonum multiflorum*)
Wild Oats	(*Avena sativa*)
Yohimbe bark	(*Corynanthe yohimbe*)

Concentration:	4:1 Herb strength ratio
Dosage:	Liquid Phyto-Caps™: 1 capsule, 3 times daily
Duration of use:	2-3 months
Best taken:	Between meals, with warm water

DESCRIPTION OF FORMULA

This formula is a powerful sexual restorative for men. For most of us who live in modern society - we are stressed beyond the natural bounds of our physiology. Stress levels affect sexual performance. Whether it's the stress of the job, or the stress of a bad diet, the effects may very well be the same. This compound takes a restorative approach to virility. We have brought together powerful nervous system restoratives that are known to enhance sexual performance and/or desire. We have not used stimulants here. To drive an already exhausted physiology with stimulants is counterproductive. While hormonal imbalances and liver dysfunction are also addressed here - it is nervous restoration that is the primary focus of this formula.

Maca is reported to have been used by native Peruvians for some 5000 years. [1] In fact, it is believed that, due to the plant's potency, the Incas traditionally restricted its use to the court of royalty. [1] Its reputation is primarily as a virility enhancer and as an aphrodisiac. [1] Early clinical reports suggest its effects are perhaps due to its regulating influence over the endocrine system - specifically, the Hypothalamus-Pituitary-Adrenal (HPA) axis. [1] One scientific researcher has stated that in animals Maca results in "significantly higher sperm production and motility rates". [1] Following the first U.S. study of this Andean Mountain herb, researchers have confirmed Macas aphrodisiac affects in animals. [2]

Tribulus is reported to be a folkloric medicine for lowering cholesterol [4] and blood pressure, [G8] as a diuretic [G8, 4] an anti-convulsant and to improve visual acuity. [G8] Traditionally, it has also been used as an aphrodisiac. [3] A small number of studies have supported this traditional use as an aphrodisiac, confirming that protodiosin (an isolated constituent of tribulus) has proerectile activity. [5] One such report suggests that protodisin "has been clinically proven to improve sexual desire and enhance erection". [6]

Epimedium is better known by its common name, Horny Goat Weed. As such a name might imply, this plant is considered an aphrodisiac. Traditionally it is also used as a tonic. [1, 7] In the Chinese system of Medicine, Epimedium is known to increase sexual desire and activity, as well as increase sperm production. [G21]

Saw Palmetto is well known for its effects with the prostate. [G16, 8] Traditionally, it was said to exert its influence over all the reproductive organs, helping to restore sexual activity after exhaustive excesses. [G6, G12] Wherever impotence is due accompanied by nervous exhaustion, Saw Palmetto is said to be useful - particularly when taken with a nervous restorative, such as Wild Oats (see below). [G6]

Sarsaparilla is an alterative (corrects cellular waste and nutrition) that is known for its anti-inflammatory affect with conditions such as psoriasis, rheumatism, and rheumatoid arthritis. [G4, G10] Liver protective action is also noted. [G3, G4, G10] It is included in this virility formula for its overall influence on metabolism.

Muira puama is also commonly known as potency wood. Said to strengthen the digestion and tonify the nervous system - particularly where nervous exhaustion is evident - [9] this rainforest botanical has a reputation as an aphrodisiac. [9, 10] At least one clinical trial has confirmed its benefits with erectile dysfunction. It has been reported that both psychological and physical aspects of sexual function were improved in this particular trial. [10]

Fo-Ti is traditionally considered to be of much value for conditions effecting the liver and kidneys. [11] It has been included here as a nervous tonic and restorative. [11] Traditional Chinese Medicine (TCM) regards Fo-Ti as one of the five major tonic herbs. [12] Chinese Fo-Ti has liver protective effects thus making it a highly valuable addition to this virility formula.[G3, G7]

Wild Oats are present here for their influence with nervous exhaustion. [G12] Often used with complaints of the digestive system where there is also physical weakness and fatigue, [13] Wild Oats may be used during convalescence from chronic disease, [G12] or from nicotine abuse. [13] This plant also combines well with Saw Palmetto where nervous exhaustion leads to impotence. [G6]

Yohimbe is a highly praised traditional aphrodisiac. [G3, 14] Scientific research focusing on the alkaloid yohimbine has shown it to improve sexual function. [15, 16] In addition to these popularized benefits with erectile dysfunction, Yohimbe has been included here for its noted antidepressant action. [G3]

THERAPEUTIC APPLICATIONS*

Note: The intention of the following information is to represent the traditional use of the individual botanicals found in these formulas and to inform the reader of any evolving scientific inquiry relevant to the formula's ingredients.

SUPPORTED BY TRADITIONAL USE

Aphrodisiac, [G3, 2, 9, 10, 14] Sexual restorative, [G6, G12] Tonic, [1, 7, 11, 12] Nervous restorative, [11] Nervous exhaustion, [G6, G12, 9] Physical weakness and fatigue, [13] Anti-inflammatory. [G4, G10]

SCOPE OF RELEVANT SCIENTIFIC INVESTIGATION

Aphrodisiac, [2] Proerectile activity, [5, 6, 10, 15, 16] Improve Sexual desire, [6, 10] Improve sexual activity, [G21] Increase sperm production, [G21, 1] Liver protective. [G3, G4, G7, G10]

CAUTIONS, CONTRA-INDICATIONS AND DRUG INTERACTIONS

Please reference Chapter 9. Do not use during pregnancy or lactation.

COMPLIMENTARY HERBS/FORMULAS
Energy & Vitality, Siberian Ginseng Tonic

REFERENCES

1. Walker M. Medical Journalist Report of Innovative Biologics. *Townsend Letter for Doctors.* 1998; Nov: 18-22.

2. Zheng BL, *et al.* Effect of a lipidic extract from *lepidium meyenii* on sexual behavior in mice and rats. *Urology.* 2000;55(4):598-602.

3. Agricultural Research Service. Dr. Duke's Phytochemical and Ethnobotanical Databases: Ethnobotanical uses Tribulus terrestris. Online. Internet. [8/23/00]. Available WWW: http://www.ars-grin.gov/cgi-bin/duke/ethnobot.pl

4. Arcasoy HB, *et al.* Effect of *Tribulus terrestris* L. saponin mixture on some smooth muscle preparations: a preliminary study. *Boll Chim Farm* 1998;137(11):473-5.

5. Adaikan PG, *et al.* Proerectile pharmacological effects of *Tribulus terrestris* extract on the rabbit corpus cavernosum. *Ann Acad Med Singapore* 2000;29(1):22-6.

6. Adimoelja A. Phytochemicals and the breakthrough of traditional herbs in the management of sexual dysfunctions. *Int J Androl.* 2000;23 Suppl 2:82-4.

7. Agricultural Research Service. Dr. Duke's Phytochemical and Ethnobotanical Databases: Ethnobotanical uses *Epimedium grandiflorum*. Online. Internet. [8/30/00]. Available WWW: http://www.ars-grin.gov/cgi-bin/duke/ethnobot.pl

8. Blumenthal M, *et al.* Ed. *The Complete German Commission E Monographs.*Austin, TX: American Botanical Council; 1998. Pg. 201.

9. Easterling J. Traditional uses of rainforest botanicals. Self Published?????

10. Werbach M, Murray M. Botanical Influences on Illness: A sourcebook of clinical research. CA: Third Line Press, 1994. Pg. 200.

11. Agricultural Research Service. Dr. Duke's Phytochemical and Ethnobotanical Databases: Ethnobotanical uses *Polygonum multiflorum*. Online. Internet. [8/30/00]. Available WWW: http://www.ars-grin.gov/cgi-bin/duke/ethnobot.pl

12. Duke J, Ayensu ES. Medicinal Plants of China. Michigan: Reference Publications, 1985. Pg. 508.

13. Blumenthal M, *et al.* Ed. *The Complete German Commission E Monographs.*Austin, TX: American Botanical Council; 1998. Pg. 356.

14. Agricultural Research Service. Dr. Duke's Phytochemical and Ethnobotanical Databases: Ethnobotanical uses *Corynanthe yohimbe*. Online. Internet. [8/30/00]. Available WWW: http://www.ars-grin.gov/cgi-bin/duke/ethnobot.pl

15. Jacobsen FM. Fluoxetine-induced sexual dysfunction and an open trial of yohimbine. *J Clin Psychiatry.* 1992;53:119-122.

16. Susset JG, *et al.* Effect of Yohimbine hydrochloride on erectile impotence: A double-blind study. *J Urol.* 1989;141:1360-1363.

MIGRA-PROFEN

*Ultimate Relief of Headache Pain & Cramps**

FORMULA

Feverfew tops	(*Tanacetum parthenium*)
Kava Kava	(*Piper methysticum*)
Chinese Skullcap root	(*Scutellaria baicalensis*)
Rosemary leaf	(*Rosmarinus officinalis*)
Ginger root	(*Zingiber officinale*)
Valerian root	(*Valeriana officinalis*)
Jamaican Dogwood bark	(*Piscidia erythrina*)

Concentration:	3:1 Herb strength ratio
Dosage:	Liquid Phyto-Caps™: 2 capsules at onset of pain. Repeat every 15 minutes until pain subsides (4-6 capsules)
Duration of use:	Use as directed above as needed
Best taken:	Between meals, with warm water

DESCRIPTION OF FORMULA

Many of the plants found in this compound have a long tradition of use with disorders of inflammation. Many have in turn been shown by modern science to inhibit the enzyme cyclooxygenase-2 (COX-2). COX-2 is known to play a major role in the process of inflammatory disease. The group of pharmaceutical drugs known as Non-Steroidal Anti-inflammatories (NSAIDs) directly inhibit COX-2. Unfortunately, most also inhibit the highly protective and beneficial enzyme, COX-1. This 'non-selective' inhibition is the reason why NSAIDs produce severe gastric bleeding and ulceration that is known to kill 16, 500 Americans, annually. As Chronic Inflammatory Diseases (CIDs) such as rheumatoid and osteo-arthritis, asthma, psoriasis, etc. increase in our culture(s), it is becoming increasingly important that we search for safe and effective medicines to relieve the suffering associated with these conditions. The medicinal plants in this formula have a long history of safe use with such inflammatory disorders. At the same time, many possess antioxidant and liver-protective affects - further adding to their diverse application with inflammatory conditions.

Feverfew has been used in systems of traditional medicine for hundreds of years to treat disorders of pain and inflammation. [G10, G12, 1, 2] Today, it most commonly finds use for the prevention of migraine headaches. [G4, 1, 2] Scientific investigation has confirmed the ability of Feverfew to inhibit the production of inflammatory mediators, such as - prostaglandins, leukotrienes and thromboxanes. [G10, 1, 2, 3] Clinical trials have also confirmed its positive effect with migraine headaches. [G4, G10, 1, 2] Recent research has shown promise for Feverfew with sensitizing breast cancer cells to chemotherapeutic drugs.[4]

Kava is highly regarded in Europe as an effective treatment for anxiety. Numerous clinical studies have verified its efficacy. A randomized placebo-controlled trial evaluated kava's effectiveness in 101 patients with anxiety of non-psychotic origin. Subjects were followed for 6 months. Symptoms were evaluated using the Hamilton Anxiety Scale (HAM-A). Significant improvements were seen at 8 weeks (reduction of HAM-A score from 30-17) and continued for another 16 weeks. At the end of the trial the HAM-A score was reduced to 9. In this study, long-term treatment had better efficacy than short-term treatment. [2]

Similar, but quicker results were seen in a placebo-controlled double blind study of 40 women with menopause-related symptoms of anxiety. However, unlike the previous study there was a significant decrease (measured by HAM-A) in symptoms after just 1 week of treatment. Improvement continued throughout the full 8 week study period. [3]

Several studies have been conducted comparing Kava with benzodiazepines. A double-blind study of 174 patients with anxiety compared kava with oxazepam and bromazepam. Patients were followed for 6 weeks. Similar improvements in HAM-A scores were seen in all 3 treatment groups. Statistically there was no difference in the outcome of the 3 therapies. Kava was well tolerated with none of the side effects associated with benzodiazepines. [4]

A recent meta-analysis reviewed several clinical trials to determine the efficacy of kava for the treatment of anxiety. The reviewers concluded that kava was superior to placebo as a symptomatic treatment for anxiety. The authors agreed that Kava is an herbal option for the treatment of anxiety. [5]

Chinese Skullcap has a long been recognized as an anti-inflammatory of noted importance. [G10] Modern science confirms its anti-inflammatory influence. [G3, G8] In fact, Chinese Skullcap is now acknowledged to selectively inhibit the enzyme known as COX-2. [8] Its value here is as an anti-inflammatory and a powerful antioxidant. [G10] As an antioxidant, Chinese Skullcap further supports the reduction of the free-radical stress that is well known to be generated at times of inflammation.

Rosemary is an antioxidant [G10] and anti-inflammatory [8] that also has a history of being used to treat headache. [8] Relief from indigestion and muscle spasms has also traditionally been noted with Rosemary. [G10] Although some conflicting reports exist [G10] - a number of compounds found in Rosemary have recently been shown to inhibit the COX-2 enzyme. [9]

Ginger is known across several continents to have traditionally been used for the treatment of a diverse range of inflammatory disorders. [8, 14] In recent times, compounds found in Ginger have been shown to be more powerful as an anti-inflammatory than the pharmaceutical drug, indomethacin. [G5] Clinical human trials have also confirmed its effectiveness in relieving the symptoms of Rheumatoid arthritis - without any adverse side effects. [G5] As digestive health has been strongly associated with various inflammatory conditions, [12, 13] Ginger is also of benefit here for its well known ability to improve gastric function. [G5, 11, 14]

Valerian root is useful here for its highly regarded antispasmodic influence. [G12, G20, 15] Also known to possess a sedative effect in disorders of the nervous system, Valerian is helpful where inflammation triggers nervous system related spasms, [15] anxiety, and insomnia. [15, 16]

Jamaican Dogwood contributes the benefits of a sedative and powerful antispasmodic to this formula. [G1, G4, 17] In addition, its ability to relieve pain [G1] and inflammation [G1, G4] are useful. Traditional use has generally applied the Jamaican Dogwood to treat gynecological disorders. [17]

THERAPEUTIC APPLICATIONS*

Note: The intention of the following information is to represent the traditional use of the individual botanicals found in these formulas and to inform the reader of any evolving scientific inquiry relevant to the formula's ingredients.

SUPPORTED BY TRADITIONAL USE

Anti-inflammatory, [G5, G10, G12, 1, 2, 6, 8, 14] Pain, [G12, 1, 2] Digestive dysfunction, [G3, G5, 5, 6, 7, 15, 16] Liver dysfunction, [G3, G5, 5, 7, 15, 16] Antispasmodic,

SCOPE OF RELEVANT SCIENTIFIC INVESTIGATION

Anti-inflammatory, [G3, G5, G8, G10, 1, 2, 3] COX-2 inhibition, [8, 9, 10] Migraine headaches, [G4, G10, 1, 2] Antispasmodic, [G20, 15, 17]

CAUTIONS, CONTRA-INDICATIONS AND DRUG INTERACTIONS

Please reference Chapter 9. Do not use during pregnancy or lactation.

COMPLIMENTARY HERBS/FORMULAS

Infla-Profen, Feverfew - Professional Strength

REFERENCES

1. Pizzorno J, Murray M. Textbook of Natural Medicine. New York: Churchill Livingstone; 1999.

2. Anonymous. Feverfew. *The Lawrence Review of Natural products.* 1994; September: 1-3.

3. Sumner H, *et al.* Inhibition of 5-lipoxygenase and cyclo-oxygenase in leukocytes by feverfew. Involvement of sesquiterpene lactones and other components. *Biochem Pharmacol.* 1992; 43(11): 2313-20.

4. Patel NM, *et al.* Paclitaxel sensitivity of breast cancer cells with constitutively active NF-kappa B is enhanced by I kappa B-alpha super-repressor and parthenolide. *Oncogene* 2000; 19(36): 4159-4169.

5. Snow JM. *Curcuma longa* L. (Zingiberaceae). *The Protocol Journal of Botanical Medicine.* 1995; Autumn: 43-46.

6. Srimal RC. Turmeric: A brief review of medicinal properties. *Fitoterapia;* 1997; 68(6): 483-493.

7. Selvam R. The antioxidant activity of turmeric (*Curcuma longa*). *Journal of Ethnopharmacology.* 1995; 47: 59-67.

8. Newmark TM, Schulick P. Beyond Aspirin. Prescott, Az. HOHM Press. 2000.

9. Kelm MA, *et al.* Antioxidant and cyclooxygenase inhibitory phenolic compounds from *Ocimum sanctum* Linn. *Phytomedicine.* 2000; 7(1): 7-13.

10. Zhang F, *et al.* Curcumin inhibits Cyclooxygenase-2 transcription in bile acid and phorbol ester treated human gastrointestinal epithelial cells. *Carcinogenesis.* 1999; 20(3): 445-451.

11. Kapoor LD. Handbook of Ayurvedic Medicinal Plants. Florida. CRC Press; 1990.

12. Astwood JD, *et al.* Stability of food allergens to digestion in vitro. *Nat Biotechnol.* 1996; 14(10): 1269-73.

13. Majamaa H, *et al.* Evaluation of the gut mucosal barrier: evidence for increased antigen transfer in children with atopic eczema. *J Allergy Clin Immunol.* 1996; 97(4): 985-90.

14. Schulick P. Ginger, common spice or wonder drug. Herbal Free Press, Vermont. USA.

15. Morazzoni P, Bombardelli E. *Valeriana officinalis:* traditional use and recent evaluation of activity. *Fitoterapia.* 1995; 66(2): 99-112.

16. Brown D. Valerian: Clinical Overview. *Townsend Letter for Doctors.* 1995; May: 150-151.

17. Della Loggia R, *et al.* Isoflavones as spasmolytic principles of *Piscidia erythrina. Progress in clinical and biological research.* 1988; 280: 366-368.

18. Piscopo G. Kava Kava. Gift to the islands. *Alt Med Rev.* 1997; 2(5): 355-364.

19. Voltz HP and Kieser M. Kava Kava extract WS 1490 versus placebo in anxiety disorders- a randomized placebo-controlled 25 week outpatient trial. *Phamacopsychiat.* 1997; 30:1-5.

20. Warnecke G. [Psychosomatic dysfunctions in the female climacteric. Clinical effectiveness and tolerance of kava extract WS 1490]. *Fortschr Med.* 1991; 109 (4): 119-122. [in German]

21. Woelk H, *et al.* The treatment of patients with anxiety. A double blind study: kava extract WS 1490 vs benzodiazepine. *Zitschrift for Allgemenie Medizine.* 1993; 69: 271-277. [in German]

22. Pittler MH, *et al.* Efficacy of kava extract for treating Anxiety: Systematic review and meta-analysis. *J Clin Psychopharmacology.* 2000; 20: 84-89.

PHYTO-ESTROGEN

Support for the Peri-Menopausal and Menopausal Years *
FORMULA

Chaste tree berry	(*Vitex agnus-castus*)
Alfalfa leaf	(*Medicago sativa*)
Black Cohosh root	(*Cimicifuga racemosa*)
Blue Vervain herb	(*Verbena hastata*)
Dandelion root	(*Taraxacum officinalis*)
Red clover tops	(*Trifolium pratense*)
St. John's Wort buds	(*Hypericum perforatum*)
Wild Oats	(*Avena sativa*)
Sage leaf	(*Salvia off.*)

Concentration:	3:1 Herb strength ratio
Dosage:	Liquid Phyto-Caps™: 1 capsule, Three times daily
Duration of use:	4-6 Months
Best taken:	Between meals, with warm water

DESCRIPTION OF FORMULA

This formula assists the physiological and emotional transitions associatated with peri-menopause and menopause. The formula stabilizies the hormonal functions which lead to menopausal symptoms - that may include menstrual irregularities, vaginal dryness, fatigue, depression, decreased libido, sleep disturbances, fluid retention, food cravings, and palpitations. This formula works indirectly to support the body's production of both estrogen and progesterone. In addition to supplying plant estrogen-like compounds - called isoflavones - the important transfer of estrogen production from the ovaries to the adrenal glands that accompanies menopause is also addressed by this formula, by its supportive influence over the body's nervous function.

Chaste tree has three primary pituitary functions:[G12]

1. Inhibits follicle hormone (FSH)
2. Stimulates luteal hormone (LH)
3. Inhibits prolactin hormone

Through this action upon pituitary tissue it extends the function of the corpus luteun to produce progesterone.[17] Through a positive/negative feedback mechanism, it regulates ovarian, adrenal, and liver function.[17]

Alfalfa leaf brings several influential benefits to this formula. Alfalfa leaf's reputation to be highly nutritive, [G16] It contains vitamin K_1 which aids in the maturing of the body's calcium managing proteins[5]. Alfalfa also supplies estrogen-like plant compounds. These compounds, which are reported to be hundreds of times weaker in their effect than the body's estrogens, exert their reduced influence at receptors where the body's more powerful estrogens would otherwise bind. [5,6] Thus, the addition of such weak estrogen-mimicking compounds may either reduce the overall estrogen signaling in the body (by competing with the powerful estrogens), or increase it by supplying weak estrogens where there is a shortage of the body's more powerful estrogens. [5,6]

Note: Current concerns with Alfalfa inducing a reversible Systemic Lupus Erythematosus (SLE)-like syndrome are based on toxicology studies of canavanine - an alkaloid which is only found in Alfalfa's seeds and sprouts. As canavanine is not found in the mature tops of the plant, this concern is not clinically relevant when using the leaf or blade, as is the case here.

Black Cohosh has been used by the Cherokee people to promote menstruation. [7] Modern science has shed some light on its application with such disorders of the menstrual cycle with the discovery that Black Cohosh is able to reduce levels of Luteinizing Hormone (LH), [7,8] without effecting levels of the Follicle Stimulating Hormone (FSH). [8] As LH is, in part, responsible for the release of progesterone - and FSH is, in part, responsible for the release of estrogen - it may be seen that Black Cohosh produces an overall estrogen-like affect. [8,9] Clinical research has confirmed its value in treating conditions where there is an underlying imbalance between estrogen and progesterone. [8,9]

Blue Vervain is another example of a plant remedy that has traditionally been used to restore absent menstruation. [G12] Species related to that used here are reported to have particular influence over the nervous system, being both sedative and restorative in affect. [G2] Such influence over the nervous system has lead to its use with nervous exhaustion and depression. [G2]

Dandelion Root & Leaf promotes healthy liver function enabling improved metabolism of estrogens.[18]

Red Clover has traditionally been recognized as an alterative correcting cellular waste and nutrition. [G6, G12] Red Clover is similar to Alfalfa in the fact that it too contains isoflavones that are known to produce estrogen-like effects. [G3] At least one clinical trial has shown that Red Clover is able to reduce cardiac palpitations associated with menopause. [11]

St. John's Wort has a history of use for the treatment of nerve and emotional conditions associated with menstrual imbalances. [G12] It is also a useful addition to this menopause formula for its well-known antidepressant, anti-inflammatory [11, 12, 13] and liver-protective [11] effects. In one clinical study with 111 pre and postmenopausal women, patient's psychological symptoms were improved significantly by St. John's Wort. Sexual well being was also improved. [14]

Wild Oats have long been used as a nerve tonic for individuals with nervous exhaustion. [G6, G12] German Commission E approves Wild Oats for chronic anxiety, stress and general weakness. It also is discussed as a tonic and a restorative. [15, 16]

Sage Leaf is an antispasmodic and mild antidepressant.[18] It is indicated in menopause symptoms and aids in exhausting sweats.[19]

THERAPEUTIC APPLICATIONS*
Note: The intention of the following information is to represent the traditional use of the individual botanicals found in these formulas and to inform the reader of any evolving scientific inquiry relevant to the formula's ingredients.

SUPPORTED BY TRADITIONAL USE
Estrogen balancing, [5, 6] Menstruation promoting, [G12] Nervous restorative, [G2, G6, G12] Depression, [G2] Alterative, [G6, G12]

SCOPE OF RELEVANT SCIENTIFIC INVESTIGATION

Menopausal symptoms, [11, 14] Increases progesterone,[1, 2, 3] Estrogen mimicking, [G3, 8, 9] Hot flashes associated with menopause, [2, 4] Luteinizing Hormone (LH) reduction, [8] Antidepressant, [11, 12, 13] Anti-inflammatory, [11, 12, 13] Liver-protective [11]

CAUTIONS, CONTRA-INDICATIONS AND DRUG INTERACTIONS

Please reference Chapter 9. Do not use during pregnancy or lactation.

COMPLIMENTARY HERBS/FORMULAS.

Black Cohosh Root, Phyto-Proz Supreme

REFERENCES

1. Snow JM. Vitex agnus-castus L. (Verbenaceae). The Protocol Journal of Botanical Medicine. 1996; Spring: 20-23.
2. Brown D. *Vitex agnus-castus* Clinical Monograph. *The Quarterly Review of Natural Medicine.* 1994; Summer: 111-121.
3. Anonymous. Chaste Tree. *The Lawrence Review of Natural products.* 1994; December.
4. Pizzorno J, Murray M. Textbook of Natural Medicine. New York: Churchill Livingstone; 1999. Pg. 1021.
5. Mitchell W. Plant Medicine. Seattle, Wa: Self-published; 2000. Pg. 14-15.
6. Reilly P. Clinical application Medicago sativa extracts. Journal of Naturopathic Medicine. 1 (1):
7. Brinker F. Macrotys. *The Eclectic Medical Journals.* 1996; 2(1): 2-4.
8. Snow JM. *Cimicifuga racemosa. The Protocol Journal of Botanical Medicine.* 1996; 1(4): 17-19.
9. Hudson T. A Woman's Guide to Herbal Care. Herbal Research Publications. Brevard, NC, 1998.
10. Nestel P, *et al.* Isoflavones from Red Clover improve systemic arterial compliance but not plasma lipids in menopausal women. The Journal of Clinical Endocrinology & Metabolism. 1999; 84(3): 895-898.
11. Snow JM. *Hypericum perforatum* L. (Hyperiaceae). *The Protocol Journal of Botanical Medicine.* 1996; 2(1): 16-21.
12. Gruenwald J. Standardized St. John's Wort Extract Clinical Monograph. *The Quarterly Review of Natural Medicine.* 1997; Winter: 289-298.
13. Murray M. The healing power of herbs - The enlightened persons guide to the wonders of medicinal plants. 2nd ed. Prima publishing. Rocklin, Ca. 1995.
14. Grube B, *et al.* St. John's Wort extract: efficacy for menopausal symptoms of psychological origin. *Adv Ther.* 1999; 16(4)177-186.
15. Blumenthal M, *et al.* Ed. *The Complete German Commission E Monographs.*Austin, TX: American Botanical Council; 1998.
16. Witchl M. (Bisset NG, Ed.) Herbal Drugs and Phytopharmaceuticals. Medpharm, CRC Press: Boca Raton. 1994.
17. Mills, S & Bone, K Principles and Practice of Phytotherapy. Churchill Livingston; 2000. Pg 328-333.
18. Ibid, Pg 241

PHYTO-PRŌZ SUPREME

*Ultimate Support for Emotional Well Being**

FORMULA

Kava Kava root+	(*Piper methysticum*)
St. John's Wort flower bud+	(*Hypericum perforatum*)
Passionflower vine	(*Passiflora incarnata*)
Gotu Kola leaf and root	(*Centella asiatica*)
Schizandra berry	(*Schisandra chinensis*)
Siberian Ginseng root	(*Eleutherococcus senticosus*)
Wild Oat milky seed	(*Avena sativa*)
Stinging Nettle seed	(*Urtica dioica*)
Calamus root	(*Acorus calamus*)
Prickly Ash bark	(*Xanthoxylum clava-herculis*)

+ *indicates professional strength extract*

Concentration:	4:1 Average Herb Strength Ratio; Standardized to 57.75 mg of kavalactones and 0.52 mg hypericins per three capsules
Dosage:	1 capsule, Three times daily
Duration of use:	4-6 Months
Best taken:	Between meals, with warm water

DESCRIPTION OF FORMULA

This compound synergistically enhances emotional well being through a number of different strategies. The strategic objective of the formula is to:

a. Inhibit seratonin re-uptake

b. Promote seratonin uptake at its receptors

c. Promote seratonin release

d. Elevate intra-cellular cyclic AMP levels

e. Inhibit mono-amine oxidase

f. Provide tropho-restoration to the vital nerve centers

Kava kava has been used in Polynesia and Hawaii as a social lubricant because of its mild psychotropic effects. The definition of Piper methysticum is 'intoxicating pepper'.[1] In Europe it is used for anxiety, mild insomnia, nervous tension and as a muscle relaxant.[2] The active ingredients are kavalactones. In a six month randomized placebo controlled study with 100 people with tension and anxiety produced significant results after two months with even better results in 6 months.[3] Another study showed improvement in anxiety symptoms after one week of treatment. The effect as a muscle relaxant appears to be a direct effect on the contractility of the muscle rather than a relaxing effect on the nerve conduction.[4] Kava has become a mainstream herbal product in the U.S. and holds promise as an anticonvulsant and anxiolytic actions. The mechanisms for its CNS activity is not characteristic of morphine, aspirin or other pain relievers.[5]

St. John's Wort has been used as a medicine for more than 2,000 years. It is an effective antidepressant. In several recent studies when compared to standard antidepressant drugs it proves as effective, better tolerated and has much fewer side effects.[6] St. John's Wort has been shown to be effective in Seasonal Affective Disorder(SAD).[7] It has also been shown to increase libido in contrast to conventional medications. In addition to its antidepressant effect, it also is a valuable anti-inflammatory[8], wound healing[9] and antiviral agent. [10]

Wild Oat milky seed has a reputation as a trophorestorative (builds nervous reserve).[11] It is useful in states of nervous debility, exhaustion, depression, sleeplessness and wherever convalescence is required for chronic conditions and cardiac weakness. [12,13] An acute indication for use is for a headache from over work. "It is not a remedy of great power...probably its chief value as a medicine is to energize in nervous exhaustion" Harvey W. Felter, MD.[14]

Passionflower is used as a sedative to reduce restlessness and produce rest. It has wide application as an antispasmodic for the GI and nervous system. It is indicated for the pain of neuralgia.[15] A flavonoid, vitexin acts as a anti-inflammatory and lowers blood pressure.[16]

Gotu Kola is considered to be one of the so-called 'elixirs of life'. [17,18,19] It has long been used in India to improve intelligence and mental function. [G3] Several studies suggest that Gotu Kola may be useful with improving memory, reducing fatigue and stress, increasing general mental ability, and increasing I.Q. in developmentally disabled children. [G3, 2]

Schizandra Berry is an adaptogen, enhancing resistance to external and internal stress. It increases mental alertness and athletic performance. Its effects are compared to Milk Thistle with similar mechanisms of action including antioxidant effects focused on the liver.[20] It is an effective cholagogue and is used in China for nonjaundice (chronic) hepatitis.[21]

Siberian Ginseng root has been in use in China for over 4000 years. Used regularly, it is said to increase longevity, improve general health, improve the appetite, and restore memory.[2] Today, as an adaptogen, it is known to produce improvement in overall metabolic efficiency, as well as to increase resistance to disease and stressful influences. [G3, G4]

Nettle seed is able to exert numerous effects on the signals sent by the immune system that provoke chronic inflammation. Studies have shown that nettle can block formation of pro-inflammatory cytokines[22] and prostaglandins.[23] It may even be able to convert some T-cells into forms that inhibit rather than promote inflammatory reactions.[24] Nettle leaf and seed were widely used in traditional medicine to relieve arthritis pain, help fight bladder infections, and for gout, chronic skin diseases such as eczema, autoimmune diseases such as lupus and rheumatoid arthritis, bleeding, diarrhea, kidney inflammations, wounds, and sciatica.[25]

Calamus Root (Sweet Flag) has a very long history of use. It is used worldwide by many cultures including American Indians where it was used almost universally for a very wide variety of ailments.[26] It is described as an aromatic bitter that has a powerful tonic effect of the stomach, encouraging secretory activity and increasing the appetite. It is used with people who have lost their appetite in cancer, and in cases of Anorexia nervosa.[27] In Ayurvedic medicine it is specifically indicated for sedative and analgesic properties. It lowers the blood pressure and respiration moderately.[28]

Prickly Ash bark is considered an ideal gastric stimulant when poor digestion needs assistance or constipation is present. It is a potent alterative and has a long history of use with chronic muscular rheumatism, lumbar back pain, and myalgia. Dr. Felter gave it high marks when the nerve force is low and neural irritation is present but where recuperation is possible.[29]

THERAPEUTIC APPLICATIONS*

Note: The intention of the following information is to represent the traditional use of the individual botanicals found in these formulas and to inform the reader of any evolving scientific inquiry relevant to the formula's ingredients.

SUPPORTED BY TRADITIONAL USE

Tension and anxiety,[30] nervous debility, exhaustion, <u>depression</u>, sleeplessness, [31,32] An acute indication is headache from over work, [33] sedative, reduces fatigue and restlessness, antispasmodic, neuralgia,[34] increasing general mental ability. [G3]

SCOPE OF RELEVANT SCIENTIFIC INVESTIGATION

Anxiety, insomnia, nervous tension, muscle relaxant,[35] anticonvulsant and anxiolytic actions,[36] <u>antidepressant effects</u>,[37] Seasonal Affective Disorder(SAD).[38]

CAUTIONS, CONTRA-INDICATIONS AND DRUG INTERACTIONS

Please reference Chapter 9. Do not use during pregnancy or lactation. Kava may potentiate the effect of alcohol and should not be used with it. Photosensitivity to St. John's Wort has occurred in rare instances—avoid excessive exposure to light when taking. See your physician if taking a pharmaceutical MAO-inhibitor.

Schizandra may potentiate some medications including calcium channel blockers and corticosteroids.

COMPLIMENTARY HERBS/FORMULAS

Siberian Ginseng Tonic Elixir, St. Johns Wort Professional Strength, St. John's Wort Liquid Phyto-Cap™

REFERENCES

1 Singh,Y.D. and Blumenthal, M. (1997) Kava: and overview. Special review reprinted and updated from Singh, Y.D.Kava:an overview. Journal of Ethnopharmacology 1992; 37:13-45.

2 Lehmann, E., Kinzler, E. and Friedmann, J. Efficacy of a special kava extract, in patients with states of anxiety, tension, and excitedness of non-mental origin, Phytomedicine 1996; 3:113-119.

3 Volz, H.P. and Kieser, N.Kava-kava extract WS 1490 versus placebo in anxiety disorders.Pharmacopsychiatry 1997;30: 1-5.

4 Singh,Y.N. Effects of dava on meuromuscular transmissionand muscle contractility. Journal of Ethnopharmacology, 7:267-276,1983.

5 Murray M. The healing power of herbs - The enlightened persons guide to the wonders of medicinal plants. Rocklin, Ca. Prima publishing;1995.210-219.

6 Linde, K., Ramirez, G., Mulrow, C.D. et al. (1996). St. John's Wort for depression-an overview and meta analysis of randomized clinical trials. British Medical Journal 313:253-258.

7 Wheatley D. Hypericum in seasonal affective disorder (SAD). Curr Med Res Opin 1999; 15:33-37

8 Wren RC. Potter's New Cyclopaedia of Botanical drugs and preparations. Essex, UK. Saffron Walden;1988.

9 Hobbs C:St. John's Wort, Hypericum perforatum L. Herbalgram 18/19, 24-33, 1989.

10 Leung A, Foster S. Encyclopedia of Common Natural Ingredients. NY: Wiley;1996, 310-312.

11 Priest AW, Priest LR. Herbal medication. A clinical dispensary handbook. 1982.

12 Wren RC. Potter's New Cyclopaedia of Botanical drugs and preparations. Essex, UK. Saffron Walden;1988.

13 Witchl M. Herb drugs and phytopharmaceuticals. CRC Press.1994

14 Felter HW. The Eclectic Materia Medica, Pharmacology and Therapeutics. Portland, Oregon: Eclectic Medical publications. 1985.235.

15 Felter H, Lloyd JU. King's American Dispensatory. Portland. Eclectic medical Publications; 1983.1140.

16 Brinker, Francis ND. Formulas for Healthful Living. Sandy, OR: Eclectic Medical Publications;1995.120.

17 Duke J. CRC Handbook of Medicinal Herbs. Boca Raton. CRC Press. 1985. Murray M. The healing power of herbs - The enlightened persons guide to the wonders of medicinal plants. 2nd ed. Prima publishing. Rocklin, Ca. 1995.

18 Leung A, Foster S. Encyclopedia of Common Natural Ingredients. NY: Wiley;1996.

19 Murray M. The healing power of herbs - The enlightened persons guide to the wonders of medicinal plants. 2nd ed. Prima publishing. Rocklin, Ca. 1995.173-183.

20 Bensky and Gamble. Chinese Herbal Medicine: Materia Medica. Seattle, Eastland Press,1986,541-2

21 Huang KC. The Pharmacology of Chinese Herbs. CRC Press: Boca Raton. 1993,201.

22 Obertreis B, Ruttkowski T, Teucher T, et al. Ex-vivo in-vitro inhibition of lipopolysaccharide stimulated tumor necrosis factor-_ and interleukin-1_ secretion in human whole blood by extractum Urticae dioicae foliorum. Arzneim Forsch 1996;46:389-94.

23 Obertreis B, Giller K, et al. (1996) Antiphlogistic effects of Urtica dioica folia extract in comparison to caffeic malic acid. Arzneim Forsch 1996;46:52-6 [in German].

24 Klingelhoefer S, Obertreis B, Quast S, Behnke B. Antirheumatic effect of IDS 23, a stinging nettle leaf extract, on in vitro expression of T helper cytokines. J Rheumatol 1999;26:2517-22.

25 Yarnell E. Stinging nettle: A modern view of an ancient healing plant. Altern Complem Ther 1998;4:180-6.

26 Motley T, The Ethnobotany of Sweet Flag, Acorus calamus. Economic botany, Vol. 48, No.4,1994, pp.397-412

27 Weiss R. Herbal medicine. Beaconsfield, UK. Beaconsfield Publishers;1985.45-6.

28 Kapoor LD. *Handbook of Ayurvedic Medicinal Plants.* CRC Press: Boca Raton. 1990,18-19.

29 Felter HW. The Eclectic Materia Medica, Pharmacology and Therapeutics. Portland, Oregon: Eclectic Medical publications. 1985.697-8

30 Volz, H.P. and Kieser, N.Kava-kava extract WS 1490 versus placebo in anxiety disorders.Pharmacopsychiatry 1997;30: 1-5.

31 Wren RC. Potter's New Cyclopaedia of Botanical drugs and preparations. Essex, UK. Saffron Walden;1988.

32 Witchl M. Herb drugs and phytopharmaceuticals. CRC Press.1994

33 Felter HW. The Eclectic Materia Medica, Pharmacology and Therapeutics. Portland, Oregon: Eclectic Medical publications. 1985.235.

34 Felter H, Lloyd JU. King's American Dispensatory. Portland. Eclectic medical Publications; 1983.1140.

35 Lehmann, E., Kinzler, E. and Friedmann, J. Efficacy of a special kava extract, in patients with states of anxiety, tension, and excitedness of non-mental origin, Phytomedicine 1996; 3:113-119.

36 Murray M. The healing power of herbs - The enlightened persons guide to the wonders of medicinal plants. Rocklin, Ca. Prima publishing;1995.210-219.

37 Linde, K., Ramirez, G., Mulrow, C.D. *et al.* (1996). St. John's Wort for depression-an overview and meta analysis of randomized clinical trials. British Medical Journal 313:253-258.

38 Wheatley D. Hypericum in seasonal affective disorder (SAD). Curr Med Res Opin 1999; 15:33-37

PMS - DAY 1-14
Ultimate Support of the
Follicle Phase of the Menstrual Cycle*
FORMULA

Dong Quai	(*Angelica sinensis*)
Black Cohosh	(*Cimicifuga racemosa*)
Partridgeberry	(*Mitchella repens*)
Saw Palmetto berry	(*Serenoa repens*)
Licorice root	(*Glycyrrhiza glabra*)
Dandelion root	(*Taraxacum officinalis*)
Ginger root	(*Zingiber officinale*)

Concentration:	3:1 Herb strength ratio
Dosage:	Liquid Phyto-Caps™: 1 capsule, Twice Daily
Duration of use:	Days 1-14 of monthly cycle - immediately following menses. Discontinue at ovulation. Following ovulation commence use of the formula PMS DAY 14-28.
Best taken:	Between meals, with warm water

DESCRIPTION OF FORMULA

This formula works to correct the alterations of hormone release and metabolism that lead to the symptoms of PMS. Its primary focus is to normalize the progesterone to estrogen balance, by promoting optimal circulation and liver metabolism - and by regulating the hormonal triggers that underly their production and release. It also tonifies and nourishes the ovarian tissues and encourages normal development of the ovarian follicles.

Note: This formula represents part 1 of a two-part approach. For best results, this formula should be taken with the product PMS DAY 14-28.

Dong Quai is an ancient remedy of the Traditional Chinese system of Medicine (TCM). Considered to be a 'blood tonic', [G5, 1, 2, 3] its traditional use represented a range of disorders that had, as an underlying factor, varying degrees of circulatory insufficiency. [G5, 1, 3]

Such use included depression and fatigue, poor memory [3] - and absent or delayed menstruation. [G5, 1, 2, 3] It is principally known here in the west for its application with gynecological conditions. Dong Quai has been shown to relax uterine muscle, [G5, 3] improve uterine blood flow, [3] reduce pain [3] and inflammation, [G5, 3] improve liver metabolism, [G5, 1, 2, 3] as well as protect the liver from chemical poisoning. [G5, 1, 2, 3]

Due to its liver protective properties, Dong Quai may exhibit a broader effect of the modification of hepatic oxidation of glutamic acid and L-cysteine. Along with the amino acid L-glycine, these two compounds form the molecule glutathione (GSH). As most phase-2 hepatic biotransformation is GSH dependant, this key metabolic effect may be responsible for hepatoprotection against carbon tetrachloride induced oxidative damage to hepatocytes - along with noted increases in hepatic haemoglobin. This theory may further be extended in that increases in GSH would reduce the metabolic load of the phase-1 CP450 system - as has already been well established in the literature. As hepatic biotransformation of the 3-ketosteroids takes place via phase-1, improved metabolism of progesterone may result in the encouragement of the favored 5-alpha reduction of progesterone, versus the alternate cytoplasmic 5-beta reduction.[1,2,3]

Black Cohosh has been used by the Cherokee people to stimulate menstruation. [4] It was also known to the Eclectic medical doctors for use with painful menstruation, [G12, 4] considering it 'surpassed by no other drug'. [G12] Although much is yet to be understood regarding the exact processes through which Black Cohosh operates, modern science has shed some light on its application with menstrual disorders with the discovery that it is able to reduce levels of Luteinizing Hormone (LH), [4, 5] without effecting levels of the Follicle Stimulating Hormone (FSH). [5] As LH is, in part, responsible for the release of progesterone, and FSH is, in part, responsible for the release of estrogen - it may be seen that Black Cohosh produces an overall estrogen-like affect. [5, 6] Clinical research has confirmed its value in treating conditions where there is an underlying imbalance between estrogen and progesterone. [5, 6]

Partridgeberry is highly regarded in traditional herbalism as a women's tonic [G12, 7, 8] with value in treating a wide range of uterine complaints, [8] including painful and irregular menstruation. [G12, 7]

Saw Palmetto is often mislabeled as a man's herb. While it certainly has many benefits for men, it holds an important place in this formula for women. Traditionally considered a uterine tonic, [G3] Saw Palmetto has long been used for painful menstruation, [G6] and ovarian pain and inflammation. [G12] Scientific understanding of its influence in the body also suggests its use for the reduction of androgen (male hormones) excess in women.[13]

Licorice root is present in this formula for its anti-inflammatory influence, [G21, 9, 10] along with its liver-protective effect. [G3, 9] Licorice most protect liver cells against toxin-induced free radical damage (as well as its influence on the hormones produced by the adrenal glands).

Dandelion Root is present in this formula in that it targets the liver and promotes correct liver metabolism. In this respect it is valuable to facilitate the metabolism of estrogens.[15]

Ginger root is anti-inflammatory [2, 11, 12] and antispasmodic, [G1, G5, 11, 12] and as such, is of great use in this formula. Traditionally, Ginger has also been recognized as having use with painful menstruation [G12] and uterine cramping. [2]

THERAPEUTIC APPLICATIONS*

Note: The intention of the following information is to represent the traditional use of the individual botanicals found in these formulas and to inform the reader of any evolving scientific inquiry relevant to the formula's ingredients.

SUPPORTED BY TRADITIONAL USE

Absent or delayed menstruation, [G5, G12, 1, 2, 3, 4, 7, 13] Painful menstruation, [G6, G12, 4, 7] Blood tonic, [G5, 1, 2, 3] Circulatory insufficiency, [G5, 1, 3] Depression, [3] Fatigue, [3] Poor memory [3]

SCOPE OF RELEVANT SCIENTIFIC INVESTIGATION

Menopause, [5, 6] Reduction in Luteinizing Hormone (LH), [4, 5] Estrogen-like influence, [5, 6] LH/FSH ratio imbalance, [5, 6] Uterine muscle relaxant, [G5, 3] Antinflammatory, [G5, G21, 3, 9, 10, 11, 12] Improve uterine blood flow, [3] Improve liver metabolism, [G5, 1, 2, 3] Liver protective, [G3, G5, 1, 2, 3, 9] Improve uterine blood flow, [3] Anodyne [3]

CAUTIONS, CONTRA-INDICATIONS AND DRUG INTERACTIONS

Please reference Chapter 9. Do not use during pregnancy or lactation.

COMPLIMENTARY HERBS/FORMULAS
PMS Day 14-28, Liver Health, Anti-Oxidant Supreme, Cell Wise

REFERENCES

1. Noe JE. *Angelica sinensis*: A Monograph. *The Journal of Naturopathic Medicine*. 1997; Winter: 66-72.

2. Willard T. Wild Rose Scientific Herbal. Wild rose College of Natural Healing; Alberta; 1991.

3. Belford-Courtney R. Comparison of Chinese and Western uses of *Angelica sinensis*. *The Australian Journal of Medical Herbalism*. 1993; 5(4): 87-91.

4. Brinker F. Macrotys. *The Eclectic Medical Journals*. 1996; 2(1): 2-4.

5. Snow JM. *Cimicifuga racemosa*. *The Protocol Journal of Botanical Medicine*. 1996; 1(4): 17-19.

6. Hudson T. A Woman's Guide to Herbal Care. Herbal Research Publications. Brevard, NC, 1998.

7. Gladstar R. Herbal Healing for Women. ??????

8. Grieve M, Mrs. A Modern Herbal. New York. Dover; 1982.

9. Snow JM. *Glycyrrhiza glabra*. *The Protocol Journal of Botanical Medicine*. 1996; Winter: 9-14.

10. Kapoor LD. Handbook of Ayurvedic Medicinal Plants.Florida. CRC Press; 1990.

11. Bisset NG. Herbal Drugs and Phytopharmaceuticals. Ann Arbor. CRC Press;1994.

12. Schulick P. Ginger, common spice or wonder drug. Herbal Free Press, Vermont. USA.

13. Newmark T, Schulick P. Beyond aspirin. Prescott.Hohm Press; 2000.

14. Magdy El-Sheikh M. The effect of permixon on androgen receptors. *Acta Obstet Gynacol Scand*. 1998; 67: 397-399.

15. Mills, S & Bone, K Principles and Practice of Phycothorapy. Churchill Livingston, 2000. Pg. 241.

PMS - DAY 14-28

Ultimate Support of the
Luteal Phase of the Menstrual Cycle*

FORMULA

Dong Quai root	(*Angelica sinensis*)
Chaste-tree berry	(*Vitex agnus-castus*)
Black Cohosh	(*Cimicifuga racemosa*)
Wild Yam root	(*Dioscorea villosa*)
Kava Kava root	(*Piper methysticum*)
St. John's Wort buds	(*Hypericum perforatum*)
Licorice root	(*Glycyrrhiza glabra*)
Motherwort herb	(*Leonurus cardiaca*)
Ginger root (Dried)	(*Zingiber officinale*)

Concentration:	3:1 Herb strength ratio
Dosage:	Liquid Phyto-Caps™: 1 capsule, Twice Daily
Duration of use:	3-4 Months
Best taken:	Between meals, with warm water

DESCRIPTION OF FORMULA

This compound should be used collaberatively with PMS Day 1-14. Working to correct the metabolic imbalances that lead to many of the symptoms of PMS, this formula specifically addresses dysfunction in the release and metabolism of progesterone and estrogen. This is, in part, achieved by its regulating influence on the release of both Leuteinizing Hormone (LH) and Follicle Stimulating Hormone (FSH). By taking this compound following the use of PMS Day 1-14, a co-operative influence is invoked to reduce the symptoms of PMS associated with dysfunction during days 15-28 of the menstrual cycle (the luteal phase). Such symptoms include - uterine and ovarian spasms and inflammation, anxiety, transient depression, confusion, mood

swings, irritability, sleep disturbances, food cravings, bloating and gastric upset.

Note: This formula represents part 2 of a two-part approach. For best results, this formula should be taken with the product PMS DAY 1-14.

Chaste tree has three primary pituitary functions:[G12]

1. Inhibits follicle hormone (FSH)

2. Stimulates luteal hormone (LH)

3. Inhibits prolactin hormone

Through this action upon pituitary tissue it extends the function of the corpus luteun to produce progesterone.[17] Through a positive/negative feedback mechanism, it regulates ovarian, adrenal, and liver function.[17]

Black Cohosh has been noted, traditionally, for its effect on the nervous system. [G12] Reputedly possessing marked influence with muscular pain, Black Cohosh was said to be unsurpassed for treating painful menstruation. [G12] Its ability to restore delayed or suppressed menses was also highly valued. [G12] In addition, Black Cohosh is also of benefit here to assist with digestive disturbances that may accompany disorders of menstruation. [G12] The team of modern experts that comprise the German commission E approve Black Cohosh for use with pre-menstrual discomfort and dymenorrhea (painful menstruation). [6]

Wild Yam has traditionally been regarded as being effective with flatulent digestive complaints. [G15] It is also considered to be an antispasmodic which has particular use with painful ovarian complaints and menstruation. [G16] No credible support could be found for the highly speculative DHEA and progesterone stimulating claims that are often made for commercial products containing Wild Yam. In fact, a small number of studies have loaned support for disproving such claims. [G16, 7]

Kava Kava, like Wild Yam, has traditionally been used to treat both digestive disorders and painful, spasmodic menstruation.[G12] It is also of use here for its influence with nervous anxiety. [G3, 8, 9, 10] Eclectic physicians specifically used this plant for menstruation associated with emotional anxiety.

St. John's Wort has a history of use for the treatment of nervous conditions, and excessive bleeding during menses. [G12]

Antidepressant, anti-inflammatory [11, 12, 13] and liver-protective [11] effects are also of value to this formula.

Ginger has traditionally been recognized as being useful with painful menstruation [G12] and uterine cramping.[17] It is a powerful anti-inflammatory [G1, 15, 16] that engages the circulatory system and aids the delivery of the entire formula throughout the body. It is also useful for its digestive promoting[16] and antispasmodic actions.[G1, 15, 16]

Dong Quai is considered to be of use in a variety of menstrual disorders, including suppressed and painful menstruation. [G16, 18] Dong Quai has also been reported to relax uterine muscle, [G5, 19] improve uterine blood flow, [19] reduce pain [19] and inflammation, [G5, 19] and improve liver metabolism. [G5, 18, 19]

Licorice root is present in this formula for its anti-inflammatory influence, [G21, 20, 21] along with its liver-protective effect (see PMS Day 1-14). [G3, 20]

Motherwort herb is present to provide a bitter nervine with specificity for the reproductive tissues. Its bitter principles promote improved digestion while its nervine properties relieve anxiety and emotional unrest associated with cardiac tension.

THERAPEUTIC APPLICATIONS*

Note: The intention of the following information is to represent the traditional use of the individual botanicals found in these formulas and to inform the reader of any evolving scientific inquiry relevant to the formula's ingredients.

SUPPORTED BY TRADITIONAL USE

Painful menstruation (dysmenorrhea), [G12, G16] <u>PMS</u>, [G16] Anti-inflammatory, [1, 2] Menstruation promoting, [G12, G16, 1, 2] Digestive disturbances, [G12, G15, 16] <u>Ovarian pain</u>, [G16] Nervous anxiety, [G3] Antispasmodic, [G1] Uterine cramping [17]

SCOPE OF RELEVANT SCIENTIFIC INVESTIGATION

<u>PMS (Pre-Menstrual Syndrome)</u>, [G16, 1, 2, 4] Dysmenorrhea (painful menstruation), [6, 18] Inhibits FSH (Follicle Stimulating Hormone), [1, 2] Increases LH (Luteinizing Hormone), [1, 2] Increases progesterone, [1, 2, 3] Decreases prolactin, [1, 2] Antispasmodic, [15, 16] Nervous anxiety, [8, 9, 10] Antidepressant, [11, 12] Antiinflammatory [11, 12, 19, 20, 21]

CAUTIONS, CONTRA-INDICATIONS AND DRUG INTERACTIONS

Please reference Chapter 9. Do not use during pregnancy or lactation.

COMPLIMENTARY HERBS/FORMULAS
PMS Day 1-14, Liver Health, Cell Wise, Anti-Oxidant Supreme

REFERENCES

1. Snow JM. *Vitex agnus-castus* L. (Verbenaceae). *The Protocol Journal of Botanical Medicine.* 1996; Spring: 20-23.

2. Brown D. *Vitex agnus-castus* Clinical Monograph. *The Quarterly Review of Natural Medicine.* 1994; Summer: 111-121.

3. Anonymous. Chaste Tree. *The Lawrence Review of Natural products.* 1994; December.

4. Lauritzen CH, *et al.* Treatment of premenstrual tension syndrome with *Vitex agnus-castus* - Controlled, double-blind study versus pyridoxine. *Phytomedicine.* 1997; 4(3): 183-189.

5. Mitchell W. Plant Medicine. Seattle, Wa: Self-published; 2000. Pg. 14-15.

6. Blumenthal M, *et al.* Ed. *The Complete German Commission E Monographs.*Austin, TX: American Botanical Council; 1998. Pg. 90.

7. Araghiniknam M, *et al.* Antioxidant activity of *Dioscorea* and dehydroepiandrosterone (DHEA) in older humans. *Life Sci.* 1996; 59:147-157.

8. Singh YN, Blumenthal M. Kava - An Overview. Special Review Herbalgram: 39; 34-56.

9. Blumenthal M, *et al.* Ed. *The Complete German Commission E Monographs.*Austin, TX: American Botanical Council; 1998. Pg. 156.

10. Pittler MH, Ernst E. Efficacy of Kava extract for treating anxiety: systematic review and meta-analysis. *J Clin Psychopharmacol.* 2000; 20(1):84-89.

11. Snow JM. *Hypericum perforatum* L. (Hyperiaceae). *The Protocol Journal of Botanical Medicine.* 1996; 2(1): 16-21.

12. Gruenwald J. Standardized St. John's Wort Extract Clinical Monograph. *The Quarterly Review of Natural Medicine.* 1997; Winter: 289-298.

13. Murray M. The healing power of herbs - The enlightened persons guide to the wonders of medicinal plants. 2nd ed. Prima publishing. Rocklin, Ca. 1995.

14. NAPRALERT Search results. Program for Collaborative Research in the Pharmaceutical Sciences College of Pharmacy, University of Illinois at Chicago. October 1994.

15. Bisset NG. Herbal Drugs and Phytopharmaceuticals. Ann Arbor. CRC Press;1994.

16. Schulick P. Ginger, common spice or wonder drug. Herbal Free Press, Vermont. USA.

17. Willard T. Wild Rose Scientific Herbal. Wild rose College of Natural Healing; Alberta; 1991.

18. Noe JE. *Angelica sinensis*: A Monograph. *The Journal of Naturopathic Medicine.* 1997; Winter: 66-72.

19. Belford-Courtney R. Comparison of Chinese and Western uses of *Angelica sinensis.* The Australian Journal of Medical Herbalism. 1993; 5(4): 87-91.

20. Snow JM. *Glycyrrhiza glabra. The Protocol Journal of Botanical Medicine.* 1996; Winter: 9-14.

21. Kapoor LD. Handbook of Ayurvedic Medicinal Plants.Florida. CRC Press; 1990.

SERENITY with KAVA KAVA
Ultimate Support of Relaxation *
FORMULA

American Skullcap	(*Scutellaria lateriflora*)
Passionflower vine	(*Passiflora incarnata*)
Kava Kava	(*Piper methysticum*)
Chamomile flowers	(*Matricaria recutita*)
Hops strobile	(*Humulus lupulus*)
Wild Oats	(*Avena sativa*)
Mugwort	(*Artemesia vulgaris*)
Peppermint	(*Mentha piperita*)

Concentration:	3:1 Herb strength ratio
Dosage:	Liquid Phyto-Caps™: 1 capsule, Three times daily
Duration of use:	3-4 Months
Best taken:	Between meals, with warm water

DESCRIPTION OF FORMULA

This calming formula works not only as a nervous relaxant, but also as a nervous restorative particularly where nervous integrity has become compromised due to overwork and stress and nervous exhaustion has resulted. In addition, these botanicals that help with anxiety and digestion have been incorporated to reduce these manifestations of nervous debility.

American Skullcap was used quite extensively by the early Eclectic physicians of the last century as a tonic, nervine, and as an antispasmodic. [G12] It was said to be especially useful for nervous condition, particularly those manifesting "excitability, restlessness, or wakefulness". [G6, G12] Skullcap has been brought into this formula for its specific use with nervousness from mental or physical exhaustion. [G12] It is this highly specific use for treating nervous exhaustion that makes Skullcap an excellent addition to this stress formula.

Passionflower vine shares with American Skullcap its traditional use as an antispasmodic and as a remedy for nervous excitement and irritability. [G6] When mental worry and exhaustion are evident, the Passionflower is considered specific. [G6] The monograph published by Germany's Commission E lists Passionflower for use with nervous restlessness. [1] In addition, there is some evidence to suggest that it also possesses antianxiety activity. [G4]

Kava Kava is well known for its relaxing effect. Numerous clinical trials have supported the use of kava for the treatment of nervous anxiety.[15] German Commission E approves Kava for 'conditions of nervous anxiety, stress and restlessness'.[16] Kava is used here to remove the stress and anxiety that can often prevent someone from obtaining deep, restful sleep. Antispasmodic activity has been noted. [17, 18]

Chamomile flowers are considered antispasmodic and anti-inflammatory, with specific influence on the gastrointestinal tract. [23] *Matricaria*, a genus of chamomile comes from the root 'matrix', meaning womb or mother. This reflects the opinion that it is particularly useful with female reproductive disorders. [4] It is used as a sedative in cases of restlessness and irritability, particularly where there is disturbed digestion and flatulence. [24]

Hops strobiles are used traditionally for nervous irritation and wakefulness, chiefly where anxiety and worry are the cause. [G6] The German Commission E monograph mentions Hops for restlessness and anxiety, as well as disorders of sleep. [G4, 1, 4] Also used historically to stimulate digestion [G6] and to tonify cerebro-spinal function, [5] Hops serves this formula as a valued relaxing and restorative tonic.

Wild Oats are considered to be a nerve tonic specific for those individuals who suffer from nervous exhaustion. [G6, G12] Its noted use during convalescence, and recovery from addiction, is reflective of its traditionally espoused ability to restore the "wasted elements of nerve force". [G6] Wild Oats is another plant that has received official mention by the German Commission E, in this case for chronic anxiety stress and weakness. It also is discussed as a tonic and a restorative. [1, 4]

Mugwort also receives mention by the German Commission E as a sedative, for use with restlessness, anxiety, and insomnia. [1, 4] Similar to a number of other plants in this formula, Mugwort also stimulates digestion,[4] thereby assisting with an increase overall vitality.

Peppermint possesses antispasmodic action, aids with digestion, and helps to relief intestinal bloating and flatulence. [G16] The German Commission E has stated that Peppermint increases digestion and the flow of bile. [G16, 1] It also enhances the overall taste of this formula.

THERAPEUTIC APPLICATIONS*

Note: The intention of the following information is to represent the traditional use of the individual botanicals found in these formulas and to inform the reader of any evolving scientific inquiry relevant to the formula's ingredients.

SUPPORTED BY TRADITIONAL USE

Anxiety, [G4, G6, 1, 3, 4] Nervous exhaustion, [G6, G12] Tonic, [G6, G12, 1, 4, 5] Nervine, [G12] Antispasmodic, [G6, G12, G16, 1] Excitability, [G6, G12] Irritability, [G6] Restlessness, [G6, G12, 1, 4] Insomnia, [G4, G6, G12, 1, 4] Mental exhaustion, [G6, G12] Digestive. [G6, G16, 1, 4]

SCOPE OF RELEVANT SCIENTIFIC INVESTIGATION

Nervous anxiety. [1, 3]

CAUTIONS, CONTRA-INDICATIONS AND DRUG INTERACTIONS

Please reference Chapter 9. Do not use during pregnancy or lactation.

COMPLIMENTARY HERBS/FORMULAS

Skullcap, St. John's Wort Supreme, Melissa Supreme

REFERENCES

1. Blumenthal M, *et al.* Ed. *The Complete German Commission E Monographs.*Austin, TX: American Botanical Council; 1998.
2. Harrison T. Savage civilization New York: Alfred A. Knopf; 1937
3. Anonymous. Natural anxiolytics - Kava and L.72 antianxiety formula. *The American Journal of Natural Medicine.* 1994; 1(2): 10-14.
4. Witchl M. (Bisset NG, Ed.) Herbal Drugs and Phytopharmaceuticals. Medpharm, CRC Press: Boca Raton. 1994.
5. Priest AW, Priest LR. Herbal medication. A clinical dispensary handbook. 1982.

SOUND SLEEP
Ultimate Support for Refreshing and Revitalizing Sleep*

FORMULA

Valerian root	(*Valeriana officinalis*)
California poppy	(*Eschscholzia californica*)
Passionflower vine	(*Passiflora incarnata*)
Kava Kava	(*Piper methysticum*)
American Skullcap	(*Scutellaria lateriflora*)
Hops Strobile	(*Humulus lupulus*)
GABA	(*Gamma Amino-butyric acid*)
L-glycine	

Concentration:	3:1 Herb strength
Dosage:	Liquid Phyto-Caps™: 2 capsules with a small amount of warm water 1 hour before bed.
Duration of use:	3-4 Months
Best taken:	Before bedtime

DESCRIPTION OF FORMULA

This formula brings together a number of medicinal plants that are recognized for their beneficial application with simple disorders of sleep. This compound is not narcotic in its affect. It simply works to reduce the anxiety, irritability, restlessness, physical tension, and worry that one will often see associated with occasional sleeplessness. This compound may also be used at times when nervous excitement and anxiety restrict normal and healthy function.

Valerian root has been used to induce sleep.[1] Today, the German Commission E notes its use for restlessness and nervous disturbances of sleep.[2,3] The World Health Organization (WHO) also suggests its use as a sleep-promoting herb, stating that it is often used as a possible substitute for stronger synthetic sedatives in the treatment of nervous excitement and disturbances of sleep, when associated with anxiety.[G24] This has been further suggested by other sources.[2,4]

California poppy has received wide acknowledgement from a number of respected clinicians for use as a sleep aid. [G11, 5, 6] Dr. Weiss from Europe states that California poppy is "altogether gentle, more in the direction of establishing equilibrium, and not narcotic". [7]

Passionflower is another example of a medicinal plant that has traditionally been reported to induce sleep by its simple calming or quieting influence, and not by any narcotic affect. [G15] It has also traditionally been used to treat nervous disorders, [G3] as an antispasmodic, and for its influence with pain relief. [G15] Passionflower has been approved by the highly regarded European Scientific Co-operative on Phytotherapy (ESCOP) for "tenseness, restlessness and irritability with difficulty in falling asleep". [G2]

Hops strobiles are used traditionally for nervous irritation and wakefulness, chiefly where anxiety and worry are the cause. [G6] The German Commission E monograph mentions Hops for restlessness and anxiety, as well as disorders of sleep. [G4, 8, 11] Also used historically to stimulate digestion [G6] and to tonify cerebrospinal function, [12] Hops serves this formula as a valued relaxing and restorative tonic.

Kava Kava is well known for its relaxing effect. Numerous clinical trials have supported the use of kava for the treatment of nervous anxiety. [15] German Commission E approves Kava for 'conditions of nervous anxiety, stress and restlessness'. [16] Kava is used here to remove the stress and anxiety that can often prevent someone from obtaining deep, restful sleep. Antispasmodic activity has been noted. [17, 18]

American Skullcap was used by the Eclectic physicians of the last century as a tonic, nervine, and as an antispasmodic. [G12] It was said to be especially useful for nervous condition manifesting with "excitability, restlessness, or wakefulness". [G6, G12] Skullcap is included here for its specific use with nervousness from mental or physical exhaustion. [G12]

GABA & L-glycine have been included in this formula due to the therapeutic benefits reported by the highly respected clinician, Dr. Bill Mitchell, ND. In combination, they are reputed to possess a mild sedative quality [14] which supports the overall function of this formula. Specifically, Dr. Mitchell suggests that they help to quiet the locus ceruleus in the mid-brain. [15]

THERAPEUTIC APPLICATIONS*

Note: The intention of the following information is to represent the traditional use of the individual botanicals found in these formulas and to inform the reader of any evolving scientific inquiry relevant to the formula's ingredients.

SUPPORTED BY TRADITIONAL USE

Promote sleep, [G6, G12, G15, G24, 1, 4] Sleeplessness due to nervousness, [G6, 2, 3] Excitability, [G6, G12] Restlessness, [G6, G12] Nervous disorders, [G3] Antispasmodic, [G12, G15] Pain relief, [G15] Nervine. [G12]

SCOPE OF RELEVANT SCIENTIFIC INVESTIGATION

Promote sleep, [G2, G4, G24, 1, 2, 8, 11] Sleeplessness due to nervousness, [G24, 3] Possible substitute for synthetic sedatives, [G24, 2, 4] Nervous anxiety, [8, 10, 13] Antispasmodic, [8]

CAUTIONS, CONTRA-INDICATIONS AND DRUG INTERACTIONS

Please reference Chapter 9. Do not use during pregnancy or lactation.

COMPLIMENTARY HERBS/FORMULAS

Serenity with Kava Kava,Valerian Root

REFERENCES

1. Valpiani C. *Valeriana officinalis. Journal of the Australian Traditional Medicine Society.* 1995;1(2):57-62.

2. Houghton PJ. The Scientific Basis for the Reputed Activity of Valerian. J. *Pharm. Pharmacol.* 1999;51:505-512.

3. Blumenthal M, *et al.* Ed. *The Complete German Commission E Monographs.*Austin, TX: American Botanical Council; 1998.

4. Brown D. Valerian: Clinical Overview - Phytotherapy Review & Commentary. *Townsend Letter for Doctors.* 1995:150151.

5. Sherman, JA The complete botanical prescriber. Self Published, 1993. Pg. 101.

6. Miller JG, Murray WJ. Herbal Medicinals: A Clinician's Guide. New York: Pharma Prod Press, 1998. Pg. 222.

7. Weiss, F. Herbal Medicine. Gothenburg, Siseden: Ab Arcanium and Beaconsfield: Beaconsfield Publishers trans Meussar, 1985 Ltd. 101-2

8. Blumenthal M, *et al.* Ed. *The Complete German Commission E Monographs.*Austin, TX: American Botanical Council; 1998.

9. Harrison T. Savage civilization New York: Alfred A. Knopf; 1937

10. Anonymous. Natural anxiolytics - Kava and L.72 antianxiety formula. *The American Journal of Natural Medicine.* 1994; 1(2): 10-14.

11. Witchl M. (Bisset NG, Ed.) Herbal Drugs and Phytopharmaceuticals. Medpharm, CRC Press: Boca Raton. 1994.
12. Priest AW, Priest LR. Herbal medication. A clinical dispensary handbook. 1982.
13. Blumenthal M, *et al*. Ed. *The Complete German Commission E Monographs*.Austin, TX: American Botanical Council; 1998.
14. Mitchell W. Foundations of Natural Therapeutics - Biochemical Apologetics of Naturopathic Medicine. Tempe, Arizona. Southwest College Press. 1997. Pg. 265.
15. Mitchell W. Plant Medicine. Seattle, Wa: Self-published; 2000. Pg. 14-15. Pg. 124.

THYROID SUPPORT

*Ultimate Support for Metabolic Enhancement**

FORMULA

Bladderwrack	(*Fucus vesiculosus*)
Collinsonia	(*Collinsonia canadensis*)
Coleus	(*Coleus forskohlii*)
Kelp	(*Nerocystis luetkeana*)
L-Tyrosine	

Concentration:	3:1
Dosage:	1 Liquid Phyto-Cap two times daily
Duration of use:	3 months
Best taken:	Between meals, with warm water

DESCRIPTION OF FORMULA

The thyroid gland is one of the most important regulators of metabolism throughout the body. It is in turn regulated by the master glands of the entire endocrine system, the pituitary and the hypothalamus. The thyroid gland produces hormones from the amino acid tyrosine and iodine known appropriately as thyroid hormones. Using these signals, it can affect practically cell in the body in a wide variety of ways. Clearly it is essential to maintain normal thyroid function if one wishes to be healthy.

Unfortunately, many people suffer from thyroid difficulties. There are two general types of low thyroid function. One is the result of a variety of diseases such as infection or inflammation of the thyroid gland. This type of hypothyroidism can be diagnosed by standard laboratory tests and is usually treated by prescribing the most critical of the four thyroid hormones in drug form. The second common problem is sometimes called "subclinical hypothyroidism," though this name is misleading.[1] The truth is that the person with this condition does have symptoms of low thyroid function, thus the problem is not subclinical at all. However, standard laboratory tests do not detect any difficulty with the thyroid. Thus the most appropriate name for the condition might be "sublaboratory low thyroid function." It has also been called Wilson's syndrome. It is likely that Wilson's syndrome results from a variety of environmental insults and is not caused directly by any disease. Wilson's syndrome can manifest as excessive fatigue, inability to concentrate, depression, dry skin and hair loss, obesity, and many other seemingly unrelated problems. When one realizes that thyroid hormones affect every cell in the body, however, it becomes apparent that some problem with thyroid hormones could possibly lead to symptoms anywhere.

The Thyroid Support formula is designed to help maintain healthy thyroid gland metabolism. It is also designed to correct Wilson's syndrome. This condition can only be diagnosed by a physician knowledgeable in natural medicine, and true disease-induced hypothyroidism must be ruled out first. Anyone who thinks he or she may have a metabolic condition such as persistent obesity that does not respond to diet and exercise therapy should consult with a physician of natural medicine to determine if Wilson's syndrome might be involved.

Note: Wilson's syndrome should not be confused with an uncommon genetic disorder of copper metabolism known as Wilson's disease. The two are in no way related.

Bladderwrack is a seaweed with a long history of use for maintaining thyroid and maintaining a healthy body weight.[2, 3] It was also used in traditional medicine for rheumatism, kidney inflammation, fatty heart, and as a tonic.[4, 5] The complex carbohydrates (alginates) have been extensively studied in the laboratory and clinic and are well known as being useful for helping with heartburn and indigestion, as well as preventing absorption of various radioactive isotopes.[6,7] Bladderwrack contains a significant amount of iodine, a nutrient necessary for thyroid hormone production. Bladderwrack has not been sufficiently studied in modern research to determine its exact mechanism of action on the thyroid gland. However, animal studies suggest bladderwrack can help maintain healthy cholesterol levels and can have profound effects on the immune system, suggesting that the actions of bladderwrack are extensive and complex.[8,9]

Collinsonia is a tonic medicine used extensively by the Eclectics, based on Native American traditional medicine, to help normalize metabolism throughout the body, including by promoting optimal function of the kidneys and digestive tract.[10]

Coleus forskohlii is a mint family herb that contains forskolin. This compound increases cyclic AMP levels within most cells.[11] Cyclic AMP is one type of second messenger, that is, one that transmits the signals from water-soluble hormones into the cell. Of particular interest here is the fact that thyroid stimulating hormone (TSH) requires cyclic AMP to transmit its signal. TSH is the hormone produced by the pituitary gland that tells the thyroid gland to produce thyroid hormones. This might explain how people with normal TSH levels can still have symptoms of low thyroid function—there isn't enough cyclic AMP to transmit the message. Coleus may help avoid this problem, and forskolin has been shown to increase TSH activity in thyroid cells.[12]

Kelp is very similar to bladderwrack in most aspects. It was used traditionally for regulation of the thyroid gland and obesity and to help relieve indigestion, constipation, and urinary tract irritations.[13]

L-Tyrosine is a central component of thyroid hormones. It is important to have adequate tyrosine to maintain normal thyroid function.[14]

THERAPEUTIC APPLICATIONS*

Note: The intention of this following information is to represent the traditional use of the individual botanicals found in these formulas and to inform the reader of any evolving scientific inquiry relevant to the formula's ingredients.

SUPPORTED BY TRADITIONAL USE

Low thyroid function,[15, 16] Goiter, Fatigue, Obesity[17, 18]

SCOPE OF RELEVANT SCIENTIFIC INVESTIGATION

Failure of thyroid cells to respond to TSH,[19] Simple goiter due to iodine deficiency, Obesity

CAUTIONS, CONTRA-INDICATIONS AND DRUG INTERACTIONS

Please reference Chapter 9. Do not use during pregnancy or lactation. If symptoms of excessive thyroid activity (restlessness, anxiety, palpitations, diarrhea) occur, the formula should be discontinued and a physician knowledgeable in natural medicine should be consulted. This formula should not be used by those with hyperthyroidism, Hashimoto's thyroiditis, or Graves' disease. This formula may exacerbate acne due to its iodine content. Before combining this formula with thyroid hormone drugs, consult with a physician knowledgeable in natural medicine.

COMPLIMENTARY HERBS/FORMULAS

Cell Wise formula can further augment the benefits of Thyroid Support formula if problems with TSH signaling are suspected.

REFERENCES

1 Budd M. Mild hypothyroidism—the missed diagnosis. *Int J Alt Compl Med* 1998;16:25-27.

2 Ellingwood F. *American Materia Medica, Pharmacognosy and Therapeutics* 11th ed. Sandy, OR: Eclectic Medical Publications, 1919:382-3.

3 Mills SY. *Out of the Earth: The Essential Book of Herbal Medicine.* Middlesex, UK: Viking Arkana, 1991:514-6

4 Hoffmann D. *The Complete Illustrated Herbal.* New York: Barnes & Noble Books, 1996:94.

5 Felter HW. *Eclectic Materia Medica, Pharmacology and Therapeutics.* Sandy, OR: Eclectic Medical Publications, 1922:381.

6 Bruneton J. *Pharmacognosy Phytochemistry Medicinal Plants.* Paris: Lavoisier Publishing, 1995:44-47.

7 Schulick P. *Herbal Therapy from the Sea.* 1993.

8 Lamela M, Vázquez-Freire MJ, Calleja JM. Isolation and effects on serum lipid levels of polysaccharide fractions from *Fucus vesiculosus. Phytother Res* 1996;10(suppl):S175-6.

9 Willenborg DO, Parish CR. Inhibition of allergic encephalomyelitis in rats by treatment with sulfated polysaccharides. *J Immunol* 1988;140:3410-5.

10 Scudder JM. *Specific Medication and Specific Medicines.* Sandy, OR: Eclectic Medical Publications,1890, 1985:116.

11 Seamon KB, Daly JW. Forskolin: A unique diterpene activator of cAMP-generating systems. *J Cyclic Nucleotide Res* 1981;7:201-24.

12 Seamon KB, Daly JW. Forskolin: Its biological and chemical properties. *Adv Cyclic Nucleotide Protein Phosphorylation Res* 1986;20:1-150.

13 Schulick P. *Herbal Therapy from the Sea.* 1993.

14 Murray M, Pizzorno J. *Encyclopedia of Natural Medicine.* Rocklin, CA: Prima Publishing, 1991:386-90.

15 Ellingwood F. *American Materia Medica, Pharmacognosy and Therapeutics* 11th ed. Sandy, OR: Eclectic Medical Publications, 1919:382-3.

16 Mills SY. *Out of the Earth: The Essential Book of Herbal Medicine.* Middlesex, UK: Viking Arkana, 1991:514-6.

17 Ellingwood F. *American Materia Medica, Pharmacognosy and Therapeutics* 11th ed. Sandy, OR: Eclectic Medical Publications, 1919:382-3.

18 Mills SY. *Out of the Earth: The Essential Book of Herbal Medicine.* Middlesex, UK: Viking Arkana, 1991:514-6.

19 Seamon KB, Daly JW. Forskolin: Its biological and chemical properties. *Adv Cyclic Nucleotide Protein Phosphorylation Res* 1986;20:1-150.

VISION ENHANCEMENT

*Anti-Oxidant Support for Healthy Vision and Eye Function**
FORMULA

Bilberry	(*Vaccinium myrtillus*)
Lutein	
Astaxanthin	(*Haematococcus pluvialis*)
Grape seed	(*Vitis vinifera*)

Concentration:	3:1
Dosage:	1 Liquid Phyto-Cap two times daily
Duration of use:	4-6 months or longer
Best taken:	With food, particularly containing some type of healthy fat such as olive oil.

DESCRIPTION OF FORMULA

Everyone wants to protect and even optimize their vision. For the many who have compromised vision, they wish to improve it. The eyes undergo numerous challenges, however, that make maintaining optimal vision difficult. The constant strain of use is one most people are familiar with, exacerbated by insufficient light (particularly natural light), flickering fluorescent lights, and computer screens. This is believed to contribute to near sightedness, the most common visual defect. Free radical excess is another serious problem in the eyes; it can promote glaucoma, cataracts, and macular degeneration. Not only do they have to handle the usual free radical burden resulting from normal metabolism by healthy cells and free radicals that are introduced in the diet, from the air, and in the water, but also the eyes are bathed in the ultraviolet portion of sunlight that can also cause damage. Luckily there are several herbal medicines that can help compensate for all these challenges and thus help maintain healthy eyes.

Bilberry, rich in anthocyanosides (similar to flavonoids), has been shown helpful in promoting optimal night vision.[1] Though there are some studies that have not found it helpful in this regard,[2] the bulk of the evidence seems to be favorable. Bilberry has also proven useful in reducing problems associated with excessive oxidation in the eye and retina.[3] Bilberry protects small blood vessels all over the body, particularly in the eye. Historically bilberry was eaten as a food and used to fight scurvy, urinary tract infections, diabetes, diarrhea, and ulcers.[4]

Lutein is a carotenoid related to beta-carotene. Large studies have confirmed that lutein is a protective antioxidant in the eyes.[5][6] Lutein is best absorbed when taken with a fatty meal.[7]

Astaxanthin is another carotenoid. It acts as an antioxidant in the retina, similar to lutein.

Grape seed proanthocyanidins have been shown in European studies to help relieve eye strain and to help maintain normal vision.[8] It may also help with adaptation after glare exposure and may help maintain normal night vision.[9] Grapes are widely eaten and used in traditional herbalism around the world for eye diseases, varicose veins, hemorrhoids, skin inflammations, asthma, and a host of other conditions.[10]

THERAPEUTIC APPLICATIONS*

Note: The intention of this following information is to represent the traditional use of the individual botanicals found in these formulas and to inform the reader of any evolving scientific inquiry relevant to the formula's ingredients.

SUPPORTED BY TRADITIONAL USE

Poor visual dark adaptation,[11] Eye ailments,[12] Indigestion,[13] Constipation, Diarrhea,[14] Venous insufficiency, Urinary tract disorders

SCOPE OF RELEVANT SCIENTIFIC INVESTIGATION

Near sightedness, Night blindness,[15] Diabetic Retinopathy,[16 17] Antioxidant, Glaucoma, Reduced risk of need for surgery to remove cataracts,[18 19] Cataracts,[20] Macular degeneration,[21] Hypertensive retinopathy, Retinitis,[22] Capillary fragility,[23] Hemorrhoids, Varicose veins

CAUTIONS, CONTRA-INDICATIONS AND DRUG INTERACTIONS

Please reference Chapter 9. Do not use during pregnancy or lactation. There are no known contraindications or problems with Vision Enhancement.

COMPLIMENTARY HERBS/FORMULAS

Anti-Oxidant Supreme complements Vision Enhancement well in people concerned about cataracts and macular degeneration. Vein Strength may be combined with Vision Enhancement for people with retinopathy due to diabetes, hypertension, or any other condition.

REFERENCES

1 Cunio L. *Vaccinium myrtillus. Australian J Med Herbalism* 1993;5:81-85.

2 Muth ER, Laurent JM, Jasper P. The effect of bilberry nutritional supplementation on night visual acuity and contrast sensitivity. *Alt Med Rev* 2000;5:164-73.

3 Murray M. Bilberry (*Vaccinium myrtillus*). *Am J Nat Med* 1997;4:18-22.

4 Cunio L. *Vaccinium myrtillus. Australian J Med Herbalism* 1993;5:81-85.

5 Chasan-Taber L, Willett WC, Seddon JM, *et al.* A prospective study of carotenoid and vitamin A intakes and risk of cataract extraction in US women. *Am J Clin Nutr* 1999;70:509-16.

6 Brown L, Rimm EB, Seddon JM, *et al.* A prospective study of carotenoid intake and risk of cataract extraction in US men. *Am J Clin Nutr* 1999;70:517-24.

7 Roodenburg AJC, Leenen R, van het Hof KH, *et al.* Amount of fat in the diet affects bioavailability of lutein esters but not of alpha-carotene, beta-carotene, and vitamin E in humans. *Am J Clin Nutr* 2000;71:1187-93.

8 Bombardelli E, Morazzoni P. *Vitis vinifera L. Fitoterapia* 1995;66:291-317.

9 Corbe C, Boissin JP, Siou A. Light vision and chorioretinal circulation. Study of the effect of procyanidolic oligomers (Endotelon). *J Fr Ophtalmol* 1988;11:453-60 [in French].

10 Bombardelli E, Morazzoni P. *Vitis vinifera L. Fitoterapia* 1995;66:291-317.

11 Brown D. *Herbal Prescriptions for Health and Healing.* Roseville, CA: Prima Health, 2000:47-54.

12 Bombardelli E, Morazzoni P. *Vitis vinifera L. Fitoterapia* 1995;66:291-317.

13 Leung AY, Foster S. *Encyclopedia of Common Natural Ingredients Used in Food, Drugs and Cosmetics* 2nd ed. New York: John Wiley & Sons Inc., 1996:84-5.

14 Weiss RF. *Herbal Medicine.* Gothenberg, Sweden: Ab Arcanum and Beaconsfield: Beaconsfield Publishers Ltd, trans. Meuss AR, 1985:101-2.

15 Brown D. *Herbal Prescriptions for Health and Healing.* Roseville, CA: Prima Health, 2000:47-54.

16 Yarnell E. Review of clinical trials on oligomeric proanthocyanidins. *HealthNotes Review of Complementary and Integrative Medicine* 1999;6:92-4.

17 Fromantin M. OPC in the treatment of capillary weakness and retinopathy in diabetics. *Méd Int* 1981;16:432-4 [in French].

18 Chasan-Taber L, Willett WC, Seddon JM, *et al.* A prospective study of carotenoid and vitamin A intakes and risk of cataract extraction in US women. *Am J Clin Nutr* 1999;70:509-16.

19 Brown L, Rimm EB, Seddon JM, *et al.* A prospective study of carotenoid intake and risk of cataract extraction in US men. *Am J Clin Nutr* 1999;70:517-24.

20 Murray M. Bilberry (*Vaccinium myrtillus*). Am J Nat Med 1997;4:18-22.

21 Murray M. Bilberry (*Vaccinium myrtillus*). Am J Nat Med 1997;4:18-22.

22 Vérin MMP, Vildy A, Maurin JF. Therapeutic essay: Retinopathy and OPC. *Bordeaux Med* 1978;11:1467-73 [in French].

23 Yarnell E. Review of clinical trials on oligomeric proanthocyanidins. *HealthNotes Review of Complementary and Integrative Medicine* 1999;6:92-4.

WOMAN'S LIBIDO
Enhancement of Fertility and Libido*
FORMULA

Damiana	(*Turnera diffusa*)
Sarsaparilla	(*Smilax officinalis v. ornata*)
Horney Goat Weed	(*Epimedium grandiflorum*)
Wild Oats	(*Avena sativa*)
Chuchuhuasi	(*Maytenus krukovit*)
Catuaba	(*Juniperus brasiliensis*)
Ginger root	(*Zingiber officinale*)
Suma root	(*Pfaffia paniculata*)
Helonias root	(*Chamaelirium luteum*)

Concentration:	3:1 Herb strength ratio
Dosage:	Liquid Phyto-Caps™: 1 capsule, Twice daily
Duration of use:	2-3 Months
Best taken:	Between meals, with warm water

DESCRIPTION OF FORMULA

This powerful formula helps restore a woman's libido where it has become lessened, or altogether lost. Any long-lasting approach to libido enhancement must include an effective strategy for building nervous reserve. No stimulants have been used here. To drive an already exhausted physiology with stimulants is counterproductive. The primary focus of this formula is simple nervous restoration. Often, individuals who live in modern society become stressed beyond the natural bounds of a healthy physiology. Regardless of the origin of the stress, the effects may very well be the same - nervous exhaustion, sexual disinterest and fatigue. In this formula we bring together powerful nervous system restoratives that are also known to enhance sexual performance and/or desire.

Damiana is reported to be a tonic, [G3, G6, 2] that is used in traditional cultures as an aphrodisiac. [G3, 1] In fact, the plant was formally given the species name, *aphrodisiaca*. It is a tonic that is said to improve sexual function in both women and men, specifically where sexual weakness and debility are associated with nervousness and depression. [G12] In the tradition of physiomedicalism, Damiana is considered to be an aphrodisiac, with particular influence as a trophorestorative (builds nervous reserve). [2] At least one scientific study with animals supports its use for enhancement of sexual performance. [3]

Sarsaparilla is an alterative (and blood tonic) that is also known for its anti-inflammatory effect with conditions such as psoriasis, rheumatism, and rheumatoid arthritis. [G4, G10] Liver protective action is also noted. [G3, G4, G10] It is included in this virility formula for its tonifying influence combined with its ability to restore correct metabolism.

Epimedium is better known by its common name, Horny Goat Weed. As such a name might imply, this plant is considered an aphrodisiac. Traditionally it is also used as a tonic. [4, 5] In the Chinese system of Medicine, epimedium is known to increase sexual desire and activity. [G21]

Wild Oats are present here for the same reason that they appear in our Male Libido formula - for their valued influence with nervous exhaustion. [G6, G12] Often used with complaints of the digestive system where there is also physical weakness and fatigue, [6] Wild Oats may be used during convalescence from chronic disease, [G12] or from nicotine abuse. [6]

Chuchuhuasi and its related species have found long traditional application with matters relating to fertility. [7, 8] It is a tonic [8] which is well known to strengthen a wide array of digestive processes. [9] It is present in this formula, primarily for its noted tonic effect, and for its reputation for enhancing virility. [12]

Catuaba is regarded as a nervous system tonic [10] that is used to relieve fatigue and nervous exhaustion. [11] Its reputation as an aphrodisiac [10, 11] is perhaps chiefly the result of this nervous system influence.

Ginger is well known as an anti-inflammatory [13, 14, 15, 16] and antispasmodic. [G1, G5, 14, 15] Traditionally, Ginger has also been recognized as having use with painful menstruation [G12] and uterine cramping. [13] It has been included in this Women's Libido formula for its traditional use as an aphrodisiac. [16, 17]

Suma is known to be used traditionally for the treatment of sterility.[18] Its benefits as a tonic have lead it to be commonly known as Brazilian Ginseng.[19] Suma's indigenous name is Para Todo, meaning "for everything".[20] Reports also suggest that Suma and its related species have been used as aphrodisiacs for some 300 years.[19, 21]

Helonias Root promotes pelvic circulation and relieves pelvic congestion. By promoting better blood supply to the reproductive organs, it facilitates improved vitality to those tissues.

THERAPEUTIC APPLICATIONS*

Note: The intention of the following information is to represent the traditional use of the individual botanicals found in these formulas and to inform the reader of any evolving scientific inquiry relevant to the formula's ingredients.

SUPPORTED BY TRADITIONAL USE

Aphrodisiac,[G3, 1, 10, 11, 16, 17, 19, 21] Tonic,[G3, G6, 2, 4, 5, 8] Improves sexual function,[G12, 12] Sexual weakness and debility associated with nervousness and depression,[G12] Nervous exhaustion,[G6, G12, 11] Trophorestorative (builds nervous reserve),[2, 10] Anti-inflammatory,[G4, G10, 13, 14, 15, 16] Strengthens digestion,[6, 9] Antispasmodic.[G1, G5, 14, 15]

SCOPE OF RELEVANT SCIENTIFIC INVESTIGATION

Sexual performance enhancing,[G21, 3] Liver protective.[G3, G4, G10]

CAUTIONS, CONTRA-INDICATIONS AND DRUG INTERACTIONS

Please reference Chapter 9. Do not use during pregnancy or lactation.

COMPLIMENTARY HERBS/FORMULAS

Siberian Ginseng Tonic

REFERENCES

1. Agricultural Research Service. Dr. Duke's Phytochemical and Ethnobotanical Databases: Ethnobotanical uses *Turnera Diffusa*. Online. Internet. [8/23/00]. Available WWW: http://www.ars-grin.gov/cgi-bin/duke/ethnobot.pl

2. Priest AW, Priest LR. Herbal medication. A clinical dispensary handbook. 1982. Pg. 80.

3. Arletti R, *et al.* Stimulating property of *Turnera diffusa* and *Pfaffia paniculata* extracts on the sexual-behaviour of male rats. *Psychopharmacology.* 1999;143(1):15-19.

4. Walker M. Medical Journalist Report of Innovative Biologics. *Townsend Letter for Doctors.* 1998; Nov: 18-22.

5. Agricultural Research Service. Dr. Duke's Phytochemical and Ethnobotanical Databases: Ethnobotanical uses *Epimedium grandiflorum.* Online. Internet. [8/30/00]. Available WWW: http://www.ars-grin.gov/cgi-bin/duke/ethnobot.pl

6. Blumenthal M, *et al.* Ed. *The Complete German Commission E Monographs.*Austin, TX: American Botanical Council; 1998. Pg. 356.

7. NAPRALERT Search results for *Maytenus ilicifolia* (ethnomedical information). Program for Collaborative Research in the Pharmaceutical Sciences College of Pharmacy, University of Illinois at Chicago. September 15, 1994.

8. Agricultural Research Service. Dr. Duke's Phytochemical and Ethnobotanical Databases: Ethnobotanical uses *Maytenus ilicifolia.* Online. Internet. [8/30/00]. Available WWW: http://www.ars-grin.gov/cgi-bin/duke/ethnobot.pl

9. Schwontkwoski D. Herbs of the Amazon: Traditional and common uses. Salt Lake City: Science Student Braintrust Pub, 1993. Pg. 19.

10. Schwontkwoski D. Herbs of the Amazon: Traditional and common uses. Salt Lake City: Science Student Braintrust Pub, 1993. Pg. 16.

11. Easterling J. Traditional uses of rainforest botanicals. Self Published. Pg. 20.

12. Easterling J. Traditional uses of rainforest botanicals. Self Published. Pg. 21.

13. Willard T. Wild Rose Scientific Herbal. Wild rose College of Natural Healing; Alberta; 1991.

14. Bisset NG. Herbal Drugs and Phytopharmaceuticals. Ann Arbor. CRC Press;1994.

15. Schulick P. Ginger, common spice or wonder drug. Herbal Free Press, Vermont. USA.

16. Newmark TM, Schulick P. Beyond Aspirin. Prescott, Az. HOHM Press. 2000. Pg. 244.

17. Qureshi S, *et al.* Studies on herbal aphrodisiacs used in Arab system of medicine. *Am J Chin Med.* 1989;17(1-2):57-63.

18. Agricultural Research Service. Dr. Duke's Phytochemical and Ethnobotanical Databases: Ethnobotanical uses *Pfaffia tuberosa.* Online. Internet. [8/30/00]. Available WWW: http://www.ars-grin.gov/cgi-bin/duke/ethnobot.pl

19. Schwontkwoski D. Herbs of the Amazon: Traditional and common uses. Salt Lake City: Science Student Braintrust Pub, 1993. Pg. 38.

20. Easterling J. Traditional uses of rainforest botanicals. Self Published. Pg. 34.

21. NAPRALERT Search results for *Pfaffia paniculata* (ethnomedical information). Program for Collaborative Research in the Pharmaceutical Sciences College of Pharmacy, University of Illinois at Chicago. November 4, 1994.

GENERAL REFERENCES

G1. Wren RC. Potter's New Cyclopaedia of Botanical drugs and preparations. Essex, UK. Saffron Walden;1988.

G2. Bartram T. Encyclopedia of Herbal Medicine. Dorset. Grace Publishers; 1995.

G3. Leung A, Foster S. Encyclopedia of Common Natural Ingredients. NY: Wiley;1996.

G4. Bradley P (Ed.). British herbal Compendium. Dorset. British Herbal Medical Assoc.; 1992.

G5. Mills S, Bone K. Principles and practice of Phytotherapy. New York. Churchill Livingstone; 2000.

G6. Ellingwood F. American Materia Medica, Therapeutics and Pharmacognosy. Portland. Eclectic Medical Publications;1985.

G7. Tang W, Eisenbrand G. Chinese Drugs of Plant Origin. New York. Springer-Verlag;1992.

G8. Huang KC. The Pharmacology of Chinese Herbs. Ann Arbor. CRC Press;1993.

G9. McGuffin M, et al. Ed. AHPA's Botanical Safety Handbook. Boca Raton: CRC Press, 1997.

G10. Newall CA, et al. Herbal Medicines: A Guide for Health-Care Professionals. London: Pharmaceutical Press; 1996.

G11. Weiss R. Herbal medicine. Beaconsfield, UK. Beaconsfield Publishers;1985.

G12. Felter H, Lloyd JU. King's American Dispensatory. Portland. Eclectic medical Publications; 1983.

G13. Duke J. Handbook of Medicinal Herbs. Boca Raton. CRC Press;1985.

G14. Hoffman D. The Holistic Herbal. Moray. The Findhorn Press;1984.

G15. Felter HW. The Eclectic materia Medica, Pharmacology and Therapeutics. Portland, Oregon. Eclectic Medical publications;1985.

G16. Boon H, Smith M. The Botanical Pharmacy. Quebec, Canada. Quarry press;1999.

G17. Mills S. The Essential Book of Herbal medicine. London. Penguin;1991.

G18. Brinker, Francis ND. Herb Contraindications and Drug Interactions. Sandy, OR: Eclectic Medical Publications;1997.

G19. Miller L. Herbal Medicinals: Selected Clinical Consideration Focusing on Known or Potential Drug-Herb Interactions. Arch Intern Med.1998;158: 2200-11.

G20. Newall C, Phillipson JD. "Interactions of Herbs with Other Medicines." Online. Internet. [4/26/00]. Available WWW: http://www.ex.ac.uk/phytonet/phytojournal/

G21. Bensky D, Gamble A. Chinese Herbal Medicine: Materia Medica. Seattle: Eastland, 1986.

G22. DeSmet PAGM. Adverse Effects of Herbal Drugs. Berlin: Springer-Verlag. 1993

G23. Bergner P. "Herb-drug Interactions." Medical Herbalism. 1997. Online. Internet. [5/20/99]. Available WWW: http://medherb.com/92DRGHRB.HTM

G24. WHO monographs on selected medicinal plants. Volume 1. Geneva: World Health Organization. 1999.

CHAPTER 7
FULL SPECTRUM
LIQUID EXTRACT FORMULAS

The following chapter represents over 50 formulas that have been developed as liquid extracts and supported by the enclosed references. Each formula is discussed followed by uses of each ingredient contained within the formula. Also the Therapeutic Applications section provides "Traditional Uses", "Scientific Investigation", "Cautions/Contra-Indications/Drug Interactions", and "Complementary Herbs/Formulas".

ARTEMESIA/QUASSIA SUPREME
An Anti-Parasitic Formula *
FORMULA

Sweet Annie herb	(*Artemesia annua*)
Quassia bark	(*Picrasma excelsa*)
Black Walnut Green Hulls	(*Juglans nigra*)
Neem leaves	(*Azadirachta indica*)
Bilva herb	(*Aegle marmelos*)
Embelia Herbs	(*Embelia ribes*)
Eclipta herb	(*Eclipta alba*)
Phyllanthus herb	(*Phyllanthus amarus*)
Gentian root	(*Gentiana lutea*)
Fresh Ginger root	(*Zingiber officinale*)

Concentration:	1:1.5 Herb strength ratio
Dosage:	15-30 drops, 3-4 times daily
Duration of use:	No longer than 3 weeks at a time
Best taken:	Between meals, with warm water

DESCRIPTION OF FORMULA

This formula has been carefully compounded to support the safe destruction and removal of intestinal parasites. In addition, it tonifies and promotes the realignment of those digestive processes that may contribute to such an invasion.

Sweet Annie - The various species of Wormwood have long been used for expelling parasitic worms from the intestine.[G1-G3] Anti-protozoal action has also been described.[G5] The species used in this formula possess fewer of the side-effects associated with the other Wormwoods.[1] As a bitter digestive tonic, Sweet Annie has traditionally found use in liver and gall-bladder congestion.[G2, G3]

Quassia bark is another bitter tonic that is known for its effect upon the expulsion and destruction of parasitic worms.[G1, G2, G4, G6]

Black Walnut (Green Hulls) are employed here for their general alterative properties[G2] and their ability to expel and/or destroy parasitic worms.[G5, 2]

Neem, like the botanicals above, is anthelmintic in its action.[G2] It is also known as an alterative with specific use with 'blood disorders'.[3]

Bilva is also an alterative.[3] The role of the alteratives in this formula is to correct the inner metabolic environment that yields to parasitic infection.

Embelia has long been recognized for its anthelmintic action.[4]

Eclipta has traditionally been used as an alterative and liver tonic.[3]

Phyllanthus is described traditionally as being effective as a liver protective herb.[G5]

Gentian is included in this formula for its traditional use as a digestive bitter which restores tone to the G.I. tract.[G4]

Ginger is included here for its well established anti-inflammatory and antispasmodic activity.[G5, 5]

THERAPEUTIC APPLICATIONS*

Note: The intention of the following information is to represent the traditional use of the individual botanicals found in these formulas and to inform the reader of any evolving scientific inquiry relevant to the formula's ingredients.

SUPPORTED BY TRADITIONAL USE

The destruction and removal of parasites, digestive bitter, liver and gallbladder disorders.[G1-G4, G6, 5, 6]

SCOPE OF RELEVANT SCIENTIFIC INVESTIGATION

Malaria.[6-9]

CAUTIONS, CONTRA-INDICATIONS AND DRUG INTERACTIONS

Please reference Chapter 9. Do not use during pregnancy or lactation. Not intended for prolonged use.

COMPLIMENTARY HERBS/FORMULAS

Candida Supreme Vital Cleanse Kit

REFERENCES

1. Mitchell W. The Eclectic Therapeutic categories. Medicines from the Earth Symposium. Black Mountain, NC. May 30 to June 1st, 1998.

2. Willard T. Wild Rose Scientific Herbal. Wild rose College of Natural Healing; Alberta; 1991.

3. Kapoor LD. Handbook of Ayurvedic Medicinal Plants.Florida. CRC Press; 1990.

4. Nadkarni AK. Indian Materia Medica. Bombay. Popular Prakashan; 1992.

5. Newmark T, Schulick P. Beyond aspirin. Prescott.Hohm Press; 2000.

6. Trigg P. Qinghaosu (Artemisinin) as an Antimalarial Drug. *Economic and Medicinal Plant Research.* 1989; 3:19-55.

7. Hien T, White N. Qinghaosu. *The Lancet.*1993; 341:603-608.

8. Foster S, *et al.* Peterson Field guides, Eastern/Central medicinal plants.

9. NAPRALERT Search results for *Artemesia annua* (ethnomedical information). Program for Collaborative Research in the Pharmaceutical Sciences College of Pharmacy, University of Illinois at Chicago. September 15, 1994.

10. Brown D. Common Drugs and Their Potential Interactions with Herbs or Nutrients. *HNR.*1999; 6(2): 124-41.

11. Kapoor LD. *Handbook of Ayurvedic Medicinal Plants.* Boca Raton. CRC Press; 1990.

ASTRAGALUS SUPREME

Strengthens Immunity and Stamina*

FORMULA

Astragalus root   (*Astragalus membranaceus*)
Schizandra berry   (*Schisandra chinensis*)
Ligustrum   (*Ligustrum lucidum*)

Concentration:	1:1.5 Herb strength ratio
Dosage:	30-40 drops, 3-4 times daily
Duration of use:	4-6 mths, or longer
Best taken:	Between meals, with warm water

DESCRIPTION OF FORMULA

This tonic formula enhances immunity by targeting the body's deepest levels of defense. Astragalus Supreme is an immune system builder, whereas Echinacea Supreme is more of an immune system activator. This compound also supports detoxification by improving liver function, and as such, is particularly useful when blood sugar abnormalities and chronic gastrointestinal dysfunction are an influence.

Astragalus has a long history as an immune enhancing tonic.[G3, G21] It assists with overcoming the debility, weakness,[G3, G21] and loss of appetite [G3] often associated with chronic disease. It is listed in the Chinese Pharmacopoeia as a tonic for the treatment of nephritis (kidney inflammation) and diabetes.[G7] There is also some evidence to suggest that Astragalus increases the production of stem cells.[5] In addition, it has been shown to increase leukocytes, interleukin-2, macrophage (immune cell) numbers and activity,[G7, 1-4] and the general immune response.[1-4]

Schizandra increases resistance[G8] to stress at all levels of the physiology. It is a powerful antioxidant that is highly specific for protecting liver tissue.[G8]

It is highly adaptogenic in nature supporting all organ systems.

Ligustrum has been shown to affect the immune system in ways similar to Astragalus.[G3, G8] It has traditionally been considered as a fortifying tonic for the liver and kidneys.

THERAPEUTIC APPLICATIONS*

Note: The intention of the following information is to represent the traditional use of the individual botanicals found in these formulas and to inform the reader of any evolving scientific inquiry relevant to the formula and its ingredients.

SUPPORTED BY TRADITIONAL USE

Chronically <u>lowered immune status</u> [G3] (characterized by frequent colds), fatigue, general weakness,[G3, G7, G8] chronic liver disorders [G3, G7, G8] (particularly where immunity is an issue), shortness of breath, swelling,[G3] to promote urination.[G3]

SCOPE OF RELEVANT SCIENTIFIC INVESTIGATION

<u>Low general immunity</u>,[G3, 1-4] stomach ulcers, glomerulonephritis, normalizing blood pressure,[G8] vasodilator,[G3, G8] modulation of cAMP,[G3, G7, G8] blood sugar stabilization,[G3, G7] restore immune function to cancer patients, AIDS,[G3] enhancing Natural Killer cell cytotoxicity,[G7] liver protection against CCl4,[G3, G7, G8] antioxidant.[G7, G8]

CAUTIONS, CONTRA-INDICATIONS AND DRUG INTERACTIONS

Please reference Chapter 9. Do not use during pregnancy or lactation. Do not take during acute infection; including cold and flu.

COMPLIMENTARY HERBS/FORMULAS

Ginseng/Schizandra Supreme, Siberian Ginseng, Reishi/Bupleurum Supreme, Siberian Ginseng Tonic, Anti-Oxidant Supreme, Cell Wise

REFERENCES

1. Halstead B, Hood L. Bulletin of the Oriental Healing Arts Institute of USA. Special Issue: *Natural Methods to Enhance Immunity*.1984; 9 (8): 391-394.
2. Wang Y, *et al.* Phytochemicals potentiate interleukin-2 generated lymphokine-activated killer cell cytotoxicity against murine renal cell carcinoma. *Mol Biother.* 1992; 4(3): 143-6.
3. Rittenhouse JR, *et al.* Chinese medicinal herbs reverse macrophage suppression induced by urological tumors. *J Urol.* 1991; 146 (2): 486-90.
4. Zhao KS, *et al.* Enhancement of the immune response in mice by Astragalus membranaceus extracts. *Immunopharmacology.* 1990; 20 (3): 225-33.
5. McCaleb R. Immune system stimulation from Astragalus. *Herbalgram.* 1998;17.

BLOODROOT/CELANDINE SUPREME

An Anti-Retro-Viral Formula*

FORMULA

Bloodroot	(*Sanguinaria canadensis*)
Celandine tops and roots	(*Chelidonium majus*)
Prickly Ash bark	(*Xanthoxylum clava-herculis*)

Concentration:	1:1.25 Herb strength ratio
Dosage:	15-30 drops, 3-4 times daily
Duration of use:	No longer than 2 weeks at a time. Discontinue for 2 weeks before resuming program
Best taken:	Between meals, with warm water

DESCRIPTION OF FORMULA

This formula supports the body's overall ability to resist and respond to viral invasion. It is particularly suited for those conditions related to respiratory and/or liver disorders. It effectively increases the vital force by optimizing liver and circulatory function. This compound contains an alkaloid known as sanguinarine that has been shown to have reverse-transcriptase inhibition activity during retro-viral infections.

Bloodroot has a reputation as a blood alterative with antiviral, anti-microbial, and anti-tumor actions.[G1, G5, G6, 1, 4, 8-10] Traditionally it has found use with respiratory disorders, such as asthma, bronchitis, croup, laryngitis, and pharyngitis.[G2, G6, G10, G13] Its use with asthma and bronchitis is particularly appropriate when weak peripheral circulation is an influence.[G10]

Celandine tops and roots have long been used for conditions of the liver and gall bladder.[G11, 2] Like the other herbs in this formula, Celandine is an alterative.[G1, G12] As such, it promotes the removal of cellular wastes and the supply of nutrition to the tissues. Antiviral, antitumour,[G1, G3, G13, 4] and anti-microbial properties have also been reported.[3-6, 9]

Prickly Ash bark is a circulatory stimulant that helps to deliver the entire formula throughout the body.[G1, G3, G4] Traditionally, it was said that its ability to 'increase tonicity and functional activity' will 'sustain the vital force through any crisis that occurs'.[G6]

THERAPEUTIC APPLICATIONS*

Note: The intention of the following information is to represent the traditional use of the individual botanicals found in these formulas and to inform the reader of any evolving scientific inquiry relevant to the formula's ingredients.

SUPPORTED BY TRADITIONAL USE

<u>Antiviral</u>, sluggish liver and/or gallbladder function, respiratory disorders, [G2, G6, G13] weak peripheral circulation (particularly when related to respiratory disorders).[G10]

SCOPE OF RELEVANT SCIENTIFIC INVESTIGATION

<u>Antiviral</u>,[4, 8] Antitumor,[G1, G3, G13, 4, 8-10] antimicrobial,[G10, 5, 6] gingivitis.[7]

CAUTIONS, CONTRA-INDICATIONS AND DRUG INTERACTIONS

Please reference Chapter 9. Do not use during pregnancy or lactation. This formula should not to be used in large amounts.[G9]

COMPLIMENTARY HERBS/FORMULAS

Astragalus Supreme, St. John's Wort, Licorice Solid Extract, Lomatium Supreme, Cell Wise

REFERENCES

1. Pizzorno J, Murray M. Textbook of Natural medicine. New york. Churchill Livingstone;1999.
2. Ritter R, *et al.* Clinical trial on standardized celandine extracts in patients with functional epigastric complaints: results of a PCDB trial. *Comp Ther Med.*1993;1:189-193.
3. Colombo ML, Bosisio E. Pharmacological activities of *Chelidonium majus* L. (Papaveraceae). *Pharmacol Res.* 1996;33(2):127-34.
4. Yance D. Herbal and Natural Strategies and Treatments for HIV and AIDS. Medicines from the Earth Symposium. Black Mountain, NC. 1997.
5. Dzink JL, Socransky SS. Comparative in vitro activity of sanguinarine against oral microbial isolates. *Antimicrob Agents Chemother.* 1985;27(4):663-65.
6. Hannah J, *et al.* Long-term clinical evaluation of toothpaste and oral rinse containing *sanguinaria* extract in controlling plaque, gingival inflammation, and sulcular bleeding during orthodontic treatment. *Am J Orthod Dentofacial Orthop.* 1989;96(3):199-207.
7. Munro IC, *et al.* Viadent usage and oral leukoplakia: a spurious association. *Regul Toxicol Pharmacol.* 1999;30(3):182-96.

8. Chaturvedi M, *et al.* Sanguinarine (pseudochelerythrine) is a potent inhibitor of NF-kappaB activation, IkappaBalpha phosphorylation, and degradation. *J Biol Chem.* 1997;272(48):30129-34.

9. Ahmad N, *et al.* Differential antiproliferative and apoptotic response of sanguinarine for cancer cells versus normal cells. *Clin Cancer Res.* 2000;6(4):1524-8.

10. Faddeeva MD, Beliaeva TN [Sanguinarine and ellipticine cytotoxic alkaloids isolated from well-known antitumor plants. Intracellular targets of their action]. [Article in Russian] *Tsitologiia* 1997;39(2-3):181-208.

BUGLEWEED/MOTHERWORT SUPREME

*For Support of Thyroid and Metabolic Enhancement**

FORMULA

Bugleweed herb	(*Lycopus virginica*)
Motherwort flowering tops	(*Leonurus cardiaca*)
Lemon Balm leaves	(*Melissa officinalis*)

Concentration:	1:1.25 Herb strength ratio
Dosage:	30-40 drops, 3-4 times daily
Duration of use:	3-4 months, then discontinue for 1 month before resuming
Best taken:	Between meals, with warm water

DESCRIPTION OF FORMULA

This calming formula influences metabolism of thyroid hormones, resulting in an overall lowering of thyroid function. It is particularly suited where hyperactivity and nervous disturbance affect heart and/or gastrointestinal function, or when auto-immune antibodies play a role in thyroid dysfunction.

Bugleweed herb has traditionally been used for a variety of disorders, including heart palpitations, hyperthyroidism and Grave's disease. [G1, G11, G14, 1]

Motherwort flowering tops has long been recognized as a sedative and cardiac tonic with particular use where there is autonomic nervous disturbance. [G1, G4, G10, G11, G15]

Lemon Balm leaves have traditionally been used for their ability to inhibit thyroid stimulating hormone. In addition, they have long been used as a sedative,[G17] an antispasmodic, carminative (relieves gas and intestinal colic), and are often employed in present times for their antiviral properties.[G3, G16]

THERAPEUTIC APPLICATIONS*

Note: The intention of the following information is to represent the traditional use of the individual botanicals found in these formulas and to inform the reader of any evolving scientific inquiry relevant to the formula's ingredients.

SUPPORTED BY TRADITIONAL USE

Cardiac tonic, [G10, G11] Heart palpitations,[1, G1, G14] hyperthyroidism,[1, G1, G11, G14] and <u>Grave's disease</u>.[1, G1, G11, G14]

SCOPE OF RELEVANT SCIENTIFIC INVESTIGATION

<u>Thyroid hormone inhibition</u>,[1, G1] <u>Grave's disease</u> (inhibits IgG thyroid receptor binding),[1, G1, G16] Leuteinizing Hormone (LH) and Testosterone inhibiton,[1] activates adenylate cyclase.[G1]

CAUTIONS, CONTRA-INDICATIONS AND DRUG INTERACTIONS

Please reference Chapter 9. Do not use during pregnancy or lactation. Due to the ability of ingredients in this formula to lower thyroid function it should not be used with hypothyroidism (underactive thyroid) or enlargement of the thyroid. [G9, G18, 2] Ingredients in this formula may interfere with radioactive iodine uptake. [G9, G18]

COMPLIMENTARY HERBS/FORMULAS

Melissa Supreme, cAMP - Coleus forskohlii Supreme, Cell Wise

REFERENCES

1. Harvey R. *Lycopus europaeus* L. and *Lycopus virginicus* L.: A Review of Scientific Research. *British Journal of Phytotherapy*.1995;4(2):55-65.
2. Auf'mkolk M, *et al*. Inhibition by certain plant extracts of the binding and adenylate cyclase stimulatory effect of bovine thyrotropin in human thyroid membranes. *Endocrinology*.1984;115(2): 527-34.

cAMP - COLEUS FORSKOHLII SUPREME

*An Intracellular Communication Formula**

FORMULA

Coleus Forskohlii	(*Coleus forskohlii*)
Bupleurum root	(*Bupleurum falcatum*)
Feverfew herb	(*Tanacetum parthenium*)
Chinese Skullcap root	(*Scutellaria baicalensis*)
Jujube dates	(*Ziziphus jujuba*)
Licorice root	(*Glycyrrhiza glabra*)
Ginger root	(*Zingiber officinale*)

Concentration:	1:1.25 Herb strength ratio
Dosage:	Liquid Extract: 40 Drops, 4 times daily
Duration of use:	This formula may be used long term for 4-6 months consecutively
Best taken:	Between meals, with warm water

DESCRIPTION OF FORMULA

This formula activates secondary messenger systems(cyclic AMP is a most important seceondary messanger)within the cell and thus facilitates the action that hormones serve within the cell.   There are many hormones that are cyclic AMP dependant within the body. Many of these hormones regulate important metabolic functions within the cell. By restoring normal cyclic AMP levels within the cell, this compound enables the communication between intra-cellular and extra-cellular functions. Since many chronic disorders are linked to the loss of intra/extra cellular communication, this compound can serve as an adjunct in most protocols for chronic disorders. This unique formula addresses cellular dysfunction by restoring the integrity of cellular *memory*, where it has been lost. In effect, this formula helps a cell to *remember* the correct response to the body's water-soluble hormones.

Coleus Forskohlii is by far one of the world's most researched medicinal plants. The majority of research has focused on forskolin, which is believed to be the plants most active constituent. It is well know to activate an enzyme that forms cyclic AMP within cells.[2] Cyclic AMP, which is perhaps the most important cell regulating molecule, carries out the message of water soluble hormones within the cell. The plants traditional uses include: cardiovascular disease, eczema, abdominal colic, disorders of the respiratory system (ie. asthma), insomnia, convulsions and painful urination.[1]

Bupleurum root has also been shown to increase cAMP.[2] This 'liver herb' is said to be antiinflammatory and an immune stimulant that regulates and restores liver and gastrointestinal function. Its reported 'protective' properties encompass liver and kidney function.[3]

Feverfew herb, like most of the botanicals in this formula, is known to stimulate the formation of cyclic AMP.[2] As its name suggests it was traditionally used to reduce fever. It is also well known as an anti-inflammatory, used primarily for the relief and prevention of migraine headaches, arthritis, and menstrual disorders. Feverfew has also been shown to possess phospholipase A2 and COX 2 inhibition activity. [G10,4, 5]

Chinese Skullcap root possesses cyclic AMP stimulating activity.[2] It is anti-inflammatory (inhibits COX 2 enzyme), and as such has been noted for its use with allergies,[G8] specifically asthma.[G7] Antibacterial, antiviral, and antioxidant properties have also been reported.[G16]

Jujube dates are reported to possess liver protective, anti-allergic and sedative properties (with particular mention for asthma).[G1, G3] Cyclic AMP is also increased by this invigorating and nutritive plant.[G1, 2]

Licorice root is included in this formula as an excellent anti-inflammatory and antispasmodic. It is well known to be anti-allergic, immunostimulating, and soothing the mucosal lining of the respiratory tract.[G1, G4]

Ginger root is known in the Ayurvedic tradition as *vishwabhesaj*, meaning the universal medicine.[6] It is a powerful anti-inflammatory which is known for its pronounced effect upon gastrointestinal function.[G1, 6] It is also known to increase cyclic AMP.[2]

THERAPEUTIC APPLICATIONS*

Note: The intention of the following information is to represent the traditional use of the individual botanicals found in these formulas and to inform the reader of any evolving scientific inquiry relevant to the formula's ingredients.

SUPPORTED BY TRADITIONAL USE

Allergies,[G1, G3, G8] Inflammation, [G10, 4, 5] (where liver/digestive influence is evident), Asthma,[G1, G3, G7], Spasmodic cramping, Cardiovascular disease (where positive inotropic action is of benefit), Eczema, Hypothyroidism, Psoriasis, Abdominal colic, Respiratory disorders, Insomnia, Convulsions, Painful urination, and Liver toxicity.[3]

SCOPE OF RELEVANT SCIENTIFIC INVESTIGATION

Activates the formation of cyclic AMP (cyclic adenosine monophosphate),[1] antiallergic,[1, 13] mast cell stabalization,[1, 13] inhibits histamine release, [1, 13] tumor- cell growth,[11, 12] cancer metastases,[1, 12] weight loss,[1, 10] glaucoma.[9]

CAUTIONS, CONTRA-INDICATIONS AND DRUG INTERACTIONS

Please reference Chapter 9. Do not use during pregnancy or lactation.

COMPLIMENTARY HERBS/FORMULAS

cAMP/Coleus forskohlii Supreme may be used to accompany any formula or therapeutic approach that works to restore correct cellular function. Such situations include; allergies of all types, asthma, autoimmune conditions, weight loss (when used with small doses of *Corynanthe yohimbe* - under the supervision of a qualified holistic practitioner), abnormal cell growth, and endocrine disorders. The use of this formula as an adjunct in treatment protocols for most chronic disorders is essential to root out the underlying causative influences of most chronic disorders.

REFERENCES

1. Pizzorno J, Murray M. Textbook of Natural Medicine. New York: Churchill Livingstone;1999.

2. NAPRALERT Search results. Program for Collaborative Research in the Pharmaceutical Sciences College of Pharmacy, University of Illinois at Chicago. October 1994.

3. Bone K. Bupleurum: A natural steroid effect. *Canadian Journal of Herbalism.* 1996; Early Winter:22-41.

4. Anonymous. Feverfew. *The Lawrence Review of Natural products.* 1994;September:1-3.

5. Heptinstall S. Parthenolide content and bioactivity of Feverfew (*Tanacetum parthenium* (L.) Schultz-Bip.). Estimation of commercial and authenticated Feverfew Products. *J. Pharm. Pharmacol.* 1992;44:391-395.

6. Newmark T, Schulick P. Beyond aspirin. Prescott.Hohm Press; 2000.

7. Brown D. Common Drugs and Their Potential Interactions with Herbs or Nutrients. *HNR.* 1999;6(3):209-22.

8. Brown D. Common Drugs and Their Potential Interactions with Herbs or Nutrients. *HNR.* 1999; 6(2):124-141.

9. Snow JM. *Coleus forskohlii* Wild. (Lamiaceae). *PJBM.* 1995 Autumn; 1(2): 39-42.

10. Arner P, *et al.* Importance of the cyclic AMP concentration for the rate of lipolysis in human adipose tissue. *Clin Sci.*1980;59(3):199-201.

11. Verma AK, *et al.* Croton oil and benzo(a)pyrene induced changes in cyclic adenosine 3'5'-monophosphate and cyclic guanosine 3'5' monophosphate phosphodiesterase activities in mouse epidermis. *Canc Res.*1976;36:81-7.

12. Agarwal KC, *et al.* Forskolin: A potent antimetastatic agent. *Int J Cancer.*1983;32(6):801-804.

13. Marone G, *et al.* Inhibition of IgE mediated release of histamine and peptide leukotriene from human basophils and mast cells by forskolin. Biochem Pharmacol.1987;36(1):13-20.

CFS SUPREME

Support of
Healthy Energy Levels and Stamina *
FORMULA

Astragalus root	(*Astragalus membranaceus*)
Siberian Ginseng root	(*Eleutherococcus senticosus*)
Gotu Kola leaf and root	(*Centella asiatica*)
Gingko leaf	(*Gingko biloba*)
Chinese Skullcap root	(*Scutellaria baicalensis*)
Reishi Mushroom	(*Ganoderma lucidum*)
Wild Oat (milky seed)	(*Avena sativa*)
Licorice root	(*Glycyrrhiza glabra*)
Prickly Ash bark	(*Xanthoxylum clava-herculis*)

Concentration:	1.5:1 Herb strength ratio
Dosage:	40 drops, 4 times daily
Duration of use:	2-3 months
Best taken:	Between meals, with warm water

DESCRIPTION OF FORMULA

This formula works to support those functions of the body that are associated with Chronic Fatigue Syndrome. This compound addresses the following: Immunity, resistance to stress, nervous system integrity, adrenal exhaustion, detoxificaion, and circulatory imbalances.

Astragalus root is a tonic with a long history of use for increasing resistance and overcoming the debility, weakness, and loss of appetite often associated with chronic disease.[G3, G21, 1]

Siberian Ginseng root has traditionally been recognized to have the ability to stimulate 'non-specific resistance' to stress, [G3, 3, 5] promote longevity, improve general health, energy and appetite, increase work performance, and restore memory. [2, 5]

Gotu Kola leaf and root is reported to improve mental function,[4] whilst acting as a sedative, and anti-depressant.[5]

Gingko leaf is well known as an anti-oxidant[8, 9] that is also noted to improve peripheral circulation and oxygen transport.[10, 11]

Chinese Skullcap root is a powerful antioxidant herb.[G3] It is known to protect liver tissue and improve detoxification.[G10, G21] Chinese Skullcap is also reported to posses antibacterial [G8, G21] and anti-allergic properties. [G21]

Reishi Mushroom is a tonic that is well known for its affects on immune function.[G8, 12] It is also reported to increase cyclic AMP in cardiac tissue.[G8] Traditionally it was said to 'lighten weight and increase longevity'.[G8]

Wild Oat (milky seed) is highly regarded as a tonic to treat nervous exhaustion and depression.[G1, 13]

Licorice root extends the life of adrenal hormones, therefore preventing their depletion.[G3, 14] It appears to be an effective treatment for both nervous and physical exhaustion associated with CFS.[15]

Prickly Ash bark is a circulatory stimulant,[G3, G1, 16] and as such, appears in this formula to help drive the other botanicals to their target(s).

THERAPEUTIC APPLICATIONS*

Note: The intention of the following information is to represent the traditional use of the individual botanicals found in these formulas and to inform the reader of any evolving scientific inquiry relevant to the formula's ingredients.

SUPPORTED BY TRADITIONAL USE

Nervous and physical exhaustion,[2, 5, G1, 13, 15] lowered general immunity,[G3, G21, 1, 3, G3, G8] circulatory weakness.[G3, 10, 11, G1, 16]

SCOPE OF RELEVANT SCIENTIFIC INVESTIGATION

Promotes connective tissue integrity, and the formation of the connective tissues structural components.[6, 2] Improvement in capillary permeability and micro-circulation has also been noted.[7] Antioxidant properties (inhibits lipid peroxidation) [8, 9]

CAUTIONS, CONTRA-INDICATIONS AND DRUG INTERACTIONS

Please reference Chapter 9. Do not use during pregnancy or lactation.

COMPLIMENTARY HERBS/FORMULAS

Solid Extract of Siberian Ginseng, , Siberian Ginseng Tonic, Energy & Vitality and Cell Wise

REFERENCES

Foster S, Yue CX. *Herbal Emissaries: Bringing Chinese Herbs to the West.* Rochester, VT: Healing Arts Press, 1992, 27-33.

1. Murray M. The healing power of herbs - The enlightened persons guide to the wonders of medicinal plants. Rocklin, Ca. Prima publishing;1995.

2. Szolomicki S, *et al.*The influence of active components of *Eleutherococcus senticosus* on cellular defence and physical fitness in man. *Phytother Res* 2000;14(1):30-5.

3. Nalini K, *et al.* Effect of *Centella asiatica* fresh leaf aqueous extract on learning and memory and biogenic amine turnover in albino rats. *Fitoterapia.* 1992; LXIII(3):2332-7.

4. Sakina MR, Dandiya PC. A psycho-neuro-pharmacological profile of Centella asiatica extract. *Fitoterapia.*1990; LXI(4):291-6.

5. Kartnig T. Clinical Applications of *Centella asiatica* (L.) Urb. *Herbs Spices Med Plants.*1988;3:146-73.

6. Belcaro G, *et al.* Improvement of Capillary Permeability in Patients with Venous Hypertension After Treatment with TTFCA. *Angiology.*1990; 533-40.

7. Dumont E, *et al.* Protection of Polyunsaturated Fatty Acids Against Iron-Dependent Lipid Peroxidation by a *Ginkgo biloba* Extract (EGb 761). *Meth Find Exp Clin Pharmacol.*1995;17 (2):83-88.

8. Kose K, Dogan P. Lipoperoxidation Induced by Hydrogen Peroxide in Human Erythrocyte Membranes. Comparison of the Antioxidant Effect of *Ginkgo biloba* Extract (EGb 761) with those of Water-soluble and Lipid-soluble Antioxidants. *J of Int Med Res.*1995; 23: 9-18.

9. Bauer U. 6-Month Double-blind Randomised Clinical Trial of *Ginkgo biloba* Extract versus Placebo in Two Parallel Groups in Patients Suffering from Peripheral Arterial Insufficiency. *Arzneim.-Forsch.*1984; 34(I): 716-720.

10. Mouren X, *et al.* Study of the Antiischemic Action of EGb 761 in the Treatment of Peripheral Arterial Occlusive Disease by TcPo2 Determination. *Angiology.*1994; 45(6): 413-417.

11. Wagner H, Farnsworth N. Economic and Medicinal Plant Research. New york.Academic Press;1990.

12. Wichtl M. *Herbal Drugs and Phytopharmaceuticals.* Boca Raton, FL: CRC Press; 1994.

13. Soma R, Ikeda M, *et al.* Effect of glycyrrhizin on cortisol metabolism in humans. *Endocrin Regulations.*1994; 28:31-34.

14. Baschetti R. Liquorice and chronic fatigue syndrome. *NZ Med Journal* (1002): 259.1995.

15. Baranov AI. Medicinal uses of ginseng and related plants in the soviet union - recent trends in the soviet literature. J of Ethnopharmacology. 1982; 6.

16. Blumenthal M, *et al.* Ed. *The Complete German Commission E Monographs.*Austin, TX: American Botanical Council; 1998.

17. Brown D. Common Drugs and Their Potential Interactions with Herbs or Nutrients. *HNR.* 1999; 6(2):124-141.

DANDELION / FENNEL SUPREME

A Digestive Restorative *
FORMULA

Dandelion root & leaf	(*Taraxacum officinalis*)
Fennel seed	(*Foeniculum vulgare*)
Gentian root	(*Gentiana lutea*)
Peppermint leaf	(*Mentha piperita*)
Licorice root	(*Glycyrrhiza glabra*)
Ginger root	(*Zingiber officinale*)

Concentration:	1:1.25 Herb strength ratio
Dosage:	30-40 drops, 3-4 times daily before meals
Duration of use:	4-6 months consecutively
Best taken:	Between meals, with warm water

DESCRIPTION OF FORMULA

This formula helps to restore strong digestive function where it has been lost. It is ideal for individuals who are experiencing the flatulence and intestinal discomfort that is often associated with insufficient digestive secretion. As the process of digestion is considered a primary cornerstone of good health this formula may be used as a key tool to address any disorder that is associated with its malfunction.

Dandelion root & leaf has long earned a lofty reputation for its bitter and diuretic actions.[G12, G17, 1] It has been reported to stimulate digestion (stomach acid),[G3] remove obstructions of the liver, and restore correct function to various bile related disorders. Primary traditional uses include diuretic, digestive disorders, rheumatism, and various skin conditions, particularly eczema.[G12, G17, 1]

Fennel seed is a powerful carminative (relieves intestinal flatulence), anti-inflammatory, stimulant, and galactagogue (promotes the secretion of mothers milk).[G1, G3, G15, 2] Its mild stimulant effects are believed to contribute to its use as a bronchodilator and a weight loss agent.[G17] It is valuable here to both reduce intestinal flatulence and to increase intestinal transit time[3] factors which are often associated with underproduction of stomach acid.[4]

Gentian root is known to normalize gastric secretion (whether it is over or under active).[5] Traditionally it has been used for sluggish digestion, loss of appetite, and as an antiinflammatory.[G3,G4, 5, 6]

Peppermint leaf is well known as a digestive aid, being used to relieve the intestinal cramping and flatulence commonly associated with indigestion.[G4, G17] The German commission E recommends its use for spasms of the smooth muscle which influences the G.I. tract, as well as gallbladder and bile ducts.[2]

Licorice root is a well respected anti-inflammatory, that is both nutritive and soothing to the mucosal ling throughout the body.[G3, G15, 2] It has also been shown to be antiallergenic and liver protective.[7]

Ginger root engages the circulatory system and aids the delivery of the entire formula throughout the body. Here it also finds use for its digestive promoting,[9] mucosal protective,[9] anti-inflammatory[8, 9] and anti-spasmodic actions.[G1, 8, 9]

THERAPEUTIC APPLICATIONS*

Note: The intention of the following information is to represent the traditional use of the individual botanicals found in these formulas and to inform the reader of any evolving scientific inquiry relevant to the formula's ingredients.

SUPPORTED BY TRADITIONAL USE

Indigestion,[G3, G4, 1, 2, 5, 6] flatulence, intestinal colic,[G1, 2, 8, 9] loss of appetite,[G3, G4, 2, 5, 6] adjunctive for anti-inflammatory therapy,[G1, G3, G4, G15, 2, 5, 6, 8, 9] various skin disorders,[1, G12] liver congestion.[1]

SCOPE OF RELEVANT SCIENTIFIC INVESTIGATION

Hypochlohydria,[G4] indigestion,[G3] anti-inflammatory.[G3]

CAUTIONS, CONTRA-INDICATIONS AND DRUG INTERACTIONS

Please reference Chapter 9. Do not use during pregnancy or lactation.

COMPLIMENTARY HERBS/FORMULAS
Sweetish Bitters, Liver Health

REFERENCES

1. Hutchens AR. A handbook of Native American herbs. Shambhalla publications. 1992.

2. Blumenthal M, Ed. The complete German commission E monographs. Am Bot Council.1998.

3. Passalacqua G, *et al.* Anti-leukotriene agents: rationale and prospects for use. *Ann Ital Med Int.* 1996. 2:93S-96S.

4. Pizzorno J, Murray M. Textbook of Natural Medicine. New York: Churchill Livingstone;1999.

5. Willard T. Textbook of Advanced Herbology. 1992.

6. Scudder J. Specific Medications. Eclectic Med Publications.1985.

7. Werbach MR, Murray M. Botanical Influence on Illness. Third Line Press

8. Bisset NG. Herbal Drugs and Phytopharmaceuticals. Ann Arbor. CRC Press;1994.

9. Schulick P. Ginger, common spice or wonder drug. Herbal Free Press, Vermont. USA.

DEVIL'S CLAW/CHAPARRAL SUPREME

An Anti-Inflammation/Anti-Arthritic Formula*

FORMULA

Devil's Claw Root	(*Harpagophytum procumbens*)
Chaparral Leaf	(*Larrea tridentata*)
Echinacea Root	(*Echinacea angustifolia*)
Echinacea Root, Seed, Tops	(*Echinacea purpurea*)
Burdock Root and Seed	(*Arctium lappa*)
Black Cohosh Root	(*Cimicifuga racemosa*)
Licorice root	(*Glycyrrhiza glabra*)
Prickly Ash Bark	(*Xanthoxylum clava-herculis*)

Concentration:	1:1 Herb strength ratio
Dosage:	30-40 drops, 3-4 times daily
Duration of use:	6 months or longer
Best taken:	Shortly before meals with warm water

DESCRIPTION OF FORMULA

This formula assists in decreasing inflammation secondary to arthritis, muscle soreness and myalgia (muscular rheumatism). The herbs are anti-oxidant, anti-inflammatory and balance an overactive immune/inflammatory response.

Devil's Claw tuber is a plant from southern Africa long valued by the native peoples there as an anti-inflammatory, for migraines, wounds, labor pains, and as a digestive tonic.[1] Devil's Claw is well established as a protector of normal joint and muscle function in osteoarthritis.[2, 3] It is not known how devil's claw works, though it does not work like non-steroidal anti-inflammatory drugs (NSAIDs like ibuprofen).[4] Thus it does not damage the stomach like these drugs do. In fact, it may even help maintain healthy digestion.[5]

Chaparral Leaf was used by Native Americans to alleviate rheumatic pain, stomach pain and bronchitis. It was researched in the 1959 and found to contain a potent anti-oxidant NDGA, with

anti-cancer activity but its results were "weak and inconsistent".[6]
A press release from the FDA warned of a potential link between
chaparral tea and liver toxicity prompting a voluntary removal of
product from store shelves. The very low dose of chaparral in
this formula is below the dosage identified for liver toxicity.[7]

Note: In the context of this formula, *Echinacea angustifolia* and *Echinacea
purpurea* will be discussed together as their actions are similar. *E. angustifolia*
has a longer documented history of traditional use, while *E. purpurea* has been
the focus of more scientific research.

Echinacea - Research has shown that alcohol/water extracts of
Echinacea significantly enhance natural killer (NK) cell function,
and the phagocytic, metabolic and bactericidal influence of
macrophages.[8, 9] This means that Echinacea has the potential to
non-specifically activate the immune system.[10, 11, 12] It has anti-
inflammatory, antibacterial, antiviral, and wound healing properties.[13, 14] It has been said that Native Americans used Echinacea
to treat more conditions than any other remedy including colds,
coughs, sore throats, and snakebite.[15]

Burdock root & seed have long been used in traditional
herbalism for inflammatory conditions including
rheumatism(painful joints and/or muscles), arthritis, gout, and
inflammatory skin problems like eczema and psoriasis.[16, 17]
Burdock root acts as an antioxidant and interferes with a messenger chemical known as platelet-activating factor that strongly
promotes excessive inflammation.[18, 19]

Black Cohosh Root was a most valued medicine by the
Eclectic physicians. They considered it primarily for the pain of
muscles and joints described as articular rheumatism, myalgia
(muscle aching) of the whole body, muscular exhaustion.[20] It
was used for headaches and when used for painful menstruation
and uterine-related disorders, considering it 'surpassed by no
other drug'. [21, 22]

Licorice Root blocks the breakdown of the body's own
cortisol,[23] thus acting as an indirect anti-inflammatory throughout the body. The presence of higher amounts of natural cortisol would also tend to act as a break on excessive immune reactions. In particular it has been shown to support normal liver

function in people with hepatitis C as well as other forms of viral hepatitis.[24, 25] In traditional Chinese herbal formulas licorice is used to make multiple herbs work well together.[26]

Prickly Ash bark is a potent alterative and has a long history of use with "chronic muscular rheumatism," lumbar back pain and myalgia. Dr. Felter gave it high marks when the nerve force is low and neural irritation is present but where recuperation is possible.[27]

THERAPEUTIC APPLICATIONS*

Note: The intention of this information is to represent the traditional use of the individual botanicals found in these formulas and to inform the reader of any evolving scientific inquiry relevant to the formula's ingredients.

SUPPORTED BY TRADITIONAL USE

Rheumatism (painful joints and/or muscles), arthritis, gout, and inflammatory skin problems like eczema and psoriasis[28, 29] myalgia (muscle aching) of the whole body, muscular exhaustion,[30] anti-inflammatory, migraines, wounds, labor pains, digestive tonic,[31] stomach pain, bronchitis, antibacterial, antiviral, and wound healing properties,[32]

SCOPE OF RELEVANT SCIENTIFIC INVESTIGATION

Normal joint and muscle function in osteoarthritis.[34, 35] enhance natural killer (NK) cell function, phagocytic, metabolic and bactericidal influence of macrophages,[36, 37] interferes with platelet-activating factor that promotes excessive inflammation,[38, 39] potent anti-oxidant, NDGA.[40]

CAUTIONS, CONTRA-INDICATIONS AND DRUG INTERACTIONS

Please reference Chapter 9. Do not use during pregnancy or lactation. A press release from the FDA warned of a potential link between chaparral tea and liver toxicity prompting a voluntary removal of product from store shelves. The very low dose of chaparral in this formula is below the dosage identified for liver toxicity.[41]

COMPLIMENTARY HERBS/FORMULAS

As a comprehensive approach to arthritis use Turmeric/Catachu Supreme for inflammation and Red Clover Supreme for enhanced tissue alterative support. Willow bark and

Meadowsweet are herbal salicylates that are also useful. Infla-Profen and Yucca/Burdock Supreme also are useful to address pain and inflammation.

REFERENCES

1 Mills S, Bone K. *Principles and Practice of Phytotherapy: Modern Herbal Medicine*. Edinburgh: Churchill Livingstone, 2000:345-9.

2 Chantre P, Cappelaere A, Leblan D, *et al*. Efficacy and tolerance of *Harpagophytum procumbens* versus diacerhein in the treatment of osteoarthritis. *Phytomedicine* 2000;7:177-83

3 Chrubasik S, Junck H, Breitschwerdt H, *et al*. Effectiveness of *Harpagophytum* extract WS 1531 in the treatment of exacerbation of low back pain: A randomized placebo-controlled double-blind study. *Eur J Anaesthesiol* 1999;16:118-29.

4 Moussard C, Alber D, Toubin MM, *et al*. A drug used in traditional medicine, *Harpagophytum procumbens*: No evidence for NSAID-like effect on whole blood eicosanoid production in human. *Prostagland Leukotr Essential Fatty Acids* 1992;46:283-6.

5 Blumenthal M, Busse WR, Goldberg A, *et al*. (eds). *The Complete German Commission E Monographs: Therapeutic Guide to Herbal Medicines*. Austin: American Botanical Council and Boston: Integrative Medicine Communications, 1998:120-1.

6 Anonymous. Chaparal. *The Lawrence Review of Natural Products*.1986; August 93.

7 Leung A, Foster S. Encyclopedia of Common Natural Ingredients. NY: Wiley;1996, 148-50

8 Schranner I, Wurdinger M, *et al*. Modification of avian humeral immunoreactions by Influx and Echinacea angustifolia extract. Zentralbl Veterinarmed (B) 1989; 36.

9 Bukovsky M, Kostalova D, Magnusova R, Vaverkova S. Testing for immunomodulating effects of ethanol-water extracts of the above ground parts of the plants Echinaceae and Rudbeckia. Cesk Farm. 1993; 42.

10 Witchl M. (Bisset NG, Ed.) Herbal Drugs and Phytopharmaceuticals. Medpharm, CRC Press: Boca Raton. 1994.

11 Snow JM. Echinacea (Moench) Spp. Asteraceae. The Protocol Journal of Botanical Medicine. 1997; 2 (2): 18-24.

12 Bauer R, Wagner H. Echinacea species as potential immunostimulatory drugs. Economic and Medicinal Plant Research. San Diego: Academic press Ltd.; 1991.

13 Wren RC. Potter's New Cyclopaedia of Botanical drugs and preparations. Essex, UK. Saffron Walden;1988.

14 Bradley P (Ed.). British Herbal Compendium. Dorset. British Herbal Medical Assoc.; 1992.

15 Snow JM. Echinacea (Moench) Spp. Asteraceae. The Protocol Journal of Botanical Medicine. 1997; 2 (2): 18-24.

16 Newall CA, Anderson LA, Phillipson JD. *Herbal Medicines: A Guide for Health-Care Professionals*. London: Pharmaceutical Press, 1996:52-3.

17 Ellingwood F. *American Materia Medica, Pharmacognosy and Therapeutics* 11th ed. Sandy, OR: Eclectic Medical Publications, 1919:378.

18 Lin CC, Lu JM, Yang JJ, *et al*. Anti-inflammatory and radical scavenge effects of *Arctium lappa*. Am J Chin Med 1996;24:127-37.

19 Iwakami S, Wu J, Ebizuka Y, Sankawa U. Platelet activating factor (PAF) antagonists contained in medicinal plants: Lignans and sesquiterpenes. Chem *Pharm Bull (Tokyo)* 1992;40:1196-8.

20 Felter HW. The Eclectic Materia Medica, Pharmacology and Therapeutics. Portland, Oregon: Eclectic Medical publications. 1985,466-69.

21 Snow JM. *Cimicifuga racemosa* (L) Nutt. (*Ranunculaceae*). *The Protocol Journal of Botanical Medicine.*1996;1(4):17-19.

22 Felter H, Lloyd JU. King's American Dispensatory. Portland. Eclectic medical Publications; 1983.

23 Tamura Y, Nishikawa T, Yamada K, *et al.* Effects of glycyrrhetinic acid and its derivatives on 4-sulpha- and 5-beta-reductase in rat liver. Arzneim Forsch 1979;29:647-9.

24 Van Rossum TGJ, Vulto AG, Hop WCJ, *et al.* Intravenous glycyrrhizin for the treatment of chronic hepatitis C: A double-blind, randomized, placebo-controlled phase I/II trial. J Gastroenterol Hepatol 1999;14:1093-9.

25 Suzuki H, Ohta Y, Takino T, *et al.* Effects of glycyrrhizin on biochemical tests in patients with chronic hepatitis. Double blind trial. Asian Med J 1983;26:423-38.

26 Foster S, Yue CX. Herbal Emissaries: Bringing Chinese Herbs to the West. Rochester VT: Healing Arts Press, 1992:112-121.

27 Felter HW. The Eclectic Materia Medica, Pharmacology and Therapeutics. Portland, Oregon: Eclectic Medical publications. 1985.697-8

28 Newall CA, Anderson LA, Phillipson JD. *Herbal Medicines: A Guide for Health-Care Professionals.* London: Pharmaceutical Press, 1996:52-3.

29 Ellingwood F. *American Materia Medica, Pharmacognosy and Therapeutics* 11th ed. Sandy, OR: Eclectic Medical Publications, 1919:378.

30 Felter HW. The Eclectic Materia Medica, Pharmacology and Therapeutics. Portland, Oregon: Eclectic Medical publications. 1985,466-69.

31 Mills S, Bone K. *Principles and Practice of Phytotherapy: Modern Herbal Medicine.* Edinburgh: Churchill Livingstone, 2000:345-9.

32 Wren RC. Potter's New Cyclopaedia of Botanical drugs and preparations. Essex, UK. Saffron Walden;1988.

33 Snow JM. Echinacea (Moench) Spp. Asteraceae. The Protocol Journal of Botanical Medicine. 1997; 2 (2): 18-24.

34 Chantre P, Cappelaere A, Leblan D, *et al.* Efficacy and tolerance of *Harpagophytum procumbens* versus diacerhein in the treatment of osteoarthritis. *Phytomedicine* 2000;7:177-83

35 Chrubasik S, Junck H, Breitschwerdt H, *et al.* Effectiveness of *Harpagophytum* extract WS 1531 in the treatment of exacerbation of low back pain: A randomized placebo-controlled double-blind study. *Eur J Anaesthesiol* 1999;16:118-29.

36 Schranner I, Wurdinger M, *et al.* Modification of avian humeral immunoreactions by Influx and Echinacea angustifolia extract. Zentralbl Veterinarmed (B) 1989; 36.

37 Bukovsky M, Kostalova D, Magnusova R, Vaverkova S. Testing for immunomodulating effects of ethanol-water extracts of the above ground parts of the plants Echinaceae and Rudbeckia. Cesk Farm. 1993; 42.

38 Lin CC, Lu JM, Yang JJ, *et al.* Anti-inflammatory and radical scavenge effects of *Arctium lappa. Am J Chin Med* 1996;24:127-37.

39 Iwakami S, Wu J, Ebizuka Y, Sankawa U. Platelet activating factor (PAF) antagonists contained in medicinal plants: Lignans and sesquiterpenes. *Chem Pharm Bull* (Tokyo) 1992;40:1196-8.

40 Anonymous. Chaparal. *The Lawrence Review of Natural Products.*1986; August 93.

41 Leung A, Foster S. Encyclopedia of Common Natural Ingredients. NY: Wiley;1996, 148-50

DEVIL'S CLUB SUPREME

*Blood Sugar Balancing Formula**
FORMULA

Jambul Seed	(*Syzygium jambolanum*)
Devil's Club Root Bark	(*Oplopanax horridum*)
Dandelion root and Leaf	(*Taraxacum officinalis*)
Uva Ursi Leaf	(*Arctostaphylos uva ursi*)
Turmeric Root	(*Curcuma longa*)

Concentration:	1:1 Herb strength ratio
Dosage:	30-40 drops, 3 times daily
Duration of use:	3-4 months for best results
Best taken:	Shortly before meals, with warm water

DESCRIPTION OF FORMULA

This formula assists in normalizing blood sugar levels in hypoglycemia and mildly elevated blood sugar. It may do this by facilitating the function of insulin on the cell membrane receptor sites for insulin. By improving the effectiveness of insulin the pancreas does not secrete excessive insulin in order to normalize the blood sugar.

Jambul Seed/Syzygium is a frequently used Ayurvedic medicine and is reported to be very effective for diabetes mellitus and for rapidly reducing sugar in the urine.[1] It has a significant hypoglycemic effect in animals.[2]

Devil's Club Root Bark has been reported to have a hypoglycemic effect for diabetics but several studies showed inconsistent results. The hypoglycemic effects have been reported to be extracted by an acid or vinegar extract while water extracts of the bark produce an element that raises blood sugar.[3]

Dandelion Leaf and Root: The root in this formula targets the liver and promotes liver function that enhances glucose metabolism. The leaf has long earned a lofty reputation for its bitter and diuretic actions. Primary traditional uses include diuretic, digestive disorders, rheumatism, and various skin conditions, particularly eczema.[4, 5]

Uva Ursi Leaf contains arbutin that is a urinary antiseptic effective against E.coli and Proteus bacteria. The high tannin content causes an astringent action. Its effect as a diuretic has been frequently reported but contradicted in at least one study.[6, 7] Arbutin is converted to hydroxyquinone in the urine with a toxicity that may occur at doses equivalent to 1/2 ounce of fresh leaf.[8]

Turmeric root is one of the most powerful inhibitors of prostaglandins and thromboxanes that promote inflammation.[9, 10] Turmeric has been shown to not interfere with beneficial prostaglandins, such as those that protect the stomach, unlike aspirin.[11] Turmeric is traditionally used in Ayurvedic medicine for rheumatoid arthritis and a wide variety of other inflammatory diseases as well for wounds, upset stomach, liver problems, and eczema.[12, 13] Turmeric has systemic antioxidant,[14] anti-inflammatory, and liver protective effects.[15,16] The volatile oils and curcumin are the most active components. Curcumin is a potent antioxidant and combats free radicals better than vitamin E.[17] Curcumin is an effective analgesic as it depletes the nerve endings of substance P, the neurotransmitter of pain receptors.[18]

THERAPEUTIC APPLICATIONS*

Note: The intention of this information is to represent the traditional use of the individual botanicals found in these formulas and to inform the reader of any evolving scientific inquiry relevant to the formula's ingredients.

SUPPORTED BY TRADITIONAL USE

Diabetes mellitus, reducing sugar in the urine,[19] hypoglycemic effect for diabetics,[20] diuretic,[21, 22] digestive disorders, rheumatism, skin conditions, particularly eczema.[23, 24] systemic antioxidant,[25] anti-inflammatory, liver protective.[26,27]

SCOPE OF RELEVANT SCIENTIFIC INVESTIGATION

Inhibits prostaglandins and thromboxanes that promote inflammation.[28, 29]

CAUTIONS, CONTRA-INDICATIONS
AND DRUG INTERACTIONS

Please reference Chapter 9. Do not use during pregnancy or lactation. Arbutin in Uva Ursi is converted to hydroxyquinone in the urine with a toxicity that may occur at doses equivalent to 1/2 ounce of fresh leaf. [30]

COMPLIMENTARY HERBS/FORMULAS

Sweetish Bitters

REFERENCES

1 Kapoor LD. CRC Handbook of Ayurvedic Medicinal Plants. CRC Press Boca Raton. 1990,179-80.

2 Wren RC. Potter's New Cyclopaedia of Botanical drugs and preparations. Essex, UK. Saffron Walden;1988.158-9.

3 Brinker, Francis ND. *Formulas for Healthful Living.* Sandy, OR: Eclectic Medical Publications;1995.101.

4 Felter H, Lloyd JU. King's American Dispensatory. Portland. Eclectic medical Publications; 1983.

5 Mills S. The Essential Book of Herbal medicine. London. Penguin;1991.

6 Leung A, Foster S. Encyclopedia of Common Natural Ingredients. NY: Wiley;1996.505-6.

7 Bradley P (Ed.). British herbal Compendium. Dorset. British Herbal Medical Assoc.; 1992.211.

8 Merck Index, 10th ed. Merck &Co. Rahway,NJ,1983, 796-7.

9 Srivastava R, Dikshit M, Srimal RC, Dhawan BN. Anti-thrombotic effect of curcumin. *Thromb Res* 1985;404:413-7.

10 Shah BH, Nawaz Z, Pertani SA, *et al.* Inhibitory effect of curcumin, a food spice from turmeric, on platelet-activating factor- and arachidonic acid-mediated platelet aggregation through inhibition of thromboxane formation and $Ca2+$ signaling. *Biochem Pharmacol* 1999;58:1167-72.

11 Srivastava R, Puri V, Srimal RC, Dhawan BN. Effect of curcumin on platelet aggregation and vascular prostacyclin synthesis. *Arzneim Forsch* 1986;36:715-7.

12 Deodhar SD, Sethi R, Srimal RC. Preliminary study on antirheumatic activity of curcumin (diferuloyl methane). *Indian J Med Res* 1980;71:632-4.

13 Nadkarni AK, Nadkarni KM. *Indian Materia Medica vol 2.* Bombay: Popular Prakashan. 1976:414-18.

14 Snow JM. *Curcuma longa* L. (Zingiberaceae). The Protocol Journal of Botanical Medicine. 1995; 1(2):43-46.

15 Wren RC. Potter's New Cyclopaedia of Botanical drugs and preparations. Essex, UK. Saffron Walden;1988.

16 Bartram T. Encyclopedia of Herbal Medicine.Dorset. Grace Publishers;1995.

17 Shama OP: Antioxidant properties of curcumin and related compounds. Biochem Pharmacol 25,1811-18-1825, 1976.

18 Patacchini R, Maggi CA, and Meli A: Capsaicin-like activity of some natural pungent substances on peripheral ending of visceral primary afferents. Arch Pharmacol 342, 72-77,1990

19 Kapoor LD. CRC Handbook of Ayurvedic Medicinal Plants. CRC Press Boca Raton. 1990,179-80.

20 Brinker, Francis ND. *Formulas for Healthful Living.* Sandy, OR: Eclectic Medical Publications;1995.101.

21 Leung A, Foster S. Encyclopedia of Common Natural Ingredients. NY: Wiley;1996.505-6.

22 Bradley P (Ed.). British herbal Compendium. Dorset. British Herbal Medical Assoc.; 1992.211.

23 Felter H, Lloyd JU. King's American Dispensatory. Portland. Eclectic medical Publications; 1983.

24 Mills S. The Essential Book of Herbal medicine. London. Penguin;1991.

25 Snow JM. *Curcuma longa* L. (Zingiberaceae). The Protocol Journal of Botanical Medicine. 1995; 1(2):43-46.

26 Wren RC. Potter's New Cyclopaedia of Botanical drugs and preparations. Essex, UK. Saffron Walden;1988.

27 Bartram T. Encyclopedia of Herbal Medicine.Dorset. Grace Publishers;1995.

28 Srivastava R, Dikshit M, Srimal RC, Dhawan BN. Anti-thrombotic effect of curcumin. *Thromb Res* 1985;404:413-7.

29 Shah BH, Nawaz Z, Pertani SA, *et al.* Inhibitory effect of curcumin, a food spice from turmeric, on platelet-activating factor- and arachidonic acid-mediated platelet aggregation through inhibition of thromboxane formation and Ca^{2+} signaling. *Biochem Pharmacol* 1999;58:1167-72.

30 Merck Index, 10th ed. Merck &Co. Rahway,NJ,1983, 796-7.

DONG QUAI SUPREME

A Woman's Hormone-Balancing Formula*

FORMULA

Dong Quai root	(*Angelica sinensis*)
Helonias root	(*Chamaelirium luteum*)
Black Cohosh root	(*Cimicifuga racemosa*)
Partridge berry	(*Mitchella repens*)
Saw Palmetto berry	(*Serenoa repens*)
Licorice root	(*Glycyrrhiza glabra*)
Ginger root	(*Zingiber officinale*)

Concentration:	1:1 Herb strength ratio
Dosage:	30-40 drops, 3-4 times daily
Duration of use:	At least 4-6 months
Best taken:	Take between meals, with a small amount of warm water during follicular phase of menstrual cycle (days 1-14). For additional support, use the Vitex Elixir during luteal phase (days 14-28).

DESCRIPTION OF FORMULA

This formula has been compounded to address key metabolic processes that ultimately influence female hormone regulation. By selecting medicinal plants that influence and tonify functions of the nervous, digestive, and endocrine systems, symptoms may be addressed, and correct hormone metabolism may be encouraged. For best results, use as directed above.

Dong Quai root has traditionally been recognized as a blood tonic. Its specific use with gynecological disorders, is clearly defined by traditional literature, and modern usage and research. Dong Quai's highly regarded ability to regulate the female reproductive cycle is enhanced by its liver protective effect. It is clearly recognized as a uterine toner and contraction regulator. Importantly, Dong Quai does not engage the reproductive system via any proven estrogenic effect.[G5, G21, 1, 2]

Helonias root is another reproductive remedy of renowned importance. It is useful to promote pelvic circulation and to relieve pelvic congestion. It is an excellent uterine tonic that has been widely used for painful and/or absent menstruation.[G4, G12, G6]

Black Cohosh root was used by Native Americans to treat a number of uterine-related disorders, including menstrual pain and uterine spasm.[G3, 4, 5]

Partridge berry is a uterine tonic that is still in use today by native West African women. Like other ingredients in this formula, the Partridge berry is well known as a uterine tonic, for the relief of painful uterine spasms.[G2, G14]

Saw Palmetto berry may be used by women to reduce an excess of secondary male hormones.[6] Although it is all too often considered to be 'a mans herb', Saw Palmetto was traditionally used as a uterine and vaginal tonic, as well as to tonify ovaries and regulate ovarian functions.[G3]

Licorice root holds a key place in this formula. It is an anti-inflammatory [G1, G4, G21, 7] that helps to spare certain compounds that are vital to the metabolism of several primary hormones (the 3-ketosteroids). In addition, Licorice is liver protective and promotes detoxification.[G1, G4, G21, 7]

Ginger root engages the circulatory system and assists by delivering the entire formula throughout the body. Here, it also finds use for its antiinflammatory[G4] and antispasmodic actions.[G1, G4]

THERAPEUTIC APPLICATIONS*

Note: The intention of the following information is to represent the traditional use of the individual botanicals found in these formulas and to inform the reader of any evolving scientific inquiry relevant to the formula's ingredients.

SUPPORTED BY TRADITIONAL USE

Regulate menstruation,[G3, G4, G5, G6, G21, 1, 2, 4] blood tonic,[G5, G21, 1, 2] antispasmodic.[G3, G4, G5, G6, G21, 1, 2, 4]

SCOPE OF RELEVANT SCIENTIFIC INVESTIGATION

Dysmenorrhea (painful menstruation),[G4,1,2,3,5] liver protection[G1,G4,G21,7]

CAUTIONS, CONTRA-INDICATIONS AND DRUG INTERACTIONS

Please reference Chapter 9. Do not use during pregnancy or lactation. **Important note:** If excessive bleeding is present, do not continue to take this formula for any extended period, until the presence of an ovarian cyst or other pathology has been ruled out by a licensed health-care practitioner.

COMPLIMENTARY HERBS/FORMULAS

Vitex Elixir (during luteal phase; days 14-28), Feverfew/Jamaican Dogwood Supreme (when pain is present) PMS Day 1-14 and PMS Day 14-28, Phyto-Estrogen.

If diagnosis of a cyst has definitely been ruled out, then this compound may be taken with Yarrow (*Achillea millefolium*) or Shepherd's Purse (*Capsella bursa-pastoris*) to slow heavy menstrual bleeding.

REFERENCES

1. Belford-Courtney R. Comparison of Chinese and Western uses of Angelica sinensis. *Australian Journal of Medical Herbalism.* 1993; 5(4): 87-91.

2. Noe JE. *Angelica sinensis:* A Monograph. *Journal of Naturopathic Medicine.* 1997; Winter: 66-72.

3. Zhu D. Dong Quai. *American Journal of Chinese Medicine.* 1986;15(3-4):117-125.

4. Snow JM. *Cimicifuga racemosa* (L) Nutt. (*Ranunculaceae*). *The Protocol Journal of Botanical Medicine.*1996;1(4):17-19.

5. Blumenthal M, Malone D. Black cohosh. *Whole Foods.*1998; April: 32-34.

6. Murray M. The healing power of herbs - The enlightened persons guide to the wonders of medicinal plants. Rocklin, Ca. Prima publishing; 1995.

7. Snow JM. Glycyrrhiza glabraL. (Leguminaceae). The Protocol journal of botanical Medicine.1996; 1(3): 9-14.

ECHINACEA GOLDENSEAL PROPOLIS THROAT SPRAY

For symptomatic relief of sore throat, colds and upper respiratory infections*

FORMULA

Fresh Echinacea root	(*Echinacea angustifolia*)
Fresh Echinacea root, flower & ripe seed	(*Echinacea purpurea*)
Goldenseal Root	(*Hydrastis canadensis*)
Oregon Grape Root	(*Berberis aquifolium*)
Propolis	*Bee harvested tree resin*
Peppermint Leaf	(*Mentha piperita*)
Licorice Root	(*Glycyrrhiza glabra*)
Thyme leaf	(*Thymus vulgaris*)

Concentration:	1:1 Herb strength ratio
Dosage:	4-6 sprays in throat, every 2 hours
Duration of use:	Up to 8 days
Best taken:	Between meals with warm water

DESCRIPTION OF FORMULA

This throat spray contains natural antibiotics, immune stimulants and soothing herbs for the treatment of bacterial and viral infections of the throat, and upper respiratory membranes.

Note: In the context of this formula, *Echinacea angustifolia* and *Echinacea purpurea* will be discussed together. Simply, *E. angustifolia* has a much longer documented history of traditional use, while *E. purpurea* has been the focus of more scientific research. Clinically (in practice), their actions are similar. Both species have been included in this formula to offer the full benefit of their collective chemistry, and individual subtleties.

Echinacea - It has been said that Native Americans used Echinacea to treat more conditions than any other remedy. It is an immune-stimulant, whose anti-inflammatory, antibacterial, antiviral, and wound healing properties have been widely reported.[1,2] Traditionally, Echinacea has been used by Native Americans to treat colds, coughs, sore throats, and snakebite.[3] The Eclectic medical doctors, from the first half of the last century, also praised Echinacea for its benefits with various chronic catarrhal (congestive) conditions of the respiratory tract. [4]Today, modern science is beginning to support much of its established traditional use, by showing that extracts of Echinacea spp. have the ability to increase antibody production, along with resistance to various infections.[5,6] Research has further shown that alcohol/water extracts of Echinacea significantly enhance natural killer cell function, and have phagocytic, metabolic and bactericidal influence on macrophages.[7,8] This simply means that Echinacea has the potential to non-specifically activate your immune system, enhancing its ability to deal with a threat, if one should arise.[9]

Goldenseal root is native to North America. It has traditionally been used with allergic/inflammatory or infectious conditions that require soothing of the mucous membranes.[10, 11] Like several other ingredients of this formula (i.e. Oregon Grape root and Barberry root), Goldenseal contains the antibiotic[1] and immunostimulatory[1] alkaloid, berberine. Along with one other key alkaloid (hydrastine), berberine has also been shown to be antispasmodic. [12]

Oregon Grape root has a history of traditional use closely resembling and synergizing with Goldenseal. Oregon Grape has distinguished itself by its therapeutic effect with skin conditions, such as psoriasis, eczema, and acne.[13]

Propolis extract has been reported to be an immune stimulant with anti-inflammatory effects (particularly when the mucous membranes are involved). [14, 15]

Peppermint has uses as a topical analgesic, and a nasal decongestant in colds and sore throats. Traditionally been used as a digestive stimulant. The oil from the plant is also reported to be antispasmodic, via its ability to relax smooth muscle. [16, 17, 18] Peppermint, of course, also improves the taste of the formula.

Licorice Root is used for cough and bronchitis because of its expectorant qualities especially in the area of the trachea.[19,20] It has anti-inflammatory and anti-allergy properties. Licorice enhances the immune response and has antiviral properties by stimulating the body to produce interferon.[21]

Thyme is used for laryngitis, acute bronchitis, and whooping cough. It is an expectorant, antispasmodic and carminative.[22]

THERAPEUTIC APPLICATIONS*

Note: The intention of this information is to represent the traditional use of the individual botanicals found in these formulas and to inform the reader of any evolving scientific inquiry relevant to the formula's ingredients.

SUPPORTED BY TRADITIONAL USE

Laryngitis, acute bronchitis, expectorant, antispasmodic and carminative.[23] Immune-stimulant,[G1, G4, 4, 5, 6] anti-inflammatory,[G1, G4] antibacterial,[G1, G4] antiviral,[G1, G4] wound healing,[G1, G4] respiratory catarrh,[G12] alterative,[G1] blood purifier.[G6] topical analgesic, nasal decongestant in colds and sore throats.[24, 25, 26]

SCOPE OF RELEVANT SCIENTIFIC INVESTIGATION

Enhance natural killer cell function and the phagocytic, metabolic and bactericidal influence on macrophages.[27, 28]

CAUTIONS, CONTRA-INDICATIONS AND DRUG INTERACTIONS

Please reference Chapter 9. Do not use during pregnancy or lactation.

COMPLIMENTARY HERBS/FORMULAS

Echinacea Supreme, Lomatium Supreme, Wild Cherry Supreme, Lomatium/Osha Supreme

REFERENCES

1 Wren RC. Potter's New Cyclopaedia of Botanical drugs and preparations. Essex, UK. Saffron Walden;1988.

2 Bradley P (Ed.). British herbal Compendium. Dorset. British Herbal Medical Assoc.; 1992.

3 Snow JM. Echinacea (Moench) Spp. Asteraceae. The Protocol Journal of Botanical Medicine. 1997; 2 (2): 18-24.

4 Felter H, Lloyd JU. King's American Dispensatory. Portland. Eclectic medical Publications; 1983.

5 Snow JM. Echinacea (Moench) Spp. Asteraceae. The Protocol Journal of Botanical Medicine. 1997; 2 (2): 18-24.

6 Bauer R, Wagner H. Echinacea species as potential immunostimulatory drugs. Economic and Medicinal Plant Research. San Diego: Academic press Ltd.; 1991.

7 Schranner I, Wurdinger M, *et al*. Modification of avian humeral immunoreactions by Influx and Echinacea angustifolia extract. Zentralbl Veterinarmed (B) 1989; 36.

8 Bukovsky M, Kostalova D, Magnusova R, Vaverkova S. Testing for immunomodulating effects of ethanol-water extracts of the above ground parts of the plants Echinaceae and Rudbeckia. Cesk Farm. 1993; 42.

9 Witchl M. (Bisset NG, Ed.) Herbal Drugs and Phytopharmaceuticals. Medpharm, CRC Press: Boca Raton. 1994.

10 Wren RC. Potter's New Cyclopaedia of Botanical drugs and preparations. Essex, UK. Saffron Walden;1988.

11 Murray M. The healing power of herbs - The enlightened persons guide to the wonders of medicinal plants. Rocklin, Ca. Prima publishing; 1995,230-234.

12 Bradley P (Ed.). British herbal Compendium. Dorset. British Herbal Medical Assoc.; 1992.

13 Murray M, op sit.

14 Balch JF, Balch PA. Prescription for Nutritional Healing. New York; Avery Publishing

15 Anonymous. Propolis. *The Lawrence Review of Natural Products*.1986; FEB: 1-2.

16 Leung A, Foster S. Encyclopedia of Common Natural Ingredients. NY: Wiley;1996.

17 Bradley P (Ed.). British herbal Compendium. Dorset. British Herbal Medical Assoc.; 1992.

18 Mills S, Bone K. Principles and practice of Phytotherapy. New York. Churchill Livingstone; 2000.

19 Bradley P (Ed.). British herbal Compendium. Dorset. British Herbal Medical Assoc.; 1992.145-7

20 Hikano H. Economic and Medicinal Plant Research, Volume 1, London, Academic Press. 1985,53-85.

21 Murray M. op sit.

22 Leung A, Foster S. Encyclopedia of Common Natural Ingredients. NY: Wiley;1996.492-4.

23 Leung A, Foster S. Encyclopedia of Common Natural Ingredients. NY: Wiley;1996.492-4.

24 Leung A, Foster S. Encyclopedia of Common Natural Ingredients. NY: Wiley;1996.

25 Bradley P (Ed.). British herbal Compendium. Dorset. British Herbal Medical Assoc.; 1992.

26 Mills S, Bone K. Principles and practice of Phytotherapy. New York. Churchill Livingstone; 2000.

27 Schranner I, Wurdinger M, *et al*. Modification of avian humeral immunoreactions by Influx and Echinacea angustifolia extract. Zentralbl Veterinarmed (B) 1989; 36.

28 Bukovsky M, Kostalova D, Magnusova R, Vaverkova S. Testing for immunomodulating effects of ethanol-water extracts of the above ground parts of the plants Echinaceae and Rudbeckia. Cesk Farm. 1993; 42.

ECHINACEA SUPREME

A Surface Immune Activating Formula*

FORMULA

Fresh Echinacea root   (*Echinacea angustifolia*)
Fresh Echinacea root,   (*Echinacea purpurea*)
tops & ripe seed

Concentration:	1:1 Herb strength ratio (Standardized to 1.5% Isobutylamide Tetranoic Acid using Full Spectrum ProcessTM)
Dosage:	40-60 drops of extract at the onset of Cold or Flu symptoms and repeat every 1-2 hours for up to 5 days
Duration of use:	High doses of Echinacea Supreme (for immune activation at the onset of cold or flu symptoms) are best limited to short-term use (5 days); whereas low doses (as a lymphatic alterative) may be taken judiciously over longer periods (3-6 months)
Best taken:	Between meals, with warm water

DESCRIPTION OF FORMULA

Echinacea Supreme is an alterative formula that may be of assistance when immune stimulation is necessary. The many actions of this formula make it an appropriate choice for invasive and inflammatory conditions; specifically congestive disorders of the mucous membranes, upper and lower respiratory system and the lymphatic system.

Note: In the context of this formula, *Echinacea angustifolia* and *Echinacea purpurea* will be discussed together. Simply, *E. angustifolia* has a much longer documented history of traditional use, while *E. purpurea* has been the focus of more scientific research. Clinically, their actions are similar. Both species have been included in this formula to offer the full benefit of their collective chemistry, and individual subtleties.

Echinacea - It has been said that Native Americans used Echinacea to treat more conditions than any other remedy. It is an immuno-stimulant, with anti-inflammatory, antibacterial, antiviral, and wound healing properties.[G1, G4] Traditionally, Echinacea has been used by Native Americans to treat colds, coughs, sore throats, and snakebite.[1] The Eclectic medical doctors, from the first half of the last century, also praised Echinacea for its benefits with various chronic catarrhal (congestive) conditions of the respiratory tract.[G12] Today, modern science is beginning to support much of its established traditional use, by showing that extracts of Echinacea spp. have the ability to increase antibody production, along with resistance to various infections.[3] Research has further shown that alcohol/water extracts of Echinacea significantly enhance natural killer cell function,[4] and have phagocytic, metabolic and bactericidal influence on macrophages.[5] This simply means that Echinacea has the potential to non-specifically activate your immune system,[6] enhancing its ability to deal with an immune threat, if one should arise.

THERAPEUTIC APPLICATIONS*

Note: The intention of the following information is to represent the traditional use of the individual botanicals found in these formulas and to inform the reader of any evolving scientific inquiry relevant to the formula's ingredients.

SUPPORTED BY TRADITIONAL USE

Immuno-stimulant, [G1, G4, 4, 5, 6] Anti-inflammatory, [G1, G4] Antibacterial, [G1, G4] Antiviral, [G1, G4] Wound healing,[G1, G4] respiratory catarrh,[G12] alterative,[G1] blood purifier.[G6]

SCOPE OF RELEVANT SCIENTIFIC INVESTIGATION

Immunostimulant,[G1, G4, G10, 2, 3] anti-inflammatory, antibacterial, antiviral, [G1, G4, G10, 2] wound healing, antitumor activity.[G1, G4, G10]

CAUTIONS, CONTRA-INDICATIONS AND DRUG INTERACTIONS

Please reference Chapter 9. Do not use during pregnancy or lactation.

COMPLIMENTARY HERBS/FORMULAS

Diaphoretics (promote perspiration): Yarrow, Elder flowers, Peppermint, Ginger, Sage, and Boneset. Echinacea/Goldenseal and Echinacea/Goldenseal/Propolis Throat Spray, Composition Essence.

REFERENCES

1. Snow JM. *Echinacea* (Moench) Spp. *Asteraceae. The Protocol Journal of Botanical Medicine.* 1997;2 (2):18-24.

2. Bauer R, Wagner H. *Echinacea* species as potential immunostimulatory drugs. Economic and Medicinal Plant Research. San Diego: Academic press Ltd.;1991.

3. Schranner I,Wurdinger M, *et al.* Modification of avian humoral immunoreactions by Influx and *Echinacea angustifolia* extract. *Zentralbl Veterinarmed* (B) 1989; 36.

4. Broumand N, Sahl L, Tilles JG. The in vitro effects of *Echinacea* and ginseng on natural killer and antibody-dependent cell cytotoxicity in healthy subjects and chronic fatigue syndrome or aquired immuno-deficiency syndrome patients. *Immunopharmacology.* 1997; 35.

5. Bukovsky M, Kostalova D, Magnusova R, Vaverkova S. Testing for immunomodulating effects of ethanol-water extracts of the above ground parts of the plants *Echinaceae* and *Rudbeckia. Cesk Farm.* 1993; 42.

6. Witchl M. (Bisset NG, Ed.) Herbal Drugs and Phytopharmaceuticals. Medpharm, CRC Press: Boca Raton. 1994.

ECHINACEA/GOLDENSEAL SUPREME

*An Immune-Enhancement Formula**
FORMULA

Echinacea root	(*Echinacea angustifolia*)
Echinacea root, flower, and seed	(*Echinacea purpurea*)
Goldenseal root	(*Hydrastis canadensis*)
Oregon Grape root	(*Berberis aquifolium*)
Barberry root	(*Berberis vulgaris*)
St. John's Wort flower buds	(*Hypericum perforatum*)
Propolis extract	

Concentration:	1:1 Herb strength ratio
Dosage:	Liquid Extract: 40-60 drops every 1-2 hours during a secretory process for up to 5 days
Duration of use:	A maximum of 5 days
Best taken:	Between meals, with warm water

DESCRIPTION OF FORMULA

This formula activates secretory immunity at times of invasion. It is particularly useful with acute/secretory conditions when they are accompanied by inflammation and hyper-secretion of the mucous membranes and when the mucosal lining has become atonic. As you can see from the traditional use of this compound's ingredients (described below), it has been formulated to be broad-acting in such situations.

Echinacea is an immuno-stimulant,[G1, G4, G10, 1, 2, 3] whose anti-inflammatory, antibacterial, antiviral, and wound healing properties have been widely reported.[G1, G4]. (For additional information, please see the Echinacea Supreme description on the proceeding pages)

Goldenseal root is native to North America. It has traditionally been used with allergic/inflammatory[G1, 1] or infectious conditions that require tonification of the mucous membranes.[1] Like several other ingredients of this formula (i.e. Oregon grape root and Barberry root), Goldenseal contains the antibiotic[G4, 1] and immunostimulatory[1] alkaloid, berberine. Along with one other key alkaloid (hydrastine), berberine has also been shown to be anti-spasmodic.[G4]

Oregon Grape root has a history of traditional use closely resembling that of Goldenseal.[1] Oregon grape has distinguished itself, however, by its therapeutic effect with skin conditions, such as psoriasis, eczema, and acne.[1]

Barberry root is a bitter tonic[1] that, pharmacologically, shares many properties with Goldenseal and Oregon Grape root.[G3,1] And, as one may expect of plants with closely related chemistry, the traditional use of Barberry is also similar to other Berberine containing plants.[1] Fever-reducing (antipyretic) activity has also traditionally been associated with Barberry, making it particularly valuable here.[G3]

St. John's Wort flower buds have been used as a medicine for more than 2000 years. Beyond its widely reported antidepressant [G3,1] effect, it is utilized here for its effect with anxiety,[G1, G3] as well as to act as a valuable antiinflammatory[G1, G3] and an antiviral agent.[G3]

Propolis extract has been reported to be an immune stimulant[4, 5] with antiinflammatory[4, 5] effects (particularly when the mucous membranes are involved).[4]

THERAPEUTIC APPLICATIONS*

Note: The intention of the following information is to represent the traditional use of the individual botanicals found in these formulas and to inform the reader of any evolving scientific inquiry relevant to the formula's ingredients.

SUPPORTED BY TRADITIONAL USE

Immune enhancement, [G1, G4, G10, 1, 2, 3] antiinflammatory,[G1, G4, 1]

SCOPE OF RELEVANT SCIENTIFIC INVESTIGATION

Immune enhancement, [G1, G3, G4, G10, 1, 2, 3, 4, 5] antimicrobial [G1, G3, G4, 5, 6]

CAUTIONS, CONTRA-INDICATIONS AND DRUG INTERACTIONS

Please reference Chapter 9. Do not use during pregnancy or lactation.

COMPLIMENTARY HERBS/FORMULAS

Diaphoretic and Warming remedies may also be used, as needed (Composition Essence, Elder/Eyebright Formula, and Ginger tea).

REFERENCES

1. Murray M. The healing power of herbs - The enlightened persons guide to the wonders of medicinal plants. Rocklin, Ca. Prima publishing;1995.

2. Bauer R, Wagner H. *Echinacea* species as potential immunostimulatory drugs. Economic and Medicinal Plant Research. San Diego: Academic press Ltd.;1991.

3. Schranner I,Wurdinger M, *et al.* Modification of avian humoral immunoreactions by Influx and *Echinacea angustifolia* extract. *Zentralbl Veterinarmed* (B) 1989; 36.

4. Balch JF, Balch PA. Prescription for Nutritional Healing. New York; Avery Publishing*****

5. Anonymous. Propolis. *The Lawrence Review of Natural Products.*1986; FEB:1-2.

6. Tosi B, Donini A, *et al.* Antimicrobial Activity of Some Commercial Extracts of Propolis Prepared with Different Solvents. *Phytotherapy Research.* 1996;10:335-336.

ECHINACEA / RED ROOT SUPREME

*Lymphatic Circulation & Alterative Formula**

FORMULA

Echinacea Supreme	(*Echinacea angustifolia & purpurea*)
Red Root	(*Ceanothus americanus*)
Wild Indigo	(*Baptisia tinctoria*)
Thuja leaf	(*Thuja occidentalis*)
Blue Flag root	(*Iris versicolor*)
Stillingia root	(*Stillingia sylvatica*)
Prickly ash bark	(*Xanthoxylum clava-herculis*)

Concentration:	1:1.25 Herb strength ratio
Dosage:	30-40 drops, 3-4 times daily
Duration of use:	Not for more than 4-6 months
Best taken:	Between meals, with warm water

DESCRIPTION OF FORMULA

This formula brings together some of the most powerful botanical alteratives known. Due to the fact that alteratives encourage the removal of metabolic wastes through the lymphatic fluids and promote correct nutrition where it is lacking, alteratives are used to rectify metabolic disturbances at the most fundamental level of the physiology. This formula addresses the most basic principle of Naturopathic Botanical Medicine - which is to promote the removal of encumbrances (any obstacle to cure) and allow the Vital Force, the Healing Power of Nature, to heal. As a result, this formula may be used wherever inadequate removal of tissue wastes has resulted in tissue derangement, tissue encumbrances and congestion.   It is particularly useful where there are indication of lymphatic stasis and congestion.

Echinacea is primarily known for its immune activating properties. [G1, G4, G10, G24, 1, 2, 3] Although it is seldom mentioned as a lymphatic alterative, the Eclectic physicians from around the turn of the last century used it as such, stating that it influences the entire lymphatic system, improving absorption, assimilation, and excretion [G6] - therefore, preventing a build-up of disease causing wastes within the tissue. As it is not uncommon to encounter the need to use immune activating herbs when lymphatic circulation is disturbed, Echinacea's attributes are of great benefit to this formula.

Red Root was also noted by the Eclectic physicians to be of assistance where lymphatic circulation had become compromised, particularly when accompanied by inactivity of the liver. [G6] This plant is specific for occasions when lymphatic tissue has become congested.

Wild Indigo is another example of an alterative that efficiently exerts its influence upon the lymphatic fluids and liver function. [G6] Well-known Herbalist, David Hoffman suggests its use specifically when enlargement of the lymph nodes is evident. [6]

Blue Flag was also used by the Eclectic physicians for lymphatic stimulation, and like Red root & Wild Indigo (briefly discussed above) it was used particularly where liver insufficiency was evident. [G6] As an alterative with reported bile stimulating activity, [G6, 4] Blue flag was specifically indicated where clay-colored stool was present. [G6, 5] Although unrelated to this formula's application, an interesting Russian folkloric anecdote is that Wild Indigo may be used externally to remove freckles. [4]

Thuja further supports the alteratives that constitute this formula. Thuja may be considered a pure alterative, in that it addresses many disorders where deep-seated disturbances of metabolism are at play. Traditionally, the Eclectics used it to treat cancerous growths of multiple descriptions. Dr. Finlay Ellingwood, MD states that it has a peculiar influence over abnormal growths and tissue degeneration. [G6]

Stillingia is an alterative that has traditionally received much praise from those practitioners who used it with consistency. [G15] Said to exert its influence over the secretory and lymphatic functions, it is regarded to be unsurpassed by few, if any other of the known alteratives. [G12]

Prickly Ash bark is a well-known circulatory stimulant. [G1, G3, G4] As such, its presence in this formula is to help drive the other botanicals throughout the body. The Eclectic physicians used this plant to 'stimulate the nerve centers', through which it was said to 'increase the tonicity and functional activity' of the 'organs'. It also has a reputation for its ability to 'sustain the vital forces through any crisis that occurs'. [G6]

THERAPEUTIC APPLICATIONS*

Note: The intention of the following information is to represent the traditional use of the individual botanicals found in these formulas and to inform the reader of any evolving scientific inquiry relevant to the formula's ingredients.

SUPPORTED BY TRADITIONAL USE

Lymphatic congestion, [G6, G12] Alterative, [G6, G12] Improves liver function (clay-colored stool), [G6, 4, 5] Stimulates circulation. [G1, G3, G4]

SCOPE OF RELEVANT SCIENTIFIC INVESTIGATION

Immune activation. [G1, G4, G10, G24, 1, 2, 3]

CAUTIONS, CONTRA-INDICATIONS AND DRUG INTERACTIONS

Please reference Chapter 9. Do not use during pregnancy or lactation.

COMPLIMENTARY HERBS/FORMULAS

Echinacea / Goldenseal Supreme, Scudder's Alterative, Daily Detox, Cell Wise, Fraxinus/Ceanothus Supreme (gynecological use)

REFERENCES

1. Murray M. The Healing Power of Herbs - The enlightened persons guide to the wonders of medicinal plants. Rocklin, Ca. Prima publishing;1995.

2. Bauer R, Wagner H. *Echinacea* species as potential immunostimulatory drugs. Economic and Medicinal Plant Research. San Diego: Academic press Ltd.;1991.

3. Schranner I, Wurdinger M, *et al.* Modification of avian humoral immunoreactions by influx and *Echinacea angustifolia* extract. *Zentralbl Veterinarmed* (B) 1989; 36.

4. Hutchens A. Indian Herbology of North America. Ontario, Canada. Merco; 1973.

5. Clymer RS. Natures Healing Agents. Philadelphia. Dorrance and Company. 1963.

6. Hoffman D. Therapeutic Herbalism. Pg. 4-111

ELIM SLIM SUPREME

For Support of Weight Loss and Healthy Metabolism*

FORMULA

Green Tea	(*Camellia sinensis*)
Garcinia-Malabar Tamarind	(*Garcinia cambogia*)
Coleus Forskohlii	(*Coleus forskohlii*)
Elderberry	(*Sambucus canadensis*)
Gymnema leaf	(*Gymnema sylvestre*)
Bladderwrack fronds	(*Fucus vesiculosis*)
Licorice root	(*Glycyrrhiza glabra*)
Jujube date seed	(*Ziziphus jujuba*)
Turmeric root	(*Curcuma longa*)
Ginger root	(*Zingiber officinale*)

Concentration:	1:1 Herb strength ratio
Dosage:	40-60 drops, 3-4 times daily
Duration of use:	4-6 Months
Best taken:	Between meals, with a small amount of warm water

DESCRIPTION OF FORMULA

This formula helps to correct fat cell metabolism by promoting a state of utilization rather than storage. It is particularly useful for what is known as the classic 'Venus' body type, where fat storage is concentrated around the hips, thighs and buttocks. Likewise, for individuals who lose weight, only to have it return, this formula is of particular benefit. The herbs in this formula possess thermogenic properties (promote burning of calories and fat metabolism), alpha 2 inhibiting properties (preventing the uptake of norepinephrine at the fat cell receptors thus inhibiting fat storage), metabolic properties (enhancing the systemic metabolic functions of the endocrine system), cyclic AMP activating properties (promoting better utilization of

hormones that effect fat cell metabolism), blood sugar regulating properties, and liver metabolism properties.
Note: Dietary and lifestyle adjustments must be made in conjunction with this formulas use. The 3 Season Diet by Dr. John Douillard, D.C., Ph.D. is recommended reading.

Green Tea has traditionally been used to enhance mental function, promote digestion, reduce flatulence, and to regulate body temperature.[1] It is used here for the influence of several of its components to stimulate lipolysis (utilization of fat), by preventing the breakdown of cyclic AMP. Cyclic AMP is a molecule which affects hormonal messages within a fat cell.[10] This 'message' helps to amplify the response of a fat cell to adrenaline; the hormone that tells it to burn fat.[2, 10] Green Tea is also valuable here as an established antioxidant[1] and as a moderate stimulant, further assisting the underlying function of the formula. [G3]

Garcinia-Malabar Tamarind is a natural source of hydroxycitric acid (HCA). HCA is known to cause an increase in fat metabolism, possibly via its influence over liver function.[2]

Coleus Forskohlii is perhaps Green Tea's best friend, when it comes to weight-loss. As mentioned above, utilization of fat is in part controlled by the hormone adrenaline, via its capacity to form cyclic AMP inside a fat cell.[4, 10] Green Tea and Coleus both modify the fat burning affect of adrenaline (via modification of beta-1 adrenergic-receptor cAMP expression). [1, 2] Forskolin, one of the main active molecules in Coleus, is also antidepressive,[4] and has the ability to increase thyroid hormone production. Making it particularly well suited for weight management.[4]

Elderberries bring a number of desirable qualities to this formula. They are recognized as being diuretic, laxative[G2, G12, 5] and liver protective.[5] Through these actions, the Elderberry promotes the removal of cellular wastes and helps to correct metabolism. [G12]

Gymnema leaf is a digestive or stomach tonic with well-known diuretic properties.[6] It has been reported to "neutralize the excess of sugar present in the body in diabetes".[6] Gymnema is also known as *gur-mur* (which literally means, sugar destroying) because of its noted ability to abolish the taste of sugar.[6]

Bladderwrack fronds have been widely used, medicinally, for weight management. [G1, G2, G4] Such benefit quite possibly results from its stimulating effect on thyroid function. [G4] Bladderwrack fronds are harvested from pristine water, as they are known to absorb toxic waste metals from polluted waters. [G1, G12]

Licorice root has a history of application dating back several thousand years. [G3, 7] Traditionally, it has been used as a demulcent (membrane soothing and protective), diuretic, and mild laxative. [G3, 7] In addition to these benefits, Licorice is also useful in this formula for its ability to protect liver function, and to moderate the metabolism of hormones. [G3, G4, 7]

Jujube date seed is said to tonify the heart and brain, [8] and invigorate the body's vital energy. [G3] Traditionally, it has been used as an anti-inflammatory, and as a blood purifier. [G3]

Turmeric root serves this formula through its outstanding antioxidant, [9] anti-inflammatory, and liver protective effects. [9, G1, G3] Normalizing liver function during weight management is highly desirable, as the liver is actively involved in regulating blood sugar availability, and metabolism of the 3-ketosteroids, which is a group of hormones which in part effect fat metabolism.

Ginger root addresses indigestion. It also provides benefit as an antioxidant, [G3] anti-inflammatory, and as a carminative (reduces intestinal gas). [G3, G4] In addition, Ginger is useful here as a circulatory stimulant, [G3, G4] helping to deliver the entire formula throughout the body.

THERAPEUTIC APPLICATIONS*

Note: The intention of the following information is to represent the traditional use of the individual botanicals found in these formulas and to inform the reader of any evolving scientific inquiry relevant to the formula's ingredients.

SUPPORTED BY TRADITIONAL USE

Diuretic, [6, G2, G12, 5] Sugar taste reducer, [6] Digestive tonic[6]

SCOPE OF RELEVANT SCIENTIFIC INVESTIGATION

Weight management, [G2, G4, 1, 2, 3, 10] Antioxidant, [1, 9] Anti-inflammatory, [G1, G3, G4, 7, 9] Cyclic AMP activation, [1, 2, 4, 10]

CAUTIONS, CONTRA-INDICATIONS AND DRUG INTERACTIONS

Please reference Chapter 9. Do not use during pregnancy or lactation.

COMPLIMENTARY HERBS/FORMULAS

Diet Slim, Cell Wise, Supreme Cleanse, Sweetish Bitters, Yohimbe (*Corynanthe yohimbe*) in small doses (5-15 drops, twice daily) specifically helps to redirect adrenaline toward the receptors on a fat cell that burn fat (Beta-1), by blocking those that result in fat storage (Alpha-2). [1, 10]

Important Note: If elevated blood pressure, or a tendency toward it, exists - Yohimbe must not be used.

REFERENCES

1. Snow JM. *Camellia sinensis* (L.) Kuntze (Theaceae). The Protocol Journal of Botanical Medicine. 1995; 1(2):47-51.

2. Fredholm BB, Lindgren E. The effect of alkylxanthines and other phosphodiesterase inhibitors on adenosine-receptor mediated decrease in lipolysis and cyclic AMP accumulation in rat fat cells. *Acta Pharmacol Toxicol (Copenh)*. 1984; 54(1):64-71.

3. McCarty MF, Gustin JC. Pyruvate and hydroxycitrate/carnitine may synergize to promote reverse electron transport in hepatocyte mitochondria, effectively 'uncoupling' the oxidation of fatty acids. *Med Hypothese*. 1999; 52(5):407-16

4. Murray M. The unique pharmacology of Coleus Forskohlii. *The American Journal of Natural Medicine*. 1994; 1(3):10-13.

5. Anonymous. Elderberry. *The Lawrence Review of Natural Products*.1992; Jul.

6. Kapoor LD. Handbook of Ayurvedic Medicinal Plants. Florida. CRC Press; 1990.

7. Snow JM. *Glycyrrhiza glabra* L. (Leguminaceae). The Protocol Journal of Botanical Medicine. 1995; 1(3):9-14.

8. Kapoor LD. Handbook of Ayurvedic Medicinal Plants. Florida. CRC Press; 1990.

9. Snow JM. *Curcuma longa* L. (Zingiberaceae). The Protocol Journal of Botanical Medicine. 1995; 1(2):43-46.

10. Mitchell W. Foundations of Natural Therapeutics - Biochemical Apologetics of Naturopathic Medicine. Tempe, Arizona. Southwest College Press. 1997.

EYEBRIGHT/BAYBERRY SUPREME

*An Allergy and Sinus Formula**
FORMULA

Eyebright herb	(*Euphrasia officinalis*)
Bayberry root bark	(*Myrica cerifera*)
Goldenseal root	(*Hydrastis canadensis*)
Calamus root	(*Acorus calamus*)
Stinging Nettle leaf	(*Urtica dioica*)

Concentration:	1:1.5 Herb strength ratio
Dosage:	15-30 drops, 3-4 times daily
Duration of use:	No longer than 3 weeks
Best taken:	Between meals, with warm water

DESCRIPTION OF FORMULA

This formula addresses allergies from three viewpoints. It works to reduce inflammation, relieve sinus congestion, and to tonify hyper-secretive and atonic mucosal membranes. These are all considered to be key points of leverage in restoring healthy sinus function and relief from the discomfort caused by allergies that congest the mucous membranes.

Eyebright herb is a tonic astringent[G1, G12] that works to tonify soggy and congested mucous membranes. It has been reported to be of use with catarrhal (mucous) conditions,[G12] such as allergies.[G3] It is well recognized as being particularly suited to relieve nasal/sinus congestion.[G12]

Bayberry root bark is also a tonic astringent.[G1, G3, 1] It constringes, contracts and condenses mucous membranes that are hyper-secretive. In addition to having a tonifying effect upon the mucous membranes, Bayberry is also reported to possess the properties of a circulatory stimulant, diaphoretic (promotes perspiration),[G10] and fever-reducing agent.[G1, G10]

Goldenseal root - Due to its profound influence upon the mucous membranes of the body, Goldenseal's role in this formula cannot be overstated. It is a mucous membrane normalizer, *par excellence.* Traditional uses are many; including indigestion,[G1, G3, G4, G12] eczema, and inflammation.[G1, G12, 3] It has also traditionally been used as a bitter tonic,[G1, G3, G12] as an alterative, and a mild laxative.[G1, G3] Goldenseal alkaloid's have been researched for their immune enhancing,[G10] and antimicrobial actions.[G1, G3, G4, G10]

Calamus root has a traditional use that spans as many centuries as it does continents. Many cultures have historically used this plant to improve digestion, relieve intestinal flatulance, and to reduce spasmodic contraction of the smooth muscles (i.e. intestinal, bronchial contraction).[G10, 3]

Stinging Nettle leaf has a long history of use with inflammatory disorders, including rheumatism, and skin disorders.[4, G10] Recent research has highlighted its use with allergic rhinitis (hayfever).[5]

THERAPEUTIC APPLICATIONS*

Note: The intention of the following information is to represent the traditional use of the individual botanicals found in these formulas and to inform the reader of any evolving scientific inquiry relevant to the formula's ingredients.

SUPPORTED BY TRADITIONAL USE

Mucous membrane tonic/astringent (with congestion),[G1, G3, G12, 1] allergies,[G3] antiinflammatory,[G1, G10, G12, 1, 3, 4] fever-reducing,[G1, G10]

SCOPE OF RELEVANT SCIENTIFIC INVESTIGATION

Antimicrobial,[G3, G10] fever-reducing,[G10] allergic rhinitis,[5]

CAUTIONS, CONTRA-INDICATIONS AND DRUG INTERACTIONS

Please reference Chapter 9. Do not use during pregnancy or lactation.

COMPLIMENTARY HERBS/FORMULAS

Turmeric/Catechu Supreme, Nettle Liquid Phyto-Cap, Echinacea/Goldenseal Supreme (if discoloration/yellowing of the mucous is present), Feverfew Professional Strength, Milk Thistle.

REFERENCES

1. Grieve M, Mrs. A Modern Herbal. New York. Dover; 1982.
2. Foster S. Goldenseal: *Hydrastis canadensis*. Botanical Series #309. Austin, TX. American Botanical Council.
3. Motley TJ. The Ethnobotany of Sweet Flag (Araceae). *Economic Botany*. 199; 48(4): 397-412.
4. Bombardelli E, Morazzoni P. *Urtica dioica* L. *Fitoterapia*. 1997; 48(5): 387-402.
5. Mittman P. Randomized, Double-Blind Study of Freeze-Dried *Urtica dioica* in the treatment of Allergic Rhinitis. *Planta Medica*. 1990; 56(1):44-47.

FENNEL/WILD YAM SUPREME

*A Gallbladder and Fat Digestion Formula**
FORMULA

Fennel seed	(*Foeniculum vulgare*)
Wild Yam root	(*Dioscorea villosa*)
Mayapple root	(*Podophylum peltatum*)
Dandelion root & leaf	(*Taraxacum officinalis*)
Celandine root	(*Chelidonium major*)
California poppy	(*Eschscholzia californica*)
Peppermint oil	(*Mentha piperita*)

Concentration:	1:1.5 Herb strength ratio
Dosage:	30-40 drops, 3-4 times daily
Duration of use:	3-4 months
Best taken:	Between meals, with a little warm water

DESCRIPTION OF FORMULA

Fennel/Wild Yam Supreme has been formulated to reduce painful spasms of the gastrointestinal tract. This compound contains principles that have choleretic and spasmolytic properties that promote the release and flow of congested bile through the gall system, and that relax the muscles and membranes to alleviate cramps associated with gallbladder colic. It is particularly of value with states of excessive flatulence, particularly where gallbladder and/or liver dysfunction contribute to the condition.

Fennel seed has traditionally been used as a digestive tonic,[G1, G3] capable of relieving gastrointestinal colic, when it is present.[G1, G3, G17, 1] It is also known to be antispasmodic[G1, G3, 1] and antiinflammatory.[G1, G17, 1]

Wild Yam root is highly valued for its use with flatulent colic and gastrointestinal spasms.[G1, G6, 2, 4] It is also present in this formula due to its known anti-inflammatory action.[G1, 2]

Mayapple root is an alterative with specific application where excessive flatulence is due to liver and gastrointestinal insufficiency.[G6]

Note: The key to using Mayapple in a formula such as this, is that it must be extracted in water, not alcohol. This guarantees that any unfavorable laxative compounds present in the plant are not extracted along with those that are highly desired.

Dandelion root & leaf is reported to increase the flow of bile into the upper intestine.[G6] In fact, it has traditionally been said to possess a cleansing effect on the liver, encouraging its renewal and repair. Furthermore, it is said to be particularly recommended for gallbladder inflammation and gallstones.[G17]

Celandine root is said to possess an antispasmodic action[G1, G11] which is directed, specifically, at the bile ducts of the gallbladder.[G11] It is widely reported to be useful when liver dysfunction is present.[G12, 5]

California poppy has been included here for its reported pain relieving and antispasmodic influence.[6, 7]

Peppermint oil reduces intestinal flatulence, and is reported to be antispasmodic, via its ability to relax smooth muscle.[G3, G4] It also improves the taste of the formula (a valuable commodity in a culture that appears to have a strong aversion to anything that does not taste either salty or sweet).

THERAPEUTIC APPLICATIONS*

Note: The intention of the following information is to represent the traditional use of the individual botanicals found in these formulas and to inform the reader of any evolving scientific inquiry relevant to the formula's ingredients.

SUPPORTED BY TRADITIONAL USE

Gastrointestinal spasms, [G1, G6, G11, 2, 4] gastrointestinal colic,[G1, G3, G6, G17, 2, 4] Digestive debility,[G1, G3, G6, G17] antiinflammatory, [G1, G6, G17, 1, 2] liver insufficiency,[G6, G12, 5]

SCOPE OF RELEVANT SCIENTIFIC INVESTIGATION

Antispasmodic,[G3, G4] antiinflammatory,[G1, G3]

CAUTIONS, CONTRA-INDICATIONS AND DRUG INTERACTIONS

Please reference Chapter 9. Do not use during pregnancy or lactation.

COMPLIMENTARY HERBS/FORMULAS

Sweetish Bitters, Milk Thistle

REFERENCES

1. Tierra M. Planetary Herbology. Twin Lakes, WI. Lotus Press; 1998.
2. Hoffmann, D. Therapeutic Herbalism
3. Hutchens A. Indian Herbology of North America. Ontario, Canada. Merco; 1973.
4. Willard T. Wild Rose Scientific Herbal. Wild rose College of Natural Healing; Alberta; 1991.
5. Brinker F. Chelidonium majus. The Journal of Naturopathic Medicine. 1992; 3(1):93.
6. Duke, J. Handbook of Medicinal Herbs. CRC Boca Raton. 1955
7. Hoffman D. The Holistic Herbal. Moray. The Findhorn Press; 1984.

FEVERFEW/JAMAICAN DOGWOOD SUPREME

For Relief of Headache Pain, Cramps, and Inflammation *
FORMULA

Feverfew herb	(*Tanacetum parthenium*)
Jamaican Dogwood	(*Piscidia erythrina*)
Black Haw bark	(*Viburnum prunifolium*)
St. John's Wort flower buds	(*Hypericum perforatum*)
Butterbur root	(*Petasites frigida*)
Meadowsweet herb	(*Filipendula ulmaria*)
Willow bark	(*Salix nigra*)
Ginger root	(*Zingiber officinale*)

Concentration:	1:1.5 Herb strength ratio
Dosage:	40-60 drops at the onset of pain and repeat every 15 minutes until pain subsides
Duration of use:	This formula may be taken as needed
Best taken:	Between meals, with warm water

DESCRIPTION OF FORMULA

This compound is an excellent pain formula. Its primary affect is to reduce the inflammation and spasms involving nerve and muscular tissue. It is useful with headaches, intestinal spasms, pain and spasms of the muscular/skeletal system, as well as pain associated with disorders of menstruation. Current research on COX-2 inhibition suggests that this formula is effective agent at inhibiting the COX-2 and phospholipase A2 enzymes that are associated with pain and inflammation.

Feverfew herb is a powerful COX-2 inhibiting botanical. It has been used, since the middle-ages, as a carminative (flatulence relieving) tonic. Its traditional use has also encompassed numerous disorders that are clearly characterized by pain and inflammation[G1, G3, 1] (i.e. rheumatism,[G1, G3, 1] headache,[G1] migraines,[G4] etc.). Present day interest, however, generally centers around its use with preventing migraines.[G1, G3, G4]

Jamaican Dogwood is one of nature's most highly praised pain remedies and uterine anti-spasmodics. Herbal tradition has also found it to be a nerve sedative, with anti-inflammatory and anti-spasmodic qualities.[G6] Not surprisingly, scientific inquiry has loaned support to these traditional uses.[G3, G4] Jamaican Dogwood is also said to enhance the effectiveness of Black Haw, the following herb in this formula.[2]

Black Haw bark has traditionally been praised as a pain relieving antispasmodic, having had popular application when such a remedy was required for gynecological conditions.[G6, 3, 4] It is present here for its reported effects with nervous disorders of varying kind, along with those listed uses above.[G6]

St. John's Wort flower buds are said to be "for the nervous system, what arnica is for the muscular".[1] It is widely known for its use with depression. St. John's Wort has also traditionally been used as a herb with positive effect upon digestion and liver function, although such use is seldom mentioned.[2] Anxiety and inflammation are also reported to be relieved with use of this herb.[G1]

Butterbur root is a pain remedy[8] that is antispasmodic,[5] as well as being both gastro-protective and antiinflammatory.[5, 7] A recent report has discussed those uses of the plant that have been supported by science, including, migraine headaches, inflammation, and muscular spasms.[6]

Meadowsweet herb is the original source of salicylic acid, the molecule that would later be converted into aspirin (acetyl salicylic acid).[G5] Traditionally, it has been used for urinary and gastrointestinal disorders,[G5] as well as for painful joint disorders.[G4]

Willow bark shares similar chemistry to Meadowsweet.[G4] As such, its uses are closely allied to those mentioned above. Traditional use includes painful,[G1, G4] inflammatory disorders, including headache, toothache, [G4] and joint disorders.[G1, G4]

Ginger root engages the circulatory system and aids the delivery of the entire formula throughout the body. It is also a powerful

COX 2 inhibitor thus greatly reducing pain and inflammation. Here it also finds use for its digestive,[G4, 4, 9] antiinflammatory [G4, G5, 9] and antispasmodic actions.[G1, G4, G5]

THERAPEUTIC APPLICATIONS*

Note: The intention of the following information is to represent the traditional use of the individual botanicals found in these formulas and to inform the reader of any evolving scientific inquiry relevant to the formula's ingredients.

SUPPORTED BY TRADITIONAL USE

Headaches,[G1] migraines,[G3, G4] inflammatory conditions,[G1, G3, G4, G6, 4] antispasmodic,[G3, G6, 4, 8] pain,[G6, 8]

SCOPE OF RELEVANT SCIENTIFIC INVESTIGATION

Migraines,[G1, G3, G4, 6] inflammatory conditions,[G1, G3, G4, 1, 5, 6, 7, 9] antispasmodic,[G1, G3, G4, G5, 5, 6]

CAUTIONS, CONTRA-INDICATIONS AND DRUG INTERACTIONS

Please reference Chapter 9. Do not use during pregnancy or lactation.

COMPLIMENTARY HERBS/FORMULAS

Feverfew Professional Strength, Migra-Profen, Infla-Profen.

REFERENCES

1. Milspaugh C. American Medicinal Plants. New York. Dover Publications.1974.
2. Clymer RS. Natures Healing Agents. Philadelphia. Dorrance and Company. 1963.
3. Coon N. Using plants for healing. Philadelphia, Pa. Rodale Press. 1979.
4. Bisset NG. Herbal Drugs and Phytopharmaceuticals. Ann Arbor. CRC Press; 1994.
5. Bickel D. Identification and characterization of inhibitors of peptido-leukotriene-synthesis from *Petasites hybridus*. *Planta Med*. 1994; 60(4): 318-22.
6. Eaton J. Butterbur - Herbal help for Migraine. *Natural pharmacy*. 1998; 2(10): 23-24.
7. Brune K, *et al*. Gastro-protective effects by extracts of Petasites hybridus: the role of inhibition of peptido-leukotriene synthesis. *Planta Med*. 1993 Dec;59(6):494-6.
8. Grieve M, Mrs. A Modern Herbal.New York. Dover. 1982.
9. Schulick P. Ginger, common spice or wonder drug. Herbal Free Press, Vermont. USA.

FRAXINUS/CEANOTHUS SUPREME

A Uterine and Ovarian Corrective Formula*

FORMULA

White Ash bark	(*Fraxinus americana*)
Red Root	(*Ceanothus americanus*)
Life Root	(*Senecio aureus*)
Mayapple root	(*Podophylum peltatum*)
Helonias root	(*Chamaelirium luteum*)
Goldenseal root	(*Hydrastis canadensis*)
Lobelia herb & seed	(*Lobelia inflata*)
Ginger root	(*Zingiber officinale*)

Concentration:	1:1.25 Herb strength ratio
Dosage:	30-40 drops, 3-4 times daily
Duration of use:	3-4 months
Best taken:	Between meals, with warm water

DESCRIPTION OF FORMULA

This formula is an alterative formula that addresses the uterine and ovarian tissues. As such, it promotes the removal of catabolic wastes at the cellular level. It is particularly suited to promoting change within ovarian and uterine tissue when stagnancy of the lymphatic fluids and poor elimination are an influence. Eclectic physicians used many of the herbs in this formula to address uterine fibroids, and cysts, endometriosis, and prolapse.

White Ash bark is an astringent, hemostatic herb[2-4] (reduces bleeding) that promotes the shedding and regeneration of the tissues of the uterus and cervix.[1,4] It has a long history of use as a tonic with a variety of uterine diseases.[1-5]

Red Root promotes lymphatic circulation.[G6] As such it promotes the removal of cellular wastes and the supply of nutrition, thus it supports the overall aim of this formula that is to restore integrity to degenerated uterine and ovarian tissue.

Life Root is a uterine tonic,[6,7] astringent[7] and hemostatic[8] (reduces bleeding) that has a long history of use with gynecological complaints.[6,8]

Mayapple root is a valuable alterative.[10] It has traditionally been used as a gynecological remedy for 'fullness of the tissue'.[9]

Helonias root is highly esteemed as a uterine tonic.[6,11] It relieves pelvic congestion and pelvic tissue tension and promotes blood supply to the pelvic tissues.

Goldenseal root is an astringent, alterative[7] and hemostatic[7,11] (reduces bleeding) herb that has effect on the nervous as well as the reproductive tissue.[11]

Lobelia herb & seed is used here as an antispasmodic.[11]

Ginger root engages the circulatory system and aids the delivery of the entire formula throughout the body. Here it also finds use for its antiinflammatory[11] and antispasmodic actions.[7,11]

THERAPEUTIC APPLICATIONS*

Note: The intention of the following information is to represent the traditional use of the individual botanicals found in these formulas and to inform the reader of any evolving scientific inquiry relevant to the formula's ingredients.

Supported by Traditional Use

Tissue regenerative and alterative. It may be used for <u>uterine complaints</u> where there is excessive bleeding accompanied by a congestive influence of the lymphatic fluids. Gynecological complaints where deranged tissue has taken hold and must be replaced by healthy tissue.

Scope of Relevant Scientific Investigation

None relevant.

Cautions, Contra-Indications and Drug Interactions

Please reference Chapter 9. Do not use during pregnancy or lactation.

Complimentary Herbs/Formulas

Scudder's Alterative, Echinacea/Red Root Supreme, Daily Detox, Cell Wise

REFERENCES

1. Ellingwood F. American Materia Medica, Therapeutics and Pharmacognosy. Portland. Eclectic Medical Publications;1985.

2. Duke J. "Dr. Dukes Phytochemical and Ethnobotanical Databases" 3 Nov 1998. Online. Internet.[11/3/98]. Available at www.ars-grin.gov/cgi-bin/duke/ethnobot.pl

3. Grieve M, Mrs. A Modern Herbal. New York. Dover; 1982.

4. Duke J. Handbook of Northeastern Indian Medicinal Plants.

5. Wood H, Osol A. The Dispensatory of the United States of America. Philadelphia. JB Lippincott Co;1943.

6. Hoffman D. The Holistic Herbal. Moray. The Findhorn Press. 1984.

7. Wren RC. Potter's New Cyclopaedia of Botanical drugs and preparations.Essex, UK: Saffron Walden;1988.

8. Bisset NG. Herbal Drugs and Phytopharmaceuticals. Ann Arbor. CRC Press. 1994.

9. Felter H, Lloyd JU. King's American Dispensatory. Portland. Eclectic medical Publications; 1983.

10. Scudder J. Specific Medication and Specific medicines. Portland. Eclectic Medical Publications; 1985.

11. Bradley P (Ed.). British herbal Compendium. Dorset. British Herbal Medical Assoc.; 1992.

12. Brinker F. *Herb Contraindications and Drug Interactions.* Portland, OR: Eclectic Inst., 1997.

13. Miller, L. Herbal Medicinals: Selected Clinical Consideration Focusing on Known or Potential Drug-Herb Interactions. Arch Intern Med. 1998; 158: 2200-11.

GINKGO/GOTU KOLA SUPREME

Promotes Memory and Mental Energy *
FORMULA

Gotu Kola leaf & root	(*Centella asiatica*)
Siberian Ginseng root	(*Eleutherococcus senticosus*)
Ginkgo leaf	(*Ginkgo biloba*)
Wild Oats milky seed	(*Avena sativa*)
Chinese Fo-Ti root	(*Polygonum multiflorum*)
Peppermint leaf	(*Mentha piperita*)
Rosemary leaf	(*Rosmarinus officinalis*)

Concentration:	1:1 Herb strength ratio
Dosage:	Liquid Extract: 30-40 drops, 3-4 times daily
Duration of use:	3-4 months for best results
Best taken:	Between meals, with warm water

DESCRIPTION OF FORMULA

This formula specifically focuses on enhancing mental function and circulation, particularly where such processes have become enfeebled due to stress and nervous exhaustion. This formula is adaptogenic and as such, it promotes overall health and stamina, along with the overall ability to deal with stress, both physical and emotional. The herbs in this formula contain compounds now shown to have anti-oxidant properties that slow down degredation of tissues.

Gotu Kola leaf & root is considered to be one of the so-called 'elixirs of life'.[1,2] It has long been used in India to improve intelligence and mental function.[G3] Several studies suggest that Gotu Kola may be useful with improving memory, reducing fatigue and stress, increasing general mental ability, and increasing I.Q. in developmentally-disabled children.[G3,2]

Siberian Ginseng root has been in use in China for over 4000 years. Used regularly, it is said to increase longevity, improve general health, improve the appetite, and restore memory.[2] Today, as an adaptogen, it is known to produce improvement in overall metabolic efficiency, as well as to increase resistance to disease and stressful influences.[G3, G4]

Ginkgo leaf is a plant that derives the majority of its medicinal support from modern science, not from established traditional use. Ginkgo leaf has been shown to reduce symptoms related to Cerebral Vascular Insufficiency (CVI), including impaired mental performance, dizziness, headache, depression, ringing in the ears, and short-term memory loss.[2, 3] Many studies today focus on its influence with repairing short-term memory loss.[3]

Wild Oat milky seed has a reputation as a trophorestorative (builds nervous reserve).[5] It is useful in states of nervous debility, exhaustion, depression, sleeplessness and wherever convalescence is required.[G1, 4]

Chinese Fo-Ti root is traditionally said to replenish the vital essence of the kidneys and the liver.[G8] It is an excellent tonic to include in any formula that endeavours to support the functions of both kidney and liver.

Peppermint has traditionally been used as a digestive stimulant, and to provide relief from intestinal flatulence.[G3, G4, G5, 6] The oil from the plant is also reported to be antispasmodic, via its ability to relax smooth muscle.[G3, G4] Peppermint, of course, also improves the taste of the formula.

Rosemary leaf is a natural antioxidant[G3] and anti-inflammatory.[G1] It has been proposed that natural antioxidants, such as Rosemary, may be useful to help reduce the free-radical damage that occurs with Alzheimer's disease.[7] Rosemary has been used for centuries as a tonic and stimulant, and as remedy for intestinal flatulence, indigestion, and nervous disorders.[G3] Known as the 'herb of remembrance', Rosemary has a long history as a memory-enhancing medicine.[7]

THERAPEUTIC APPLICATIONS*

Note: *The intention of the following information is to represent the traditional use of the individual botanicals found in these formulas and to inform the reader of any evolving scientific inquiry relevant to the formula's ingredients.*

SUPPORTED BY TRADITIONAL USE

Improve mental function,[G3, 2, 7] Tonic [G1, G3, G4, 1, 2, 4, 5]

SCOPE OF RELEVANT SCIENTIFIC INVESTIGATION

Improve mental function,[G3, G4, 2, 3] Reduce fatigue and stress,[G3, G4]

CAUTIONS, CONTRA-INDICATIONS AND DRUG INTERACTIONS

Please reference Chapter 9. Do not use during pregnancy or lactation.

COMPLIMENTARY HERBS/FORMULAS

Hawthorn Supreme, Ginkgo Liquid Phyto-Caps™, Anti-Oxidant Supreme

REFERENCES

1. Duke J. CRC Handbook of Medicinal Herbs. Boca Raton. CRC Press. 1985.
2. Murray M. The healing power of herbs - The enlightened persons guide to the wonders of medicinal plants. 2nd ed. Prima publishing. Rocklin, Ca. 1995.
3. Snow JM. *Ginkgo biloba* L. (Ginkgoaceae). *The Protocol Journal Of Botanical Medicine.* 1996; 2(1):9-15.
4. Witchl M. Herb drugs and phytopharmaceuticals. CRC Press.1994
5. Priest AW, Priest LR. Herbal medication. A clinical dispensary handbook. 1982.
6. Hutchens AR. A handbook of Native American herbs. Shambhalla publications. 1992.
7. Duke J. The Green pharmacy. Emmaus, Pa. Rodale Press. 1997.

GINSENG SUPREME

Promotes Energy and Resistance to Stress*
FORMULA

American Ginseng	(*Panax quinquifolium*)
Siberian Ginseng	(*Eleutherococcus senticosus*)

Concentration:	1:1.5 Herb strength ratio
Dosage:	20 drops, 3-4 times daily
Duration of use:	3-4 months
Best taken:	Between meals, with warm water

DESCRIPTION OF FORMULA

This formula may be used to increase energy and stamina, as well as resistance to physical and mental/emotional stress. It is particularly useful when energy is low, or when stress or overwork has resulted in fatigue and low adrenal function. Individuals who consume caffeinated beverages to excess will also benefit from this formula. This compound is a classic adaptogenic formula that helps the body adapt to stressful environments and situations. The eleutherosides and ginsenosides in this compound have a positive influence upon all major organs and glands, improving the vitality and stamina of the entire system.

American Ginseng belongs to a genus (a sub-group of a family) named Panax, which is derived from the word panacea, meaning 'cure-all'. The common name also distinguishes this highly regarded herb, as Ginseng means 'wonder of the world'.[1] American Ginseng is said, energetically speaking, to be cooler than Asian Ginseng.[G3] Traditionally used as a yin tonic, it is used to build condensed energy which nourishes the body fluids and 'essence', in the most debilitated of conditions.[G5] Western medicine has also held this plant in high regard, as it was used in medical practice, here in the U.S. as a mild sedative and a tonic to the nerve centers, which was said to improve their tone with its use.[G6] Ginseng was also in the United States Pharmacopoeia from 1842 to 1882, as a stimulant and a digestive aid.[G3] This plant is the tonic *par excellence*.

Siberian Ginseng has been used by Chinese herbalists for more than 4,000 years.[2] Throughout its use in the orient, the root of this plant has achieved a reputation of being a stimulant, tonic, and a diuretic,[G3] capable of increasing longevity.[2] It has traditionally been used to treat insomnia, lower back or kidney pain, and rheumatoid arthritis[G3] Perhaps its most profound use is as an adaptogen. Adaptogens increase overall resistence to fatigue,[2] as well as disease and stress, whether it be of physical or emotional origin.[G3] One European government regulatory report suggests Siberian Ginseng as a tonic for 'fatigue and debility or declining capacity for work and concentration, and also in convalescence'.[G3, G4] Recent studies have highlighted its ability to enhance cellular immunity,[6] defense and physical fitness,[3] normalize certain blood parameters, increase work capacity, and rehabilitation of athletes.[4] Scientific research also reports antioxidant activity.[G3, 5]

THERAPEUTIC APPLICATIONS*
Note: The intention of the following information is to represent the traditional use of the individual botanicals found in these formulas and to inform the reader of any evolving scientific inquiry relevant to the formula's ingredients.

SUPPORTED BY TRADITIONAL USE
Tonic,[G3, G5, G6] resistance to stress and/or fatigue,[G3, G4, 2] convalescence.[G5]

SCOPE OF RELEVANT SCIENTIFIC INVESTIGATION
Improve mental performance,[G4, 2] improve physical performance,[G4, 2, 3] enhance cellular immunity[G4, 6]/defense,[2] enhance resistance to stress.[G3, G4, 2]

CAUTIONS, CONTRA-INDICATIONS AND DRUG INTERACTIONS
Please reference Chapter 9. Do not use during pregnancy or lactation.

COMPLIMENTARY HERBS/FORMULAS
Siberian Ginseng Tonic Elixir, Serenity with Kava Kava Herbal Elixir (where stress is an issue), Vitality Herbal Elixir, Ginkgo/Gotu Kola Supreme (where mental fatigue is present), Energy & Vitality.

REFERENCES

1. Coon N. Using plants for healing. Philadelphia, Pa. Rodale Press. 1979.
2. Murray M. The healing power of herbs - The enlightened persons guide to the wonders of medicinal plants. 2nd ed. Prima publishing. Rocklin, Ca. 1995.
3. Szolomicki J. The influence of active components of *Eleutherococcus senticosus* on cellular defence and physical fitness in man. *Phytother Res.* 2000; 14(1):30-5.
4. Azizov AP, *et al.* [Effects of eleutherococcus, elton, leuzea, and leveton on the blood coagulation system during training in athletes]. *Eksp Klin Farmakol.* 1997; 60(5):58-60. Original article in Russian.
5. Bol'shakova IV, *et al.* [Antioxidant properties of a series of extracts from medicinal plants]. *Biofizika.* 1997;42(2):480-3. Original article in Russian.
6. Wildfeuer A, Mayerhofer D. [The effects of plant preparations on cellular functions in body defense]. *Arzneimittelforschung.* 1994; 44(3):361-6. Original article in German.

GINSENG/SCHIZANDRA SUPREME

An Adaptogenic Tonic for Vital Energy and Resistance *
FORMULA

Siberian Ginseng root	(*Eleutherococcus senticosus*)
Chinese Schizandra berry	(*Schisandra chinensis*)
Damiana leaf	(*Turnera diffusa*)
Cola nut	(*Cola nitida*)
Wild Oat milky seed	(*Avena sativa*)
Licorice root	(*Glycyrrhiza glabra*)
American Skullcap	(*Scutellaria lateriflora*)
Prickly Ash bark	(*Xanthoxylum clava-herculis*)

Concentration:	1:1.25 Herb strength ratio
Dosage:	3-40 drops, 3-4 times daily
Duration of use:	3-4 months for best results
Best taken:	Between meals, with warm water

DESCRIPTION OF FORMULA

This formula is useful for those individuals who suffer from fading vitality and depleted energy. Anyone who is constantly exposed to overwork, stressful environments or situations, and excess strain to mind or body, can benefit from this powerful adaptogenic (normalizing) formula. It addresses the vital functions of the nervous and the endocrine systems, countering fatigue and stress, and supporting a return of overall vitality and resistance. It may also be useful when discontinuing certain addictive foods which have a relationship to adrenal response (sugar, caffeine, food allergies, etc.)

Siberian Ginseng has a history of use dating back some 4000 years.[1] It reduces the activation of the adrenal gland's response to stress. As a result, those hormones that keep us in a physiological state of stress are also reduced. It is finding increasing use in the treatment of Chronic Fatigue Syndrome for this very reason.[2] Siberian Ginseng is also known to enhance immune status,[G5] improve mental cognition,[G3, 2] as well as increase longevity,[2] resistence,[G3, G4] and overall work capacity.[G3, G4]

Schizandra's adaptogenic ability to increase overall reflex response, physical performance, and endurance,[5] has been compared to that of Siberian Ginseng.[4] It has been found to possess anti-depressant, immuno-modulatory, and blood pressure regulating properties. It is also used as a powerful liver protectant,[G3, 3] and as an aphrodisiac[G4] with pronounced influence on both male and female sexuality.[6]

Damiana has a long history of use as a trophorestorative (builds nervous reserve) and an even longer history as an aphrodisiac.[G4] In fact, Damiana was once referred to by the latin, *Damiana aphrodisiaca* because of this reputation. The physicians of the physio-medicalist school referred to Damiana as a stimulating nervous system tonic and trophorestorative.[7]

Cola Nut was also highly regarded as a 'stimulating tonic and trophorestorative', being used to counter fatigue and aid during convalescence.[7] When extracted in its fresh form, the Cola nut is a nervous system tonic, not a nervous system stimulant; as is the case with the dried material.[G4]

Wild Oat milky seed is another botanical that has a reputation as a trophorestorative, and as such, it is used in states of nervous debility and exhaustion. It is also said to be used for depression, sleeplessness and where convalescence is required.[G1,8]

Licorice root is now considered to be a primary form of treatment in the syndrome of Chronic Fatigue.[9] Whereas Siberian Ginseng reduces the adrenal gland's hormonal response to stress, Licorice prevents the breakdown of such hormones,[G3] resulting in an overall reduction of the load that is placed on this important glandular function. Compounds isolated from licorice have been shown to be immuno-stimulating and potentially anti-depressant.[G1]

American Skullcap has traditionally been described as both a stimulating and relaxing nervine (nervous tonic).[7] It has been used to treat a variety of nervous disorders that arise from mental or physical exhaustion.[G12, 7]

Prickly Ash bark is a circulatory stimulant[G1, G3, G4] and as such, appears in this formula to help drive the other botanicals throughout the body. The Eclectic physicians used this plant to stimulate the nerve centers, through which it was said to increase the tonicity and functional activity of the organs. It also finds value in this formula for its reputation to 'sustain the vital forces through any crisis that occurs'.[G6]

THERAPEUTIC APPLICATIONS*
Note: The intention of the following information is to represent the traditional use of the individual botanicals found in these formulas and to inform the reader of any evolving scientific inquiry relevant to the formula's ingredients.

SUPPORTED BY TRADITIONAL USE

Reduce fatigue/increase stamina,[G3, G4, 5, 7] nervous system tonic/restorative,[G4, G12, 7] aphrodisiac[G4, 6]

SCOPE OF RELEVANT SCIENTIFIC INVESTIGATION

Adrenal insufficiency,[G3, G4] immuno-stimulating,[G1, G3, G4]

CAUTIONS, CONTRA-INDICATIONS AND DRUG INTERACTIONS
Please reference Chapter 9. Do not use during pregnancy or lactation.

COMPLIMENTARY HERBS/FORMULAS
Smilax/Damiana Supreme, Siberian Ginseng Tonic Elixir, Vitality Herbal Elixir, Virilty Herbal Elixir (with Ginseng), Energy & Vitality, Astragalus Supreme

REFERENCES

1. Farnsworth NR, *et al.* Siberian ginseng (*Eleutherococcus senticosis*): Current status as an adaptogen. *Econ Med Plant Res.* 1985; 1:156-215.
2. Murray M. The healing power of herbs - The enlightened persons guide to the wonders of medicinal plants. 2nd ed. Prima publishing. Rocklin, Ca. 1995.
3. Li XY. Bioactivity of neo-lignans from fructus scizandrae. *Mem Inst Oswaldo Cruz.* 1991:31-7.
4. Brekhman II, Dardymov IV. *Ann Rev Pharmacol.* 1969: 419.
5. Wang BX. Tianjin Xiyao Zazhi. 1965; 7(338).
6. Guyton AC, Hall JE. The major tonic herbs.
7. Priest AW, Priest LR. Herbal medication. A clinical dispensary handbook. 1982
8. Witchl M. Herb drugs and phytopharmaceuticals. CRC Press.1994 Baschetti R. Liquorice and chronic fatigue syndrome. *NZ Med Journal.* 1995; (1002):259.

GRINDELIA/CAMELLIA SUPREME

Promotes Improved Respiratory Functions*

FORMULA

Grindelia floral buds	(*Grindelia robusta*)
Green tea	(*Camellia sinensis*)
Licorice root	(*Glycyrrhiza glabra*)
Rosehip solid extract	(*Rosa canina*)
Lobelia herb and seed	(*Lobelia inflata*)
Chinese Ephedra	(*Ephedra sinica*)
Ginger root	(*Zingiber officinale*)

Concentration:	1:1 Herb strength ratio
Dosage:	30-50 drops, 4 times daily
Duration of use:	As needed. Use only as directed
Best taken:	Between meals, with warm water

DESCRIPTION OF FORMULA

Many of the ingredients in this formula have a history of use with asthma and other respiratory conditions. Collectively, they target a number of the key processes that underlie most of today's inflammatory disorders. This compound's therapeutic focus includes, the reduction of free-radical stress, the stabilization of mast cells (see below), the correct metabolism of Essential Fatty Acids (EFA's), and the creation of an endocrine pattern of behavior that works to reduce inflammation, as opposed to promoting it.

Grindelia floral buds have traditionally been reported to be an effective treatment for congested respiratory disorders, specifically asthma.[G1, G12] They have also been used to treat eczema, various inflammatory disorders, and to restore digestion (particularly when it is associated with sluggish liver function).[G12] David Hoffman reports that Grindelia also relaxes the smooth muscles of the chest and the heart.[2]

Green tea has traditionally been used as a stimulant, diuretic, digestive tonic, expectorant, and to reduce the effects of toxic exposure.[G3] It is also used in this formula for its antioxidant properties, along with its ability to increase cyclic AMP* within mast cells.[G8] These cells, which release many of the compounds that mediate many inflammatory diseases (such as eczema, psoriasis, and asthma[4, 5, 6, 7]) become more stable, and less inclined toward inflammation when their cyclic AMP levels are increased.[3, 4, 5]

Note: for an explanation of cyclic AMP, see cAMP - Coleus forskohlii Supreme

Licorice root is included in this formula as an excellent antiinflammatory[G1, G4] and antispasmodic. Traditionally, its use has included the treatment of liver disorders, which is certainly of benefit here.[G1] It is also well known to be anti-allergic, immunostimulating, and soothing to the mucosal lining of the respiratory tract.[G1, G4] Compounds contained in licorice have been reported to be effective with asthma.[G1]

Rosehip solid extract is included in this formula for it's nutritive affect (it is one of the best sources of natural vitamin C),[8, 9] as well as for its reputation as an excellent tonic for 'general debility and exhaustion'.[8]

Lobelia herb and seed have traditionally, been considered by some to be the ideal remedy for asthma.[G1, G4, G6, 9] In addition, it is present here for its antispasmodic reputation.[G4, G6, 9]

Chinese Ephedra has been used for more than 2,000 years[G3] in the treatment of asthma, hayfever.[G1, G3] and various other inflammatory diseases.[G3] Its use as a bronchodilator is also well established.[G1, G3]

Ginger root is included here for its ability to increase absorption of the entire formula, in addition to its well established anti-inflammatory, antioxidant, and antispasmodic activity.[G5, 10]

THERAPEUTIC APPLICATIONS*

Note: The intention of the following information is to represent the traditional use of the individual botanicals found in these formulas and to inform the reader of any evolving scientific inquiry relevant to the formula's ingredients.

SUPPORTED BY TRADITIONAL USE

Asthma,[G1, G4, G6, G12, 9] respiratory congestion,[G1, G12] inflammation[G12, 10]

SCOPE OF RELEVANT SCIENTIFIC INVESTIGATION

Asthma,[G1, 4, 6] mast cell stabalization,[3, 4, 5] inflammation,[G1, G4, G8, 3, 4, 5, 6, 10] skin disorders,[5, 7]

CAUTIONS, CONTRA-INDICATIONS AND DRUG INTERACTIONS

Please reference Chapter 9. Do not use during pregnancy or lactation. This formula should not be used to supplant asthma medication without a doctor's consent.

COMPLIMENTARY HERBS/FORMULAS

cAMP - Coleus forskohlii Supreme, Turmeric/Catechu Supreme

Note: Ensuring adequate Essential Fatty Acid (EFA) intake will enhance the effectiveness of this formula. The flavonoid quercetin should also be considered.

REFERENCES

1. Tierra M. Planetary Herbology. Santa Fe, NM. Lotus Press. 1989.
2. Hoffman D. The Herbal Handbook. Rochester, Vt. Healing Arts Press. 1988.
3. Shichijo M, *et al.* Role of cyclic 3',5'-adenosine monophosphate in the regulation of chemical mediator release and cytokine production from cultured human mast cells. *J Allergy Clin Immunol.* 1999; 103(5 Pt 2): S421-8.
4. Weston MC, Peachell PT. Regulation of human mast cell and basophil function by cAMP. *Gen Pharmacol.* 1998; 31(5): 715-9.
5. Singh LK, *et al.* Acute immobilization stress triggers skin mast cell degranulation via corticotropin releasing hormone, neurotensin, and substance P: A link to neurogenic skin disorders. *Brain Behav Immun.* 1999; 13(3): 225-39.
6. Webster EL, *et al.* Corticotropin-releasing hormone and inflammation. *Ann N Y Acad Sci.* 1998; 840:21-32.
7. Theoharides TC, *et al.* Corticotropin-releasing hormone induces skin mast cell degranulation and increased vascular permeability, a possible explanation for its proinflammatory effects. *Endocrinology.* 1998; 139(1): 403-13.

8. Hoffman D. The Holistic Herbal. Moray, Scotland. The Findhorn Press. 1984.

9. Coon N. Using plants for healing. Philadelphia, Pa. Rodale Press. 1979.

10. Schulick P. Ginger, common spice or wonder drug. Brattleboro, Vt. Herbal Free Press. 1996.

HAWTHORN SUPREME

Ultimate Support of Cardiovascular Function *
FORMULA

Hawthorn berry (Solid extract)	(*Crataegus oxycantha*)
Hawthorn flower and leaf	(*Crataegus spp.*)

Concentration:	2.5:1 Herb strength ratio
Dosage:	Liquid Extract: 40-60 drops, three times daily
Duration of use:	4-6 months or longer, for best results
Best taken:	Between meals, with warm water

DESCRIPTION OF FORMULA

A combination of the Hawthorn berry with its flower and/or leaves has traditionally been used in Europe as a highly regarded heart tonic. Its specific application includes heart weakness, particularly where nervous exhaustion is present. This nutritive plant, nourishes the entire cardiovascular system promoting connective and cardiovascular tissue integrity. Due to the absence of plant bioflavonoids from foods in the American diet, simple plant compounds, such as these, will prove to become increasingly effective with many of today's chronic degenerative disorders. This compound contains two groups of active flavonoids that exert their actions upon the cardiovascular system. One group of flavonoids has been shown to enhance rhythmical activity (Positive inotropic) of the heart while the other group has been shown to reinforce the collagen tissue of the cardiovascular system.

Hawthorn berries have been used historically to tonify the heart.[G3, G5, G6, 1, 2, 3] In fact, such use for Hawthorn has been reported since the first half of the 17th century.[2] The berries have also traditionally found use as a digestive stimulant for relief of numerous gastrointestinal disturbances.[G3, G5] Primary focus, has of course fallen predominantly upon its well established cardiovascular affect. In the tradition of the American Eclectics, Hawthorn was considered to be a specific for cardiac insufficiency of virtually any kind.[G6] Today, Hawthorn is primarily recognized in the scientific literature for its influence with congestive heart disease,[G5, 7, 8] cholesterol lowering effects, antioxidant properties, and collagen stabilizing ability.[G5, 1]

Hawthorn flowers and leaves possess similar properties and chemistry to the Hawthorn berry.[3] While the berries are higher in connective tissue flavonoids, the flower and leaf are higher in cardiovascular acting flavonoids.[2] They have been combined here in Hawthorn Supreme to offer the full spectrum of Hawthorn's chemistry and vast therapeutic effects. The German Commission E (Germany's equivalent of the FDA) endorses the use of the leaf and flower, of Hawthorn for Cardiac Insufficiency, and 'the aging heart, not yet requiring digitalis'.[9] Hawthorn is considered to be one of the most gentle heart remedies in the herbal *materia medica* (materials of medicine).[3]

THERAPEUTIC APPLICATIONS*

Note: The intention of the following information is to represent the traditional use of the individual botanicals found in these formulas and to inform the reader of any evolving scientific inquiry relevant to the formula's ingredients.

SUPPORTED BY TRADITIONAL USE

Heart tonic,[G3, G5, G6, 1, 2, 3] Antisclerotic,[G3, G6] Digestive.[G3, 2]

SCOPE OF RELEVANT SCIENTIFIC INVESTIGATION

Congestive Heart Disease,[G5, 1] High Blood Pressure,[G3, G5, 1] Elevates cyclic AMP,[G5, 1, 9] Extends refractory period,[G5] Positively inotropic,[G3, G5, 1, 2, 4, 5, 9] Cholesterol lowering,[G5] Antioxidant,[G5, 1] Collagen stabalization,[G5, 1] Increased coronary and peripheral blood flow.[G3, 1, 6, 7, 8]

CAUTIONS, CONTRA-INDICATIONS
AND DRUG INTERACTIONS

Please reference Chapter 9. Do not use during pregnancy or lactation.

COMPLIMENTARY HERBS/FORMULAS

Hawthorn Berry Solid Extract, Night Blooming Cereus (for MVP - Practitioners Only), Anti-Oxidant Supreme, Ginkgo Leaf

REFERENCES

1. Murray M. The healing power of herbs - The enlightened persons guide to the wonders of medicinal plants. 2nd ed. Prima publishing. Rocklin, Ca. 1995.

2. Hobbs C, Foster S. Hawthorn - A Literature Review. *Herbalgram.* 1990; 22:19-33.

3. Mitchell W. Plant Medicine. Seattle, Wa. Self-published. 2000.

4. Loew D. Phytotherapy in heart failure. *Phytomedicine.* 1997; 4(3): 267-71.

5. Popping S, *et al.* Effect of a Hawthorn Extract on Contraction and Energy Turnover of Isolated Rat Cardiomyocytes. *Arzneim.-Forsch.* 1995; 45(1): 1157-61.

6. Ammon H, Handel M. Crataegus, Toxikologie und Pharmakologie Teil II: Pharmakodynamik *Planta Med.* 1991; 43(3): 209-39.

7. Schussler M, *et al.* Functional and Antiischaemic Effects of Monoacetyl-vitexinrhamnoside in Different In Vitro Models. *Gen. Pharmac.* 1995; 26(7): 1565-70.

8. Al Makdessi S, *et al.* Myocardial Protection by Pretreatment with Crataegus oxyacantha. *Arzneim.-Forsch.* 1996; 46(1): 25-27.

9. Witchl M. (Bisset NG, Ed.) Herbal Drugs and Phytopharmaceuticals. Medpharm, CRC Press: Boca Raton. 1994.

HOXSEY/RED CLOVER SUPREME

A Deep Tissue Alterative*
FORMULA

Red Clover blossoms	(*Trifolium pratense*)
Buckthorn bark	(*Rhamnus cathartica*)
Barberry root bark	(*Berberis vulgaris*)
Burdock root	(*Arctium lappa*)
Stillingia root	(*Stillingia sylvatica*)
Poke root	(*Phytolacca americana*)
Cascara sagrada bark	(*Rhamnus purshiana*)
Licorice root	(*Glycyrrhiza glabra*)
Prickly Ash bark	(*Xanthoxylum clava-herculis*)

Note: Cascara amarga (*Sweetia panamensis*) is believed to be the species of Cascara used in the original Hoxsey Formula. Cascara sagrada (*Rhamnus purshiana*) shares similar chemistry, and tradition of use. They may be considered interchangeable, as we have done so here.

Concentration:	1:1 Herb strength ratio
Dosage:	40-60 drops, 3-4 times daily
Duration of use:	4-6 months or longer, for best results
Best taken:	Between meals, with warm water

DESCRIPTION OF FORMULA

The Hoxsey formula has been in use for over 100 years, for the treatment of cancer. Said to 'restore normalcy' to disturbed metabolism, this alterative compound works to remove catabolic wastes from deranged tissue, while facilitating the correct uptake of nutrition. Although a 1958 United States Senate Committee report concluded that organized medicine had indeed conspired to suppress Hoxsey therapy, this formula continues to be used for conditions where deranged tissue is the result of a longstanding inability to remove catabolic wastes from the cells of the body.

Red Clover blossoms have traditionally been used for conditions where the eliminative properties of a diuretic[G3] and alterative[G1, G12] would be of benefit, including bronchitis, skin sores and ulcers, and whooping cough.[G1, G3] This common weed has also been used extensively with cancer.[G3] In addition, it is reported that Red Clover reduces platelet aggregation (blood stickiness) and angiogenesis (development of tumor vascular-networks), inhibits leukotriene (a pro-inflammatant and inducer of cellular proliferation) production,[1] and contains compounds that may impede tumor development by blocking estrogen receptors.[G3, 2, 3] Topoisomerase-2 inhibition has also been reported.[4]

Buckthorn bark is closely related to Cascara Sagrada (see below). Both have traditionally been recognized as tonic laxatives.[G1, G6] Importantly, they both contain emodin compounds[G1, 5] that have been researched for their ability to inhibit angiogenesis (development of tumor vascular-networks).[5, 6]

Barberry root bark has found traditional use as a bitter tonic.[G3] In China, it has been used, with some success with radiation and chemotherapy induced leukopaenia.[G1] Modern medical research has also focused on the isolated alkaloid, berberine, bringing to light its antitumor and antineoplastic[G1] potential.

Burdock root is an alterative[G6, 10] (corrects cellular waste and nutrition) that is somewhat similar in action to Yellowdock.[G6] It has long been used for rheumatism, skin disorders, and to stimulate urination.[G3, G4, G6, 10] It is also well known for its ability to stimulate liver/bile related functions.[G4] It is reported to possess anti-tumor activity,[G3] along with the ability to induce cell differentiation.[7] Traditional anticancer use supports this research.[G3]

Stillingia root, like many remedies in this formula, is an alterative.[G1, G6] It has also been used as a folk remedy for cancer.[8]

Poke root is also an alterative.[G1, G6, 9] Poke root has been used for rheumatism, skin conditions, and disorders of the respiratory system.[G6, G15] It also has been used traditionally for cancer.[9]

Cascara sagrada bark, if allowed to dry and age (for at least one year), has traditionally been used as a tonifying laxative, not an irritating laxative.[G4, 10] Cascara sagrada also contains emodin compounds [G1, 5] which, as mentioned previously, have been researched for their ability to inhibit angiogenesis (development of tumor vascular-networks).[5, 6]

Licorice root has been in use as a medicine for over 3,000 years.[G4] It is a well respected anti-inflammatory[G1, G4, G21] that is both nutritive and soothing to the mucosal ling throughout the body.[G3, G15, 2] It is well known to be liver protective, and to promote detoxification.[G1, G4, G21, 7] Licorice has a history of use in many countries to treat cancer.[G3] Research has indicated that compounds in Licorice to possess antitumor properties.[11, 12, 13]

Prickly Ash bark is a circulatory stimulant[G1, G3, G4] and appears in this formula to help drive the other botanicals throughout the body. The Eclectic physicians used this plant to 'stimulate the nerve centers', and to 'sustain the vital forces through any crisis that occurs'.[G6] It also finds value in this formula as an anti-inflammatory, and for the fact that oils from Prickly Ash have shown anticarcinogenic potential.[14]

THERAPEUTIC APPLICATIONS*

Note: The intention of the following information is to represent the traditional use of the individual botanicals found in these formulas and to inform the reader of any evolving scientific inquiry relevant to the formula's ingredients.

SUPPORTED BY TRADITIONAL USE

Alterative,[G1, G6, G12, G15, 9, 10] Anticancer,[G3, 8, 9] Bronchial conditions,[G1, G3, G6, G15] Skin disorders,[G1, G3, G4, G6, G15, 10] Rheumatism,[G3, G4, G6, G15, 10] Tonic laxative,[G1, G4, G6, 10]

SCOPE OF RELEVANT SCIENTIFIC INVESTIGATION

Reduces platelet aggregation,[1] Inhibits angiogenesis,[1, 5, 6] Inhibits leukotriene production,[1] Possible estrogen receptor antagonist.[G3, 2, 3] Topoisomerase [2] inhibition,[4] Induces differentiation,[7] Antineoplastic,[G1] Radiation and chemotherapy induced leukopaenia,[G1] Antitumor,[G1, G3, 11, 12, 13] Anticarcinogenic.[14]

CAUTIONS, CONTRA-INDICATIONS AND DRUG INTERACTIONS

Please reference Chapter 9. Do not use during pregnancy or lactation.

COMPLIMENTARY HERBS/FORMULAS

Juniper Berry Supreme, Scudder's Alterative, Cell Wise, Daily Detox, Astragalus Supreme, Sheep Sorrel/Burdock Supreme

REFERENCES

1. Beckstrom-Sternberg and Duke Phytochemical Database: http://www.ars-grin.gov/~ngrlsb.

2. Hartwell JL. Plants used against cancer: A survey. *Lloydia*. 1967-1971, 30.

3. Messina M, Barnes S. The role of soy products in reducing risk of cancer. *J Natl Cancer Inst*. 1991; 83: 541-546.

4. Budavari, S, *et al*. The Merck Index: An Encyclopedia of Chemicals, Drugs, and Biologicals, 11th ed. Merck and Co., Inc., Rahway, N.J. 1989.

5. Harborne J, Baxter H. Phytochemical Dictionary: A Handbook of Bioactive Compounds from Plants. Washington, D.C., Taylor and Francis. 1993.

6. Evans, WC. Trease and Evans' Pharmacognosy. 13th ed. Philadelphia: Bailliere Tindall (The Curtis Center), 1989.

7. Boik J. Cancer and Natural Medicine: A Textbook of Basic Science and Clinical Research. Oregon Medical Press, Princeton, MN.1996.

8. Duke, JA. Handbook of Medicinal Herbs. Boca Raton, Fl. CRC Press; 1985

9. Hutchens AR. A handbook of Native American herbs. Shambhalla publications. 1992.

10. Witchl M. (Bisset NG, Ed.) Herbal Drugs and Phytopharmaceuticals. Medpharm, CRC Press: Boca Raton. 1994.

11. Agarwal R, *et al*. Inhibition of mouse skin tumor-initiating activity of DMBA by chronic oral feeding of glycyrrhizin in drinking water. *Nutrition and Cancer*. 1991; 15:187-193.

12. Wang ZY, *et al*. Inhibition of mutagenicity in Salmonella typhimurium and skin tumor initiating and tumor promoting activities in SENCAR mice by glycyrrhetinic acid: comparison of 18 alpha- and 18 beta-stereoisomers. Carcinogenesis. 1991;12(2):187-92.

13. Kim DH, *et al*. Biotransformation of glycyrrhizin by human intestinal bacteria and its relation to biological activities. Arch Pharm Res. 2000; 23(2):172-7.

14. Hashim S, *et al*. Modulatory effects of essential oils from spices on the formation of DNA adduct by aflatoxin B1 in vitro. *Nutr Cancer*. 1994; 21(2):169-75.

JUNIPER BERRY SUPREME

Promotes Healthy Urinary Function *
FORMULA

Juniper Berry	(*Juniperus communis*)
Horsetail	(*Equisetum arvense*)
Corn Silk	(*Zea mays*)
Goldenrod leaf & tops	(*Solidago odora*)
Cleavers herb	(*Galium aparine*)
Marshmallow root	(*Althaea officinalis*)

Concentration:	1:1.5 Herb strength ratio
Dosage:	30-40 drops, 3-4 times daily
Duration of use:	2-3 months
Best taken:	Between meals, with warm water

DESCRIPTION OF FORMULA

This formula soothes inflamed and irritated membranes of the urinary system. By aiding in the reduction of urinary irritation, and by supporting the removal of urinary wastes via the kidneys, it helps to restore overall integrity and function to the urinary apparatus. Its anti-inflammatory and antispasmodic influence is also useful here. The compound contains diuretic, antiseptic, and demulcent properties that act to gently stimulate renal excretions, disinfect the urinary tract and soothe irritated urinary membranes.

Juniper Berry is a soothing[G6] diuretic that medical tradition holds as being particularly suited to chronic disorders of the kidney's.[G6, 1] It was also used to restore normal action and function of the kidneys following acute, irritating disorders.[G6] This remedy also is useful for indigestion,[2, 3] bronchitis (using steam inhalation),[G3] various gastrointestinal disorders,[G3, 2] snakebites,[G3] and as a carminative,[G3, 2, 3] to treat intestinal flatulence[G3, 3] and colic.[G3] Pharmacological research reports that the oil from Juniper possesses an antispasmodic influence over smooth muscle.[G3]

Horsetail is also recognized as a soothing diuretic, being useful where there is irritation of the mucosal lining of the urinary tract.[G6] European tradition suggests its general use for promoting kidney function and digestive elimination.[G3] The respected Commission E monograph for Horsetail, suggests its use for 'bacterial and inflammatory diseases of the lower urinary tract and renal gravel'(kidney stones).[4]

Corn Silk is a non-irritating diuretic that soothes and protects irritated mucous membranes.[G6] According to American Eclectic practice, it is said to be specific for bladder irritation,[G6,2] and all congested conditions of the urinary passages.[G6]

Goldenrod leaf & tops have reportedly been used in Germany for centuries for the treatment of backache and 'diseases of the kidneys'.[G6] It is known to be used for bladder[5] and kidney inflammation, and 'urinary obstructions of any character'[G6] and weakness of the stomach.[5] Goldenrod has also been used as a carminative, to relieve intestinal flatulence, cramping, and colic.[G6, G12]

Cleavers herb is said to be one of the best lymphatic tonics available. It is also an alterative and diuretic.[G1,6] In the tradition of the American Eclectic's it is recognized as a sedative remedy in acute inflammation or irritation of the urinary tract.[G6] In general, it was considered to be a tonic for the urinary tract.[G6]

Marshmallow root is soothing to inflamed and painful mucous membranes.[G6,7] As such, it has traditionally found use with painful urinary disorders, such as cystitis (kidney inflammation),[G6,2,7] and bladder irritation.[G6] Marshmallow is also reported to possess immunostimulating properties.[4]

THERAPEUTIC APPLICATIONS*
Note: The intention of the following information is to represent the traditional use of the individual botanicals found in these formulas and to inform the reader of any evolving scientific inquiry relevant to the formula's ingredients.

SUPPORTED BY TRADITIONAL USE

Urinary irritation,[G6,1,6,7] Cystitis [G6,2,7] Chronic kidney disorders,[G6,1,6] Kidney tonic,[G6] Diuretic,[G1,G6,2,6] Restorative following acute kidney disorders,[G6,1] Promotes kidney function,[G3,G4]

Demulcent (soothing to mucous membranes),[G1, G6, 7] Promotes digestive elimination,[G3, G4] Urinary catarrh (congestion),[G6] Carminative,[G6, G12] Alterative[G1]

SCOPE OF RELEVANT SCIENTIFIC INVESTIGATION

Diuretic,[G1, G3, G4, 2] Antispasmodic,[G3] Choleretic (stimulates bile secretion)[G1]

CAUTIONS, CONTRA-INDICATIONS AND DRUG INTERACTIONS

Please reference Chapter 9. Do not use during pregnancy or lactation. Do not use if there is history of urinary disease without the consult of a physician.

COMPLIMENTARY HERBS/FORMULAS

Red Clover Supreme, Scudder's Alterative, Usnea/Uva Ursi Supreme

REFERENCES

1. Clymer RS. Natures Healing Agents. Philadelphia. Dorrance and Company. 1963.
2. Witchl M. (Bisset NG, Ed.) Herbal Drugs and Phytopharmaceuticals. Medpharm, CRC Press: Boca Raton. 1994.
3. Grieve M, Mrs. A Modern Herbal. New York. Dover; 1982.
4. Blumenthal M, *et al.* Ed. *The Complete German Commission E Monographs.*Austin, TX: American Botanical Council; 1998.
5. Hutchens AR. A handbook of Native American herbs. Shambhalla publications. 1992.
6. Hoffman D. The Holistic Herbal. Moray. The Findhorn Press;1984.
7. Coon N. Using plants for healing. Philadelphia, Pa. Rodale Press. 1979.

LINDEN/CRATAEGUS SUPREME

Promotes Healthy
*Cardio-Vascular Function**
FORMULA

Linden Flowers	(*Tilia spp*)
Hawthorn berry, leaf and flower	(*Crataegus spp.*)
Mistletoe herb	(*Viscum album*)
Valerian root	(*Valeriana officinalis*)

Concentration:	1:1 Herb strength ratio
Dosage:	40 drops, 3-4 times daily
Duration of use:	4-6 months
Best taken:	Between meals, with warm water

DESCRIPTION OF FORMULA

This formula works to restore healthy cardiovascular function, where it has been compromised. It is of particular use for those individuals who are under great stress, and who cannot reduce the tension and rigidity which is often associated with stress-related cardiovascular disorders. By promoting healthy circulation, and relaxation of the cardiovascular system, this compound restores a healthy response to the stress of modern living by the circulatory system.

Linden Flowers contribute greatly to this formula. They have traditionally been used as a nervine, to soothe excessive excitement with nervous system disorders.[G1, G4, 1] Its ability to reduce blood pressure has also been reported,[G1, G4] and early animal studies seem to verify this effect.[G4] Studies using the volatile oil from Linden Flowers have also confirmed its traditionally recognized[G4] sedative and antispasmodic properties.[G4]

Hawthorn berry, leaf and flowers have historically been used to tonify the heart.[G3, G5, G6, 2, 3, 4] In modern times, Hawthorn is known to mildly[2] reduce high blood pressure,[G3, 2, 5] perhaps via its ability to relax vascular smooth muscle,[G4, 2, 5] and/or its capacity to increase cyclic AMP in heart tissue.[2, 5] Its use with hypertension is further supported by a long history of use in the traditional herbal practices of Europe[1] and China.[G3] Importantly, Hawthorn is considered to be one of the gentlest heart tonics in the known herbal *materia medica* (materials of medicine).[4]

Mistletoe herb was recommended by the American Eclectic Physicians for the reduction of blood pressure.[G6] For point of clarity from one authority it is made clear that the American Mistletoe increases the blood pressure,[7] whereas the European Mistletoe (to which we refer here) is used for its reduction.[G11, 7] Like Hawthorn, Mistletoe has been shown to affect cyclic AMP.[G1]

Valerian root is a nerve tonic[8] which is reported to soothe excitement of the body's nervous system,[G6, 7, 8] without the negative effects of a narcotic.[G6, 7] Like Hawthorn, Valerian is also reported to be useful as an aid for disorders of digestion.[G3, 8] Preliminary studies[G3] confirm its reported ability to reduce blood pressure[G1] and its traditional use as an antispasmodic.[G3, 6]

THERAPEUTIC APPLICATIONS*

Note: The intention of the following information is to represent the traditional use of the individual botanicals found in these formulas and to inform the reader of any evolving scientific inquiry relevant to the formula's ingredients.

SUPPORTED BY TRADITIONAL USE

Hypertension,[G1, G3, G6, 1, 7] Nervine,[G1, G4, 1] Heart tonic,[G1, G3, G5, G6, 2, 3, 4] Sedative,[6] Disorders of digestion,[G3, 2, 8]

SCOPE OF RELEVANT SCIENTIFIC INVESTIGATION

Hypertension,[G3, G4, G11, 2, 5] Sedative,[G4, 6] Antispasmodic,[G4, 6] Increases cAMP,[G1, 2, 5]

CAUTIONS, CONTRA-INDICATIONS AND DRUG INTERACTIONS

Please reference Chapter 9. Do not use during pregnancy or lactation.

COMPLIMENTARY HERBS/FORMULAS

cAMP - Coleus Forskohlii Supreme, Hawthorn Supreme, Dandelion root & leaf, Rauwolfia vomitoria (Medical professionals only - Use with great care, as depression has been associated with its use)

REFERENCES

1. Messegue M. Of Men and Plants. New York, NY. The MacMillan Company.1973.

2. Murray M. The healing power of herbs - The enlightened persons guide to the wonders of medicinal plants. 2nd ed. Prima publishing. Rocklin, Ca. 1995.

3. Hobbs C, Foster S. Hawthorn - A Literature Review. *Herbalgram.* 1990; 22:19-33.

4. Mitchell W. Plant Medicine. Seattle, Wa. Self-published. 2000.

5. Pizzorno J, Murray M. Textbook of Natural medicine. New york. Churchill Livingstone;1999.

6. Witchl M. (Bisset NG, Ed.) Herbal Drugs and Phytopharmaceuticals. Medpharm, CRC Press: Boca Raton. 1994.

7. Coon N. Using plants for healing. Philadelphia, Pa. Rodale Press. 1979.

8. Hutchens AR. A handbook of Native American herbs. Shambhalla publications. 1992.

LOBELIA/CALAMUS SUPREME

An Aid in the Withdrawal From Tobacco Use *
FORMULA

Lobelia herb & seed	(*Lobelia inflata*)
Calamus root	(*Acorus calamus*)
Wild Oat milky seed	(*Avena sativa*)
St. John's Wort	(*Hypericum perforatum*)
Passionflower	(*Passiflora incarnata*)
Licorice root	(*Glycyrrhiza glabra*)

Concentration:	1:1.5 Herb strength ratio
Dosage:	20-30 drops, 3-4 times daily
Duration of use:	2-3 months
Best taken:	Between meals, with warm water

DESCRIPTION OF FORMULA

This formula is composed of a number of plants that have traditionally been used to aid withdrawal from Tobacco addiction. The approach of this compound is multi-faceted. It works to relieve tension of the smooth muscle, reduce anxiety, and improve digestive processes and overall vitality to the nerve centers. Lobelia, to a certain degree, takes the place of nicotine at the site of its cell receptors, thereby reducing craving for this highly addictive compound.

Lobelia herb & seed has traditionally been described as a nerve sedative of great power.[G6] Known also as 'Indian Tobacco', Lobelia was traditionally understood to be similar (although milder) in affect to the common Tobacco plant.[G6, 3] Importantly, the absence of any addictive qualities has also been noted.[G6] Modern pharmacological research appears to support traditional observation, with the discovery that lobeline, a primary alkaloid from Lobelia, produces similar nervous system[G3, G6] effects to nicotine,[G1, G3, G4] the highly addictive alkaloid taken from tobacco. An interesting study shows that lobeline is actually able to bind to nicotine receptor sites.[1, 2] Furthermore, it enhances the action of nicotine activated processes.[1] This suggests that less nicotine may be necessary when used conjunctively with Lobelia effectively replacing a highly addictive molecule, with one that is not.

Calamus root has been used medicinally since ancient times.[G1, 4, 5] It is reported to be one of the key ingredients of the Holy Oil imparted to Moses, as well as one of the plants that was grown in the gardens of Solomon.[5] Investigation of its traditional use spans many cultures and many centuries, highlighting disorders arising from indigestion,[G1, 4, 5] and those that require a nervous sedative and antispasmodic.[G1, 5] It has also been used to help smokers quit cigarettes.[5, 6]

Wild Oat milky seed has traditionally been used for nervous exhaustion,[G6, 7, 8] tobacco[G6, 7] and drug withdrawal and convalescence.[G6, 6] It is said to increase the nerve force and "improve the nutrition of the entire system".[G6]

St. John's Wort finds use in this formula for its restorative effect on the nerve centers, following trauma.[G6] Naturally, any assistance of the restoration of nervous integrity, following withdrawal from addiction (which is traumatic), is of benefit here. St. John's Wort is well established for its anti-depressant effects,[G3, 10] along with its reputation for use with anxiety,[G1, G3, 10] digestive and liver disorders.[9]

Passionflower is a calming sedative,[G1, G3, 9] that is known to possess antispasmodic[9] and antianxiety effects.[G3] It is also of particular benefit for sleeplessness due to withdrawal.[9]

Licorice root is an expectorant which is well established as being useful for irritation of the mucous membranes of the respiratory tract.[G3, G4, G6] Its important antioxidant, antianxiety, and liver protective properties are also of benefit here.[G3]

THERAPEUTIC APPLICATIONS*

Note: The intention of the following information is to represent the traditional use of the individual botanicals found in these formulas and to inform the reader of any evolving scientific inquiry relevant to the formula's ingredients.

SUPPORTED BY TRADITIONAL USE

Withdrawal from Tobacco,[5, 6, 7] Nerve sedative,[G1, G3, G6, 5, 6, 9] Nervous exhaustion,[G6, 7, 8] Nervous restorative,[G6, 7, 8] Antispasmodic,[G1, 5] Digestive disturbances,[G1, 4, 5, 9]

SCOPE OF RELEVANT SCIENTIFIC INVESTIGATION

Nicotinic (nicotine) receptor agonist,[1, 2] Nicotine mimicry,[G4, 2]
Nicotine synergist,[1] Sedative,[G3] Antidepressant[G3, 10]

CAUTIONS, CONTRA-INDICATIONS AND DRUG INTERACTIONS

Please reference Chapter 9. Do not use during pregnancy or lactation.

COMPLIMENTARY HERBS/FORMULAS

Serenity Elixir with Kava Kava, Calcium Supreme Elixir

REFERENCES

1. Damaj MI, *et al.* Pharmacology of lobeline, a nicotinic receptor ligand. *J Pharmacol Exp Ther.* 1997; 282(1): 410-9.

2. Flammia D, *et al.* Lobeline: structure-affinity investigation of nicotinic acetylcholinergic receptor binding. *J Med Chem.* 1999; 42(18): 3726-31.

3. Willard T. Wild Rose Scientific Herbal. Wild rose College of Natural Healing; Alberta; 1991.

4. Coon N. Using plants for healing. Philadelphia, Pa. Rodale Press. 1979.

5. Motley TJ. The Ethnobotany of Sweet Flag, Acorus calamus (Araceae). *Economic Botany.*1994; 48(4): 397-412.

6. Mitchell W. Plant Medicine. Seattle, Wa. Self-published. 2000.

7. Witchl M. (Bisset NG, Gd.) Herbal Drugs and Phytopharmacenticals Medpharm, CRC Press: Baca Raton, 1994.

8. Hutchens AR. A handbook of Native American herbs. Shambhalla publications. 1992.

9. Clymer RS. Natures Healing Agents. Philadelphia. Dorrance and Company. 1963.

10. Murray M. The healing power of herbs - The enlightened persons guide to the wonders of medicinal plants. 2nd ed. Prima publishing. Rocklin, Ca. 1995.

LOMATIUM SUPREME

An Immune-Stimulating Respiratory Formula *
FORMULA

Lomatium root	(*Lomatium dissectum*)
Echinacea root	(*Echinacea spp.*)
Spilanthes flowering buds	(*Spilanthes acmella*)
St. John's Wort	(*Hypericum perforatum*)
Chinese Skullcap root	(*Scutellaria baicalensis*)
Chinese Schizandra berry	(*Schisandra chinensis*)
Licorice root	(*Glycyrrhiza glabra*)
Essential oil of Cinnamon	(*Cinnamonum zeylanicum*)

Concentration:	1:1 Average Herb Strength Ratio
Dosage:	40-60 drops, 4-5 times daily
Duration of use:	For acute applications: up to 3 weeks
	For chronic applications: 2-3 months
Best taken:	Between meals, with warm water

DESCRIPTION OF FORMULA

This upper respiratory formula brings together an array of powerful botanicals that are well known to support respiratory function. Combining antiviral and antibacterial herbs with those that are known to be immuno-stimulating, expectorant, antitussive, and anti-inflammatory, this compound works to strengthen the physiological processes of immunity and respiratory stimulation. Important aspects of nerve integrity and liver function have also been considered in this formulation. Lomatium Supreme is for those individuals who specifically cannot shake a stubborn, invasive, and congestive disorder of the upper respiratory tract.

Lomatium root has been used by Native Americans for centuries as a lung medicine. Herbalist, Michael Moore, attributes antimicrobial action to Lomatium, saying that it is of particular assistance with "limiting the severity and number of respiratory infections", especially when so-called "slow viruses" are involved.[1] One Canadian study appears to offer some support for this clinical observation, reporting that an extract of Lomatium completely inhibited rotavirus.[2]

Echinacea is an immuno-stimulant, whose anti-inflammatory, antibacterial, antiviral, and wound healing properties have been widely reported. [G1, G4] Echinacea was used by the Eclectic medical doctors, from the first half of the last century, for its benefits with chronic catarrhal (congestive) conditions of the respiratory tract. [G12] Today, modern science is beginning to support much of its traditional use, by showing that extracts of Echinacea have the ability to increase antibody production, along with resistance to various infections. [3] Research has further shown that alcohol/water extracts of Echinacea significantly enhance natural killer cell function, [4] and have phagocytic, metabolic and bactericidal influence on macrophages. [5] Echinacea thus encourages cellular immunity.[6]

Spilanthes has enjoyed a long history of indigenous use for numerous disorders, including the removal of intestinal worms. [G12] The Eclectic physicians of North America considered it to be a useful digestive stimulant. [G12] Modern research has shown its investigative light on the anti-inflammatory properties of Spilanthes. [7] Species related to the one used here have been noted for their antibacterial activity. [8]

St. John's Wort has long been considered of value where the nerve centers have become traumatized. [G6] It has been said that it is "for the nervous system, what arnica is for the muscular". [1] This contributes greatly where the coughing reflex has left someone irritable and 'on edge'. While St. John's Wort's antidepressant activity [G16, 9, 10] has dominated discussion of its virtue in recent times, powerful antiretroviral, antibacterial, [G16, G20, 10] and antifungal properties have also been noted. [G16, G20]

Chinese Skullcap has been reported to possess antiviral and antibacterial activity. [G3, G8, G16] It has also been shown to decrease inflammation, [G8, G16] reduce the damaging effects of free radicals on cellular fats, as well as reduce the release of histamine from cells which contribute to inflammation (mast cells). [G16] The latter effect may be attributed to Chinese Skullcap's ability to increase cyclic AMP. [11]

Schizandra increases resistance to physiological stress. [G3, G8] Traditionally, it has been used with respiratory disorders. [G3] It is also a powerful antioxidant that appears to be highly specific for protecting liver tissue. [G3, G8] In addition, Schizandra berries are known to possess antibacterial, [G3] expectorant and antitussive qualities. [G3, G8]

Licorice root has traditionally been used to treat respiratory disorders. [12] This amazing plant brings anti-inflammatory, antitussive, and stimulating expectorant activity to this formula. [G16, 12] Antiviral, antibacterial, [G4, G16, 12] antifungal, and antiparasitic properties have also been attributed to this soothing liver-protective plant. [G16, 12] The German Commission E approves it for use when there is congestion of the upper respiratory tract. [13]

Essential oil of Cinnamon is a warming flavorful essential oil that is reported to have anti-inflammatory, antibacterial, antifungal, and antiviral qualities. [G3]

THERAPEUTIC APPLICATIONS*

Note: The intention of the following information is to represent the traditional use of the individual botanicals found in these formulas and to inform the reader of any evolving scientific inquiry relevant to the formula's ingredients.

SUPPORTED BY TRADITIONAL USE

Respiratory disorders, [G3, 12] Congestive conditions of the respiratory tract, [G12] Nervous tonic, [G6] Antiparasitic, [G12]

SCOPE OF RELEVANT SCIENTIFIC INVESTIGATION

Upper respiratory congestion, [13] Expectorant, [G3, G8, G16, 12] Antitussive, [G3, G8, G16, 12] Antiviral, [G1, G3, G4, G8, G16, 2] Antibacterial, [G1, G3, G4, G8, G16, G20, 10] Antiretroviral, [G16, G20, 10] Anti-inflammatory, [G1, G3, G4, G8, G16, 7] Immune enhancement, [4, 5, 6] Antifungal, [G3, G16, G20] Liver protective, [G3, G8]

CAUTIONS, CONTRA-INDICATIONS AND DRUG INTERACTIONS

Please reference Chapter 9. Do not use during pregnancy or lactation.

COMPLIMENTARY HERBS/FORMULAS

Lomatium/Osha Supreme, Osha Supreme, Ginger Tea

REFERENCES

1. Moore M. Medicinal Plants of the Pacific West. Red Crane Books. Santa Fe, NM. 1995.

2. McCutcheon Ar, *et al.* Antiviral screening of British Columbian medicinal plants. *J Ethnopharmacol.* 1995;49(2):101-10.

3. Schranner I, Wurdinger M, *et al.* Modification of avian humoral immunoreactions by Influx and *Echinacea angustifolia* extract. *Zentralbl Veterinarmed* (B) 1989; 36.

4. Broumand N, Sahl L, Tilles JG. The in vitro effects of *Echinacea* and ginseng on natural killer and antibody-dependent cell cytotoxicity in healthy subjects and chronic fatigue syndrome or acquired immuno-deficiency syndrome patients. *Immunopharmacology.* 1997; 35.

5. Bukovsky M, Kostalova D, Magnusova R, Vaverkova S. Testing for immunomodulating effects of ethanol-water extracts of the above ground parts of the plants *Echinaceae* and *Rudbeckia. Cesk Farm.* 1993; 42

6. Witchl M. (Bisset NG, Ed.) Herbal Drugs and Phytopharmaceuticals. Medpharm, CRC Press: Boca Raton. 1994.

7. Wagner H, Breu W, *et al.* In vitro Inhibition of Arachidonate Metabolism by some Alkamides and Prenylated phenols. *Planta Medica.* 1989;55:566-567.

8. Fabry W, *et al.* Activity of East African medicinal plants against *Heliobacter pylori. Chemotherapy.* 1996;42(5):315-317.

9. Ernst E. St. John's Wort, an antidepressant? A systematic, criteria-based review. *Phytomedicine.* 1995;2(1):67-71.

10. Snow JM. *Hypericum perforatum* L. (Hyperiaceae). *The Protocol Journal Of Botanical Medicine.* 1996; 2(1):16-21.

11. NAPRALERT Search results. Program for Collaborative Research in the Pharmaceutical Sciences College of Pharmacy, University of Illinois at Chicago. October 1994.

12. Snow JM. *Glycyrrhiza glabra* L. (Leguminaceae). The Protocol Journal of Botanical Medicine. 1995; 1(3):9-14.

13. Blumenthal M, *et al.* Ed. *The Complete German Commission E Monographs.* Austin, TX: American Botanical Council; 1998.

MELISSA SUPREME

*Children's Calming Formula**
FORMULA

Lemon Balm	(*Melissa officinalis*)
Chamomile Flowers	(*Matricaria recutita*)
Passionflower vine	(*Passiflora incarnata*)
Skullcap herb	(*Scutellaria lateriflora*)
Wild Oat milky seed	(*Avena sativa*)
Gotu Kola herb	(*Centella asiatica*)
Irish Moss	(*Chondrus crispus*)
Mineral salts from Kelp	(*Nerocystis luetkeana*)

Concentration:	1:1 Herb strength ratio
Dosage:	20-30 drops, 3 times daily
Duration of use:	3 months or longer
Best taken:	Between meals with apple, pear or grape juice

DESCRIPTION OF FORMULA

This formula specifically focuses on quieting the excitability and agitation of the nervous system without promoting sleepiness or lethargy. The formula and the dosage is established for children's metabolism. Research has demonstrated Attention Deficit Hyperactive Disorder (ADHD) as a dysregulation of the hypothalamic-pituitary-adrenal axis. Herbal medicines have shown an ability to effect the symptoms, hormones and effects relating to this type of imbalance.

Melissa (Lemon Balm) has traditionally been used for its ability to calm nervous irritability and agitation.[1] Research has demonstrated that Lemon balm has an inhibitory effect on excess thyroid hormone stimulation to cells[2] and decreases the behavioral activities of mice at low doses.[3] In addition, it has long been used as an antispasmodic, carminative (relieves gas and intestinal colic), and for its antiviral properties.[4][5]

Chamomile is an excellent and reliable nervine that relaxes and is a tonic to the nervous system. It produces a calming action for infants, children and adults who are restless, discontented and impatient.[6] It is a traditional remedy for nervous apprehension that is out of proportion to the actual pain suffered. Chamomile is soothing to the GI tract and effective for a simple bellyache, diarrhea or constipation.[7,8]

Passionflower is another example of a medicinal plant that has traditionally been reported to induce sleep by its calming influence, and not by any narcotic effect. It has also been used to treat nervous disorders,[9] as an antispasmodic, and for its influence with pain relief.[10] Passionflower has been approved by the European Scientific Co-Operative on Phytotherapy (ESCOP) for "tenseness, restlessness and irritability with difficulty in falling asleep".[11]

A flavonoid, vitexin acts as an anti-inflammatory and lowers blood pressure.[12]

Skullcap is a tonic to the nerves and has a long and trusted use as an antispasmodic. It is used in restlessness and nervous excitability.[13] It is helpful for physical or mental overwork, or nervous exhaustion following acute illness. Skullcap is reported to act on the cerebrospinal centers of the brain and may have a beneficial effect on epilepsy and heart symptoms of a nervous origin.[14] Skullcap has been used in teething, neuralgia and headache.[15] For insomnia it calms nervous irritability.[16]

Wild Oat milky seed has a reputation as a trophorestorative (builds nervous reserve).[17] It is useful in states of nervous debility, exhaustion, depression, sleeplessness and wherever convalescence is required for chronic conditions and cardiac weakness.[18,19] An acute indication is for a headache from over work. "It is not a remedy of great power...probably its chief value as a medicine is to energize in nervous exhaustion" Harvey W. Felter, MD.[20]

Gotu Kola is considered to be one of the so-called 'elixirs of life'.[21,22] It has long been used in India to improve intelligence and mental function.[G3] Several studies suggest that Gotu Kola may be useful with improving memory, reducing fatigue and stress, increasing general mental ability, and increasing I.Q. in developmentally disabled children.[23,24]

Irish Moss contains polysaccharides and carragheenans and is soothing to tissues and is mildly laxative.[25] It is used traditionally for dry coughs in European herbalism.[26] There has been little study of this interesting algae in modern times.

Mineral salts from Kelp include iodine and other minerals. Kelp was used traditionally for regulation of the thyroid gland and to help relieve indigestion, constipation, and urinary tract irritations.[27]

THERAPEUTIC APPLICATIONS*

Note: The intention of this information is to represent the traditional use of the individual botanicals found in these formulas and to inform the reader of any evolving scientific inquiry relevant to the formula's ingredients.

SUPPORTED BY TRADITIONAL USE

Nervous irritability and agitation,[28] calming for infants, children and adults who are restless, discontented and impatient,[29] bellyache, diarrhea, constipation,[30,31] pain relief.[32] teething, neuralgia headache,[33] insomnia,[34] nervous debility, exhaustion, depression,[35,36] used in India to improve intelligence and mental function.[G3]

SCOPE OF RELEVANT SCIENTIFIC INVESTIGATION

Inhibitory effect on excess thyroid hormone stimulation to cells,[37] decreases behavioral activities of mice,[38]

CAUTIONS, CONTRA-INDICATIONS AND DRUG INTERACTIONS

Please reference Chapter 9. Do not use during pregnancy or lactation.

COMPLIMENTARY HERBS/FORMULAS

St. John's Wort, Phyto-Proz Supreme, Calcium Supreme Elixir

REFERENCES

1 Mills S. The Essential Book of Herbal medicine. London. Penguin;1991

2 Auf'mdold M *et al.* Inhibition by certain extracts of the binding and adenylate cyclase stimulatory effect of bovine thyrotropin in human thyroid membranes. *Endocrin.,*115:527-34,1984.

3 Soulimani R *et al.* Neurotrophic action of the hydroalcoholic extract of Melissa officinalis in the mouse, Planta Med 1991;4;57(2):105-9

4 Boon H, Smith M. The Botanical Pharmacy. Quebec, Canada. Quarry press;1999.

5 Leung A, Foster S. Encyclopedia of Common Natural Ingredients. NY: Wiley;1996.

6 Felter HW. The Eclectic Materia Medica, Pharmacology and Therapeutics.

Portland, Oregon: Eclectic Medical publications. 1985.475-6.

7 Bisset N. Herbal Drugs and Phytopharmaceuticals, Medpharm Scientific Publishers, Stuttgart, 1994, 322-25.

8 Hoffman D. *The Holistic Herbal.* Moray. The Findhorn Press; 1984.185

9 Leung A, Foster S. Encyclopedia of Common Natural Ingredients. NY: Wiley;1996.

10 Felter HW. The Eclectic Materia Medica, Pharmacology and Therapeutics. Portland, Oregon. Eclectic Medical publications;1985, 515.

11 Bartram T. Encyclopedia of Herbal Medicine.Dorset. Grace Publishers;1995.

12 Brinker, Francis ND. *Formulas for Healthful Living.* Sandy, OR: Eclectic Medical Publications;1995.120.

13 Hoffman D. *The Herbal Handbook: A User's Guide to Medical Herbalism.* Rochester, VT: Healing Arts Press, 1988, 77.

14 Felter H, Lloyd JU. King's American Dispensatory. Portland, Oregon: Eclectic Medical Publications. 1983, 17339-41.

15 Grieve M. A Modern Herbal, Dover Publications NY.1971,725.

16 Ellingwood F. American Materia Medica, Therapeutics and Pharmacognosy. Portland, Oregon: Eclectic Medical Publications. 1985, 625.

17 Priest AW, Priest LR. Herbal medication. A clinical dispensary handbook. 1982.

18 Wren RC. Potter's New Cyclopaedia of Botanical drugs and preparations. Essex, UK. Saffron Walden;1988.

19 Witchl M. Herb drugs and phytopharmaceuticals. CRC Press.1994

20 Felter HW. The Eclectic Materia Medica, Pharmacology and Therapeutics. Portland, Oregon: Eclectic Medical publications. 1985.235.

21 Duke J. CRC Handbook of Medicinal Herbs. Boca Raton. CRC Press. 1985. Murray M. The healing power of herbs - The enlightened persons guide to the wonders of medicinal plants. 2nd ed. Prima publishing. Rocklin, Ca. 1995.

22 Leung A, Foster S. Encyclopedia of Common Natural Ingredients. NY: Wiley;1996.

23 Leung A, Foster S. Encyclopedia of Common Natural Ingredients. NY: Wiley;1996.

24 Murray M. The healing power of herbs - The enlightened persons guide to the wonders of medicinal plants. 2nd ed. Prima publishing. Rocklin, Ca. 1995.173-183.

25 Brown D. Encyclopedia of Herbs & Their Uses, Dorling Kindersley Publishing Inc., NY, NY, 1995

26 Weiss RF. *Herbal Medicine.* Gothenberg, Sweden: Ab Arcanum and Beaconsfield: Beaconsfield Publishers Ltd, trans. Meuss AR, 1985, 199.

27 Schulick P. *Herbal Therapy from the Sea.* 1993.

28 Mills S. The Essential Book of Herbal medicine. London. Penguin;1991

29 Felter HW. The Eclectic Materia Medica, Pharmacology and Therapeutics. Portland, Oregon: Eclectic Medical publications. 1985.475-6.

30 Bisset N. Herbal Drugs and Phytopharmaceuticals, Medpharm Scientific Publishers, Stuttgart, 1994, 322-25.

31 Hoffman D. *The Holistic Herbal*. Moray. The Findhorn Press; 1984.185

32 Felter HW. The Eclectic Materia Medica, Pharmacology and Therapeutics. Portland, Oregon. Eclectic Medical publications;1985, 515.

33 Grieve M. A Modern Herbal, Dover Publications NY.1971,725.

34 Ellingwood F. American Materia Medica, Therapeutics and Pharmacognosy. Portland, Oregon: Eclectic Medical Publications. 1985, 625.

35 Wren RC. Potter's New Cyclopaedia of Botanical drugs and preparations. Essex, UK. Saffron Walden;1988.

36 Witchl M. Herb drugs and phytopharmaceuticals. CRC Press.1994

37 Auf'mdold M *et al*. Inhibition by certain extracts of the binding and adenylate cyclase stimulatory effect of bovine thyrotropin in human thyroid membranes. *Endocrin.*,115:527-34,1984.

38 Soulimani R *et al*. Neurotrophic action of the hydroalcoholic extract of Melissa officinalis in the mouse, Planta Med 1991;4;57(2):105-9

MILK THISTLE/YELLOW DOCK SUPREME

*A Skin Corrective Formula**
FORMULA

Milk Thistle Seed	(*Silybum marianum*)
Yellow Dock Root	(*Rumex crispus*)
Burdock Root	(*Arctium lappa*)
Echinacea Root	(*Echinacea spp.*)
Sarsaparilla Root	(*Smilax officinalis*)
Oregon Grape Root	(*Berberis aquifolium*)

Concentration:	1:1 Herb strength ratio
Dosage:	30-40 drops, 3-4 times daily
Duration of use:	3-4 months for best results
Best taken:	Between meals with warm water

DESCRIPTION OF FORMULA

This formula specifically focuses on enhancing the functions of the skin through improved liver metabolism and absorption of endotoxins from the gut. The formula influences conditions such as acne, blackheads, eczema, psoriasis, dandruff, seborrhea and other skin disorders. For these chronic conditions, best results are achieved if taken over 3-4 months.

A traditional use for this formula is as a spring tonic. This alterative effect promotes an improvement in the metabolism by enhancing liver and gut function. It can be used each season for this restorative function for a duration of 2 weeks.

Milk Thistle has been extensively researched. It contains a flavonoid complex, silymarin, that is an antioxidant specific to the liver.[1] Milk Thistle protects the liver from many types of chemical insult. In lab studies it demonstrated protection against a wide variety of agents including carbon tetrachloride, hepatotoxic frog virus and poisons of the *Amanita* Mushroom.[23] Clinical studies have shown success in liver damage, fatty liver hepatitis and hepatic cirrhosis[4] caused by toxic substances or drugs accelerating normalization of impaired liver function.[1,5] Milk Thistle is an important component of this formula as a liver detoxifier.[6]

Yellow Dock Root is a gentle herb that is used as an alterative effecting the skin, gastrointestinal tract and the liver.[7] It is considered a tonic alterative with mild laxative action.[8,9] Native Americans and Eclectic physicians of the last century used Yellow Dock for the treatment of skin conditions.[10] The Eclectic physicians noted that it was particularly useful where lymphatic congestion was present. Yellow Dock improves digestion and reduces liver congestion,[8] making it particularly useful in this formula.

Burdock root is an alterative (improves cellular waste and nutrition) that is similar in action to Yellow Dock.[11,12,13] It has long been used for rheumatism, skin disorders, and to stimulate urination.[10] It is also well known for its ability to stimulate liver/bile related functions.[14] Traditional cancer research reports that is has anti-tumor activity, along with the ability to induce cell differentiation.[11,15]

Echinacea is included in this formula as an immuno-stimulant, whose anti-inflammatory, antibacterial, antiviral, and wound healing properties have been widely reported.[14] Conventional research is beginning to support much of its traditional use, by showing that extracts of Echinacea have the ability to increase antibody production, along with resistance to various infections.[3] Research has further shown that extracts of Echinacea significantly enhance natural killer cell function,[4] and have phagocytic, metabolic and bacteriacidal influence on macrophages.[5] Echinacea has been found to activate cellular immunity.[6]

Oregon Grape root has a history of traditional use closely resembling that of Goldenseal including fever, diarrhea, and arthritis[16]. It contains the alkaloid berberine, which decreases the ability of bacteria to adhere to human cells, thereby preventing infections. This effect has been demonstrated in the throat, digestive tract and urinary system[17]. Oregon Grape is effective topically as an ointment in psoriasis[18] and internally it has a anti-inflammatory effect[19] which also is helpful in psoriasis, eczema and acne.[20]

Sarsaparilla contains saponins that bind endotoxins in the gut. These endotoxins are produced by gut bacteria and can aggravate inflammation throughout the body. [21,22] Sarsaparilla's systemic effects promote the absorption of endotoxins from the gut. Dr. Felter describes its use as a blood purifier and a tonic effecting the whole system. It was used effectively for the chronic, systemic effects of syphilis and gout. In a 1942 study 92 patients with psoriasis were treated and improved with 18% reporting complete clearance and 62% greatly improved.[23]

THERAPEUTIC APPLICATIONS*
Note: The intention of this information is to represent the traditional use of the individual botanicals found in these formulas and to inform the reader of any evolving scientific inquiry relevant to the formula's ingredients.

SUPPORTED BY TRADITIONAL USE

Alterative effecting skin, gastrointestinal tract and liver,[24] treatment of skin conditions,[25] rheumatism, skin disorders, stimulates urination[10] and liver/bile functions.[26] immune-stimulant, anti-inflammatory, [G1, G4] chronic catarrhal (congestive) conditions of the respiratory tract, [G12] increase antibody production,[27] arthritis[28] absorbs endotoxins from the gut,[2930] blood purifier and tonic, for the chronic and systemic effects of syphilis and gout,[31] psoriasis.[32]

SCOPE OF RELEVANT SCIENTIFIC INVESTIGATION

Protect against carbon tetrachloride, hepatotoxic frog virus and poisons of the *Amanita* mushroom.[33,34] Protects against liver damage, fatty liver hepatitis and hepatic cirrhosis.[35] Accelerates normalization of impaired liver function.[1,36] Enhances natural killer cell function, and has phagocytic, metabolic and bactericidal influence on macrophages.[37][38]

CAUTIONS, CONTRA-INDICATIONS AND DRUG INTERACTIONS

Please reference Chapter 9. Do not use during pregnancy or lactation.

COMPLIMENTARY HERBS/FORMULAS

Milk Thistle Liquid Phyto-Cap, Supreme Cleanse, Rejuve-Powder, Red Clover Supreme, Juniper Berry Supreme

REFERENCES

1 S. Foster, Milk Thistle-*Silybum marianum,*. *Botanical Series no. 305,* Austin, Texas., American Botanical Council, 1991

2 Witchl, M. *Herbal Drugs and Phytopharmaceuticals, a Cardui Mariae Fructus,*. *Medpharm,CRC Press: Boca Raton. 1994 Cardui Mariae Fructus,*

3 K. Hruby, *Forum* 8(6), 23 (1984).

4 Feher J, Lang L, *et al.* Free radicals in tissue damage in liver diseases and therapeutic approach. *Tokai J Esp Clin Med* 1986; 11:121-34.

5 H Hikano, Y.Kiso, N.R. Farnsworth, *Economic and Medicinal Plant Research,* Vol. 2. Academic press, New York, 1968, p. 39.

6 S. Foster, ed., *Milk Thistle Bibliography and Abstracts,* American Botanical Council, in press 1995.

7 Hoffman D. *The Herbal Handbook: A User's Guide to Medical Herbalism.* Rochester, VT: Healing Arts Press, 1988,40.

8 Felter H, Lloyd JU. King's American Dispensatory. Portland, Oregon: Eclectic Medical Publications. 1983.

9 Culbreth D. A manual of materia medica and pharmacology. Philadelphia. Lea & Febiger; 1927.

10 Willard T. Wild Rose Scientific Herbal. Wild rose College of Natural Healing; Alberta; 1991.

11 Boik J. Cancer and Natural Medicine: A Textbook of Basic Science and Clinical Research. Oregon   Medical Press, Princeton, MN.1996.

12 Ellingwood F. American Materia Medica, Therapeutics and Pharmacognosy. Portland. Eclectic Medical Publications;1985.

13 Witchl M. (Bisset NG, Ed.) Herbal Drugs and Phytopharmaceuticals. Medpharm, CRC Press: Boca Raton. 1994.

14 Bradley P (Ed.). British herbal Compendium. Dorset. British Herbal Medical Assoc.; 1992.

15 Leung A, Foster S. Encyclopedia of Common Natural Ingredients. NY: Wiley;1996.

16 Duke JA. *Handbook of Medicinal Herbs.* Boca Raton, FL. CRC Press;1985, 287-8.

17 Sun D, Courtney HS, Beachey EH. Berberine sulfate blocks adherence of Streptococcus pyogenes to epithelial cells, fibronectin, and hexadecane. Antimicrob Agents Chemother 1988;32(9):1370-4.

18 Wiesenauer M, Lüdtke R. Mahonia aquifolium in patients with psoriasis vulgaris-an

intraindividual study. Phytomedicine 1996;3:231-5.

19 Galle K, Müller-Jakic B, Proebstle A, *et al.* Analytical and pharmacological studies on
Mahonia aquifolium. Phytomedicine 1994;1:59-62.

20 Murray M. The healing power of herbs - The enlightened persons guide to the wonders of medicinal plants. Rocklin, Ca. Prima publishing;1995.

21 Murray M. The healing power of herbs - The enlightened persons guide to the wonders of medicinal plants. Rocklin, Ca. Prima publishing;1995. 302-306

22 Blumenthal M, Busse WR, Goldberg A, et al, eds. The Complete Commission E Monographs: Therapeutic Guide to Herbal Medicines. Boston, MA: Integrative Medicine Communications, 1998, 372-3.

23 Thurman FM: *The treatment of psoriasis with sarsaparilla compound*, New Engl J Med 227, 128-133,1942

24 Hoffman D. *The Herbal Handbook: A User's Guide to Medical Herbalism.* Rochester, VT: Healing Arts Press, 1988,40.

25 Willard T. Wild Rose Scientific Herbal. Wild rose College of Natural Healing; Alberta; 1991.

26 Bradley P (Ed.). British herbal Compendium. Dorset. British Herbal Medical Assoc.; 1992.

27 Snow JM. Echinacea (Moench) Spp. Asteraceae. The Protocol Journal of Botanical Medicine. 1997; 2 (2): 18-24.

28 Duke JA. *Handbook of Medicinal Herbs.* Boca Raton, FL. CRC Press;1985, 287-8.

29 Murray M. The healing power of herbs - The enlightened persons guide to the wonders of medicinal plants. Rocklin, Ca. Prima publishing;1995. 302-306

30 Blumenthal M, Busse WR, Goldberg A, et al, eds. The Complete Commission E Monographs: Therapeutic Guide to Herbal Medicines. Boston, MA: Integrative Medicine Communications, 1998, 372-3.

31 Felter H, Lloyd JU. King's American Dispensatory. Portland, Oregon: Eclectic Medical Publications. 1983.

32 Thurman FM: *The treatment of psoriasis with sarsaparilla compound*, New Engl J Med 227, 128-133,1942

33 Witchl, M. *Herbal Drugs and Phytopharmaceuticals, a Cardui Mariae Fructus,.* Medpharm,CRC Press: Boca Raton. 1994 *Cardui Mariae Fructus,*

34 K. Hruby, *Forum* 8(6), 23 (1984).

35 Feher J, Lang L, *et al.* Free radicals in tissue damage in liver diseases and therapeutic approach. *Tokai J Esp Clin Med* 1986; 11:121-34.

36 H Hikano, Y.Kiso, N.R. Farnsworth, *Economic and Medicinal Plant Research,* Vol. 2. Academic press, New York, 1968, p. 39.

37 Schranner I, Wurdinger M, *et al.* Modification of avian humeral immunoreactions by Influx and Echinacea angustifolia extract. Zentralbl Veterinarmed (B) 1989; 36.

38 Bukovsky M, Kostalova D, Magnusova R, Vaverkova S. Testing for immunomodulating effects of ethanol-water extracts of the above ground parts of the plants Echinaceae and Rudbeckia. Cesk Farm. 1993; 42.

OSHA SUPREME

*An Anti-Bronchitis Formula**
FORMULA

Osha Root	(*Ligusticum porteri*)
Echinacea root	(*Echinacea angustifolia and purpurea*)
Goldenseal Root	(*Hydrastis canadensis*)
Mullein Leaf	(*Verbascum olympicum*)
Lungwort Lichen	(*Sticta pulmonaria*)
Garlic bulb	(*Allium sativum*)
Licorice root	(*Glycyrrhiza glabra*)
Elecampane root	(*Inula helenium*)
Yerba Santa Leaf	(*Eriodictyon californicum*)
Irish Moss	(*Chondrus crispus*)

Concentration:	1:1 Herb strength ratio
Dosage:	30-40 drops, 4-6 times daily
Duration of use:	2-4 weeks or as needed for an acute infection
Best taken:	Shortly before meals, with warm water

DESCRIPTION OF FORMULA

The soothing demulcent principles target the lungs and respiratory membranes. These herbs are antiviral, antibacterial, expectorant, anti-tussive(cough) and anti-inflammatory.

Oshá Root has been used traditionally as an expectorant for bronchial congestion.[1] A similar plant in China has been used for centuries as a remedy for viral infections including influenza, the common cold, rheumatism, bruises, headache and menstrual cramps.[2, 3, 4] Its active component is a ligustilide shows antispasmodic activity.[5]

This formula contains the **Echinacea Supreme** formula. More information about the immune stimulant, antiviral and antibiotic properties is available about this formula on page 201.

Goldenseal root is native to North America. It has traditionally been used with infectious, allergic and inflammatory conditions that require soothing of the mucous membranes.[6 7] Goldenseal contains the antibiotic and immunostimulant [8] alkaloids berberine and hydrastine, that are antispasmodic. [9]

Mullein leaf and flower are approved in Germany for use in supporting a healthy respiratory tract.[10] In traditional herbalism it is respected for relieving the common cold, coughs, chronic bronchitis, and ear infections.[11 12] It has shown antiviral, specifically anti-influenza, activity in test tube studies.[13]

Lungwort Lichen is a remedy for pain and cough. Irritative coughs both acute and chronic are affected. Indicated for the cough that accompanies bronchitis, hay fever, influenza and whooping cough.[14] Aids in the reduction of fever, chills and night sweats.[15]

Garlic bulb is mentioned in some of the oldest written records that exist, dating back to 2600 BC in the Middle East. It is repeatedly mentioned in traditional medicine as a remedy for coughs, the common cold, lung infections, diarrhea, worm infestations, and a large number of other problems.[16] Garlic and its various constituents have repeatedly been shown to be antibacterial and antiviral in the test tube.[17] Garlic can also stimulate immune cells in laboratory tests.[18] Garlic also helps support a healthy cardiovascular system.[19]

Licorice Root is used for cough and bronchitis. Its expectorant qualities especially in the area of the trachea.[20,21] It has anti-inflammatory and anti-allergy properties. Licorice enhances the immune response and has antiviral properties by stimulating the body to produce interferon.[22]

Elecampane Root is used in bronchitis, asthma, and whooping cough.[23] The active constituents are 1-4% volatile oils composed of sesquiterpene lactones, inulin (44%) and mucilage.[24] It provides relief by assisting expectoration of mucous. It is used in combination with other remedies when treating chronic lung problems such as asthma.[25]

Yerba Santa Leaf is effective for coughs as an expectorant. It decreases the mucous secretions and inflammation with bronchitis.[26 27]

Irish Moss is used traditionally for coughs in European herbalism.[28]

THERAPEUTIC APPLICATIONS*

Note: The intention of this information is to represent the traditional use of the individual botanicals found in these formulas and to inform the reader of any evolving scientific inquiry relevant to the formula's ingredients.

SUPPORTED BY TRADITIONAL USE

Expectorant for bronchial congestion,[29] chronic bronchitis, and ear infections.[30][31] Used for viral infections including influenza, the common cold,[32][33][34] having immune stimulant, antibiotic[35][36] and antispasmodic properties.[37] Supports a healthy respiratory tract.[38] Cough that accompanies bronchitis, hay fever, influenza and whooping cough.[39][40][41][42]

SCOPE OF RELEVANT SCIENTIFIC INVESTIGATION

Shows antiviral, specifically anti-influenza, activity in test tube studies.[43] Enhances the immune response and has antiviral properties by stimulating the body to produce interferon.[44] Antibacterial and antiviral in the test tube.[45] Garlic stimulates immune cells in laboratory tests.[46]

CAUTIONS, CONTRA-INDICATIONS AND DRUG INTERACTIONS

Please reference Chapter 9. Do not use during pregnancy or lactation.

COMPLIMENTARY HERBS/FORMULAS

Wild Cherry Supreme, Lomatium/Osha Supreme, Echinacea Goldenseal Throat Spray

REFERENCES

1 Brinker, Francis ND. *Formulas for Healthful Living.* Sandy, OR: Eclectic Medical Publications;1995, 83-4.

2 Moore M. *Medicinal Plants of the Mountain West.* Santa Fe: Museum of New Mexico Press, 1979:119-21.

3 Curtin LSM; Moore M (ed). *Healing Herbs of the Upper Rio Grande: Traditional Medicine of the Southwest.* Santa Fe: Western Edge Press, 1947, reprinted 1997:121-4.

4 Leung AY, Foster S. *Encyclopedia of Common Natural Ingredients Used in Food, Drugs and Cosmetics* 2nd ed. New York: John Wiley & Sons Inc., 1996:552-3.

5 Ko WC *et al.*, Phytochemical studies on spasmolytic constituents of Lingusticum wallichii Franch, Hua Hsueh, (3):74-6, 1978, (chem.Abs.92:37764c)

6 Wren RC. Potter's New Cyclopaedia of Botanical drugs and preparations. Essex, UK. Saffron Walden;1988.

7 Murray M. The healing power of herbs - The enlightened persons guide to the wonders of medicinal plants. Rocklin, Ca. Prima publishing; 1995,230-234.

8 Murray M. The healing power of herbs - The enlightened persons guide to the wonders of medicinal plants. Rocklin, Ca. Prima publishing;1995.

9 Bradley P (Ed.). British herbal Compendium. Dorset. British Herbal Medical Assoc.; 1992.

10 Blumenthal M, Busse WR, Goldberg A, *et al.* (eds). *The Complete German Commission E Monographs: Therapeutic Guide to Herbal Medicines*. Austin: American Botanical Council and Boston: Integrative Medicine Communications, 1998:173.

11 Felter HW. *Eclectic Materia Medica, Pharmacology and Therapeutics*. Sandy, OR: Eclectic Medical Publications, 1922, reprinted 1998:693.

12 Weiss RF. *Herbal Medicine*. Gothenberg, Sweden: Ab Arcanum and Beaconsfield: Beaconsfield Publishers Ltd, trans. Meuss AR, 1985, 197-8.

13 Zgórniak-Nowosielska I, Grzybek J, Manolova N, *et al.* Antiviral activity of flos verbasci infusion against influenza and herpes simplex viruses. *Arch Immunol Ther Exp* 1991;39:103-8.

14 Felter H, Lloyd JU. King's American Dispensatory. Portland. Eclectic medical Publications; 1983.1835-6.

15 Felter HW. The Eclectic Materia Medica, Pharmacology and Therapeutics. Portland, Oregon: Eclectic Medical publications. 1985,655.

16 Koch HP, Lawson LD (eds). Garlic: *The Science and Therapeutic Application of* Allium sativum *L and Related Species*, 2nd ed. Baltimore: Williams & Wilkins, 1996:1-24.

17 Reuter HD. *Allium sativum and Allium ursinum:* part 2. Pharmacology and medicinal application. Phytomedicine 1995;2:73-91.

18 Salman H, Bergman M, Bessler H, *et al.* Effect of a garlic derivative (alliin) on peripheral blood cell immune responses. *Int J Immunopharmacol* 1999;21:589-97.

19 Warshafsky S, Kamer RS, Sivak SL. Effect of garlic on total serum cholesterol: A meta-analysis. *Ann Intern Med* 1993;119:599-605.

20 Bradley P (Ed.). British herbal Compendium. Dorset. British Herbal Medical Assoc.; 1992.145-7

21 Hikano H. Economic and Medicinal Plant Research, Volume 1, London, Academic Press. 1985,53-85.

22 Murray M. op sit.

23 Leung AY, Foster S. Encyclopedia of Common Natural Ingredients Used in Food, Drugs, and Cosmetics. New York: John Wiley & Sons, 1996, 222-4.

24 Wichtl M. Herbal Drugs and Phytopharmaceuticals. Boca Raton, FL: CRC Press, 1994, 254-6.

25 Grieve M. A Modern Herbal, Jonathan Cape, London, 1931. 281

26 MooreM. Medicinal Plants of the Northwest, red Crane Books, Santa Fe, 265-6

27 Felter HW. The Eclectic Materia Medica, Pharmacology and Therapeutics. Portland, Oregon: Eclectic Medical publications. 1985.361.

28 Weiss RF. *Herbal Medicine*. Gothenberg, Sweden: Ab Arcanum and Beaconsfield: Beaconsfield Publishers Ltd, trans. Meuss AR, 1985, 199.

29 Brinker, Francis ND. *Formulas for Healthful Living*. Sandy, OR: Eclectic Medical Publications;1995, 83-4.

30 Felter HW. *Eclectic Materia Medica, Pharmacology and Therapeutics.* Sandy, OR: Eclectic Medical Publications, 1922, reprinted 1998:693.

31 Weiss RF. *Herbal Medicine.* Gothenberg, Sweden: Ab Arcanum and Beaconsfield: Beaconsfield Publishers Ltd, trans. Meuss AR, 1985, 197-8.

32 Moore M. *Medicinal Plants of the Mountain West.* Santa Fe: Museum of New Mexico Press, 1979:119-21.

33 Curtin LSM; Moore M (ed). *Healing Herbs of the Upper Rio Grande: Traditional Medicine of the Southwest.* Santa Fe: Western Edge Press, 1947, reprinted 1997:121-4.

34 Leung AY, Foster S. *Encyclopedia of Common Natural Ingredients Used in Food, Drugs and Cosmetics* 2nd ed. New York: John Wiley & Sons Inc., 1996:552-3.

35 Wren RC. Potter's New Cyclopaedia of Botanical drugs and preparations. Essex, UK. Saffron Walden;1988.

36 Murray M. The healing power of herbs - The enlightened persons guide to the wonders of medicinal plants. Rocklin, Ca. Prima publishing; 1995,230-234.

37 Bradley P (Ed.). British herbal Compendium. Dorset. British Herbal Medical Assoc.; 1992.

38 Blumenthal M, Busse WR, Goldberg A, *et al.* (eds). *The Complete German Commission E Monographs: Therapeutic Guide to Herbal Medicines.* Austin: American Botanical Council and Boston: Integrative Medicine Communications, 1998:173.

39 Felter H, Lloyd JU. King's American Dispensatory. Portland. Eclectic medical Publications; 1983.1835-6.

40 Koch HP, Lawson LD (eds). *Garlic: The Science and Therapeutic Application of* Allium sativum *L and Related Species,* 2nd ed. Baltimore: Williams & Wilkins, 1996:1-24.

41 Bradley P (Ed.). British herbal Compendium. Dorset. British Herbal Medical Assoc.; 1992.145-7

42 Hikano H. Economic and Medicinal Plant Research, Volume 1, London, Academic Press. 1985,53-85.

43 Zgórniak-Nowosielska I, Grzybek J, Manolova N, *et al.* Antiviral activity of flos verbasci infusion against influenza and herpes simplex viruses. *Arch Immunol Ther Exp* 1991;39:103-8.

44 Murray M. op sit.

45 Reuter HD. *Allium sativum and Allium ursinum:* part 2. Pharmacology and medicinal application. *Phytomedicine* 1995;2:73-91.

46 Salman H, Bergman M, Bessler H, *et al.* Effect of a garlic derivative (alliin) on peripheral blood cell immune responses. *Int J Immunopharmacol* 1999;21:589-97.

47 Merck Index, 10th ed. Merck &Co. Rahway,NJ,1983, 796-7.

PHYTO PRŌZ SUPREME (FORMERLY ST. JOHN'S WORT) SUPREME

A Formula to Improve the Mood and Sense of Well Being *
FORMULA

Kava Kava	(*Piper methysticum*)
St. John's Wort	(*Hypericum perforatum*)
Wild Oats Milky seed	(*Avena sativa*)
Passionflower,	(*Passiflora incarnata*)
Gotu Kola	(*Centella asiatica*)
Schizandra Berry	(*Schisandra chinensis*)
Siberian Ginseng root	(*Eleutherococcus senticosus*)
Nettle Seed	(*Urtica dioica*)
Calamus Root	(*Acorus calamus*)
Prickly Ash Bark	(*Xanthoxylum clava-herculis*)

Concentration:	1:1 Herb strength ratio
Dosage:	30-40 drops, 3-4 times daily
Duration of use:	3-4 months for best results
Best taken:	Between meals with warm water

DESCRIPTION OF FORMULA

This compound synergistically enhances emotional well being through a number of different strategies. The strategic objective of the formula is to:

a. Inhibit seratonin re-uptake

b. Promote seratonin uptake at its receptors

c. Promote seratonin release

d. Elevate intra-cellular cyclic AMP levels

e. Inhibit mono-amine oxidase

f. Provide tropho-restoration to the vital nerve centers

Is used to improve the mood and promote a feeling of wellbeing. Decreases anxiety, relaxes muscles and reduces

pain. Increases nerve impulse transmitters within the brain, which maintain emotional stability and promote a general feeling of balance and happiness. Provides liver support and restoration, strengthens nerve integrity, and promotes general adaptive integrity.

Kava kava has been used in Polynesia and Hawaii as a social lubricant because of its mild psychotropic effects. The definition of Piper methysticum is 'intoxicating pepper.'[1] In Europe it is used for anxiety, mild insomnia, nervous tension and as a muscle relaxant.[2] The active ingredients are kavalactones. In a six month randomized placebo controlled study with 100 people with tension and anxiety produced significant results after two months with even better results in 6 months.[3] Another study showed improvement in anxiety symptoms after one week of treatment. The effect as a muscle relaxant appears to be a direct effect on the contractility of the muscle rather than a relaxing effect on the nerve conduction.[4] Kava has become a mainstream herbal product in the U.S. and holds promise as an anticonvulsant and anxiolytic actions. The mechanisms for its CNS activity is not characteristic of morphine, aspirin or other pain relievers.[5]

St. John's Wort has been used as a medicine for more than 2000 years. It is an effective antidepressant. In several recent studies when compared to standard antidepressant drugs it proves as effective, better tolerated and has much fewer side effects.[6] St. John's Wort has been shown to be effective in Seasonal Affective Disorder(SAD).[7] It has also been shown to increase libido in contrast to conventional medications. In addition to its antidepressant effect, it also is a valuable anti-inflammatory[8], wound healing[9] and antiviral agent.[10]

Wild Oat milky seed has a reputation as a trophorestorative (builds nervous reserve).[11] It is useful in states of nervous debility, exhaustion, depression, sleeplessness and wherever convalescence is required for chronic conditions and cardiac weakness.[12,13] An acute indication for use is for a headache from over work. "It is not a remedy of great power...probably its chief value as a medicine is to energize in nervous exhaustion" HarveyW. Felter, MD.[14]

Passionflower is used as a sedative to reduce restlessness and produce rest. It has wide application as an antispasmodic for the

GI and nervous system. It is indicated for the pain of neuralgia.[15] A flavonoid, vitexin acts as a anti-inflammatory and lowers blood pressure.[16]

Gotu Kola is considered to be one of the so-called 'elixirs of life'. [17,1819] It has long been used in India to improve intelligence and mental function. [G3] Several studies suggest that Gotu Kola may be useful with improving memory, reducing fatigue and stress, increasing general mental ability, and increasing I.Q. in developmentally disabled children. [G3, 2]

Schizandra Berry is an adaptogen, enhancing resistance to external and internal stress. It increases mental alertness and athletic performance. Its effect is compared to Milk Thistle with similar mechanisms of action including antioxidant effects focused on the liver.[20] It is an effective cholagogue and is used in China for nonjaundice (chronic) hepatitis.[21]

Siberian Ginseng root has been in use in China for over 4000 years. Used regularly, it is said to increase longevity, improve general health, improve the appetite, and restore memory.[2] Today, as an adaptogen, it is known to produce improvement in overall metabolic efficiency, as well as to increase resistance to disease and stressful influences. [G3, G4]

Nettle seed is able to exert numerous effects on the signals sent by the immune system that provoke chronic inflammation. Studies have shown that nettle can block formation of pro-inflammatory cytokines[22] and prostaglandins.[23] It may even be able to convert some T-cells into forms that inhibit rather than promote inflammatory reactions.[24] Nettle leaf and seed were widely used in traditional medicine to relieve arthritis pain, help fight bladder infections, and for gout, chronic skin diseases such as eczema, autoimmune diseases such as lupus and rheumatoid arthritis, bleeding, diarrhea, kidney inflammations, wounds, and sciatica.[25]

Calamus Root (Sweet Flag) has a very long history of use. It is used worldwide by many cultures including American Indians where it was used almost universally for a very wide variety of ailments.[26] It is described as an aromatic bitter that has a powerful tonic effect on the stomach, encouraging secretory activity and increasing the appetite. It is used with people who have lost their appetite in cancer, and in cases of Anorexia nervosa.[27] In Ayurvedic medicine it is specifically indicated for sedative and analgesic properties. It lowers the blood pressure and respiration moderately.[28]

Prickly Ash bark is considered a ideal gastric stimulant when poor digestion needs assistance or constipation is present. It is a potent alterative and has a long history of use with chronic muscular rheumatism, lumbar back pain, and myalgia. Dr. Felter gave it high marks when the nerve force is low and neural irritation is present but where recuperation is possible.[29]

THERAPEUTIC APPLICATIONS*

Note: The intention of the following information is to represent the traditional use of the individual botanicals found in these formulas and to inform the reader of any evolving scientific inquiry relevant to the formula's ingredients.

SUPPORTED BY TRADITIONAL USE

Tension and anxiety,[30] nervous debility, exhaustion, depression, sleeplessness, [31,32] An acute indication is headache from over work, [33] sedative, reduces fatigue and restlessness, antispasmodic, neuralgia,[34] increasing general mental ability. [G3]

SCOPE OF RELEVANT SCIENTIFIC INVESTIGATION

Anxiety, insomnia, nervous tension, muscle relaxant,[35] anticonvulsant and anxiolytic actions,[36] antidepressant effects,[37] Seasonal Affective Disorder(SAD).[38]

CAUTIONS, CONTRA-INDICATIONS AND DRUG INTERACTIONS

Please reference Chapter 9. Do not use during pregnancy or lactation. Kava may potentiate the effect of alcohol and should not be used with it. Photosensitivity to St. John's Wort has occurred in rare instances—avoid excessive exposure to light when taking. See your physician if taking a pharmaceutical MAO-inhibitor.

Schizandra may potentiate some medications including calcium channel blockers and corticosteroids.

COMPLIMENTARY HERBS/FORMULAS

Siberian Ginseng Tonic Elixir, St. Johns wort Professional Strength, St. John's Wort Liquid Phyto-Cap™

REFERENCES

1 Singh,Y.D. and Blumenthal, M. (1997) Kava: and overview. Special review reprinted and updated from Singh, Y.D.Kava:an overview. Journal of Ethnopharmacology 1992; 37:13-45.

2 Lehmann, E., Kinzler, E. and Friedmann, J. Efficacy of a special kava extract, in patients with states of anxiety, tension, and excitedness of non-mental origin, Phytomedicine 1996; 3:113-119.

3 Volz, H.P. and Kieser, N.Kava-kava extract WS 1490 versus placebo in anxiety disorders.Pharmacopsychiatry 1997;30: 1-5.

4 Singh,Y.N. Effects of dava on meuromuscular transmissionand muscle contractility. Journal of Ethnopharmacology, 7:267-276,1983.

5 Murray M. The healing power of herbs - The enlightened persons guide to the wonders of medicinal plants. Rocklin, Ca. Prima publishing;1995.210-219.

6 Linde, K., Ramirez, G., Mulrow, C.D. et al. (1996). St. John's Wort for depression-an overview and meta analysis of randomized clinical trials. British Medical Journal 313:253-258.

7 Wheatley D. Hypericum in seasonal affective disorder (SAD). Curr Med Res Opin 1999; 15:33-37

8 Wren RC. Potter's New Cyclopaedia of Botanical drugs and preparations. Essex, UK. Saffron Walden;1988.

9 Hobbs C:St. John's Wort, *Hypericum perforatum L. Herbalgram* 18/19, 24-33, 1989.

10 Leung A, Foster S. Encyclopedia of Common Natural Ingredients. NY: Wiley;1996, 310-312.

11 Priest AW, Priest LR. Herbal medication. A clinical dispensary handbook. 1982.

12 Wren RC. Potter's New Cyclopaedia of Botanical drugs and preparations. Essex, UK. Saffron Walden;1988.

13 Witchl M. Herb drugs and phytopharmaceuticals. CRC Press.1994

14 Felter HW. The Eclectic Materia Medica, Pharmacology and Therapeutics. Portland, Oregon: Eclectic Medical publications. 1985.235.

15 Felter H, Lloyd JU. King's American Dispensatory. Portland. Eclectic medical Publications; 1983.1140.

16 Brinker, Francis ND. *Formulas for Healthful Living.* Sandy, OR: Eclectic Medical Publications;1995.120.

17 Duke J. CRC Handbook of Medicinal Herbs. Boca Raton. CRC Press. 1985. Murray M. The healing power of herbs - The enlightened persons guide to the wonders of medicinal plants. 2nd ed. Prima publishing. Rocklin, Ca. 1995.

18 Leung A, Foster S. Encyclopedia of Common Natural Ingredients. NY: Wiley;1996.

19 Murray M. The healing power of herbs - The enlightened persons guide to the wonders of medicinal plants. 2nd ed. Prima publishing. Rocklin, Ca. 1995.173-183.

20 Bensky and Gamble. Chinese Herbal Medicine: Materia Medica. Seattle, Eastland Press,1986,541-2

21 Huang KC. *The Pharmacology of Chinese Herbs.* CRC Press: Boca Raton. 1993,201.

22 Obertreis B, Ruttkowski T, Teucher T, et al. Ex-vivo in-vitro inhibition of lipopolysaccharide stimulated tumor necrosis factor-_ and interleukin-1_ secretion in human whole blood by extractum Urticae dioicae foliorum. *Arzneim Forsch* 1996;46:389-94.

23 Obertreis B, Giller K, *et al.* (1996) Antiphlogistic effects of *Urtica dioica* folia extract in comparison to caffeic malic acid. *Arzneim Forsch* 1996;46:52-6 [in German].

24 Klingelhoefer S, Obertreis B, Quast S, Behnke B. Antirheumatic effect of IDS 23, a stinging nettle leaf extract, on in vitro expression of T helper cytokines. *J Rheumatol* 1999;26:2517-22.

25 Yarnell E. Stinging nettle: A modern view of an ancient healing plant. *Altern Complem Ther* 1998;4:180-6.

26 Motley T, The Ethnobotany of Sweet Flag, Acorus calamus. Economic botany, Vol. 48, No.4,1994, pp.397-412

27 Weiss R. Herbal medicine. Beaconsfield, UK. Beaconsfield Publishers;1985.45-6.

28 Kapoor LD. *Handbook of Ayurvedic Medicinal Plants.* CRC Press: Boca Raton. 1990,18-19.

29 Felter HW. The Eclectic Materia Medica, Pharmacology and Therapeutics. Portland, Oregon: Eclectic Medical publications. 1985.697-8

30 Volz, H.P. and Kieser, N.Kava-kava extract WS 1490 versus placebo in anxiety disorders.Pharmacopsychiatry 1997;30: 1-5.

31 Wren RC. Potter's New Cyclopaedia of Botanical drugs and preparations. Essex, UK. Saffron Walden;1988.

32 Witchl M. Herb drugs and phytopharmaceuticals. CRC Press.1994

33 Felter HW. The Eclectic Materia Medica, Pharmacology and Therapeutics. Portland, Oregon: Eclectic Medical publications. 1985.235.

34 Felter H, Lloyd JU. King's American Dispensatory. Portland. Eclectic medical Publications; 1983.1140.

35 Lehmann, E., Kinzler, E. and Friedmann, J. Efficacy of a special kava extract, in patients with states of anxiety, tension, and excitedness of non-mental origin, Phytomedicine 1996; 3:113-119.

36 Murray M. The healing power of herbs - The enlightened persons guide to the wonders of medicinal plants. Rocklin, Ca. Prima publishing;1995.210-219.

37 Linde, K., Ramirez, G., Mulrow, C.D. *et al.* (1996). St. John's Wort for depression-an overview and meta analysis of randomized clinical trials. British Medical Journal 313:253-258.

38 Wheatley D. Hypericum in seasonal affective disorder (SAD). Curr Med Res Opin 1999; 15:33-37

PHYTO QUENCH SUPREME

A Whole Body Plant Anti-Oxidant*
FORMULA

Green Tea	(*Camellia sinensis*)
Turmeric Root	(*Curcuma longa*)
Ginkgo leaf	(*Ginkgo biloba*)
Licorice root	(*Glycyrrhiza glabra*)
Siberian Ginseng Root	(*Eleutherococcus senticosus*)
Rosemary Leaf	(*Rosmarinus officinalis*)
Thyme Leaf	(*Thymus vulgaris*)
Schizandra Berry	(*Schisandra chinensis*)
Ginger Root	(*Zingiber officinale*)

Concentration:	1:1 Herb strength ratio
Dosage:	40-50 drops, 3 times daily
Duration of use:	Used as a maintenance formula for best results
Best taken:	Between meals with warm water

DESCRIPTION OF FORMULA

Cancer is the second most common cause of death in the US. This formula has been designed to include those herbs that traditional herbal medicine and the research literature suggest are most protective against cancer. These herbs contain powerful free radical scavenging antioxidants that are also anti-inflammatory and make this an excellent health maintenance formula.

Green Tea: A growing body of research has demonstrated green tea polyphenols to be powerful antioxidants with anti-cancer properties. These compounds, which account for 30-40% of the extractable solids of green tea leaves are believe to mediate many of the cancer chemoprotective effects. Mechanism of action may include antioxidant and free radical scavenging activity and stimulation of detoxification systems. Current studies are hopeful as they show an inverse association between green tea consumption and cancer risk.[1,2] Green tea is considered to be partly responsible for the low incidence of free radical-related conditions in Japan, China, and other places where green tea is widely consumed.[3]

Turmeric Root has been show to have anticancer activity by inhibiting cancer's initiation, promotion and progression.[4,5] It has demonstrated an ability to inhibit oxidative damage to DNA, [6,7] exhibits protective effects against several chemical carcinogens[8] and its use results in decreased levels of urinary mutagens.[9] Turmeric has systemic antioxidant,[10] anti-inflammatory, and liver protective effects.[11,12] The volatile oils in Turmeric are the most active components. Curcumin is a potent antioxidant and combats free radicals better than vitamin E.[13] Turmeric inhibits leukotriene formation, platelet aggregation, and excessive neutrophil response involved in the inflammation process by stabilizing the cell membranes.[14] In one clinical trial patients with rheumatoid arthritis using curcumin were compared with those using tophenlybutazone. The improvements in activities of daily living were comparable, but without the side-effects.[15] Curcumin is an effective analgesic as it depletes the nerve endings of substance P, the neurotransmitter of pain receptors.[16]

Ginkgo leaf A great wealth of studies in the past 50 years have thoroughly documented the antioxidant activity of this versatile herb.[17,18] Ginkgo's antioxidant effects appear to be most pronounced in the brain, nerves and cardiovascular system.[19,20] In addition to quenching single oxygen free radicals, ginkgo is also able to eliminate excessive nitric oxide, another type of free radical.[21]

Ginkgo leaf has been shown to reduce symptoms related to Alzheimer's disease[22,23] and Cerebral vascular insufficiency (CVI), including impaired mental performance, dizziness, headache, depression, ringing in the ears, and short-term memory loss.[24,25]

Licorice root blocks the breakdown of the body's own cortisol,[26] producing an anti-inflammatory effect throughout the body. The presence of higher amounts of natural cortisol would also tend to act to moderate excessive immune reactions. Studies suggest that in fact part of the benefit of licorice in people with hepatitis is mediated by the immune system.[27] It has been shown to support normal liver function and prevent long-term problems in people with hepatitis C as well as other forms of viral hepatitis.[28, 29, 30] Licorice has been used in traditional Western herbalism as a demulcent and expectorant for coughs,[31] to heal stomach ulcers,[32] to relieve Addison's disease (low adrenal function),[33] and for people with asthma, diabetes, urinary tract infections, tumors, and pain.[34] In traditional Chinese herbalism, licorice was widely used to synergize formulas by making the other herbs work well together.[35]

Siberian Ginseng root has been in use in China for over 4000 years. Used regularly, it is said to increase longevity, improve general health, improve the appetite, and restore memory.[2] Today, as an adaptogen, it is known to produce improvement in overall metabolic efficiency, as well as to increase resistance to disease and stressful influences.[36, 37]

Ginseng has a protective effect against radiation in animal studies.[38] The Russian research literature suggests that Siberian ginseng has a carcinostatic effect, slowing the spread of metastasis.[39]

Rosemary leaf has been demonstrated in numerous studies to be a powerful antioxidant.[40] Traditional reports of the benefits of rosemary include improving dementia and poor memory ("weakness of the brain"), preventing and eliminating infections, headaches, digestive upset, flatulence, colic, dandruff, edema and palpitations.[41]

Thyme Leaf is an antispasmodic and expectorant and is indicated in bronchitis, laryngitis, and whooping cough. It has been used in cancer.[42]

Schizandra's adaptogenic ability to increase overall physical performance, and endurance[43] has been compared to that of Siberian Ginseng.[44] It has been found to possess anti-depressant, immuno-modulatory, and blood pressure regulating properties. It is also used as a powerful liver protectant,[G3, 45] and as an aphrodisiac[G4] with pronounced influence on both male and female sexuality.[46] Use of Schizandra has been shown to result in modification of the physiological response to stress.[47]

Schizandra berry is a valued kidney and male tonic of the Traditional Chinese system of medicine.[G3] Within this system it is often referred to as a 'king' or 'harmonizing' remedy, alluding to the broad-reaching influence of this small 'five flavored' berry.[G17] Schizandra has also been shown to increase liver cyclic AMP (see cAMP - Coleus Forskohlii Supreme).[G3]

Ginger Root is used in traditional medicine to stimulate the appetite, treat nausea, diarrhea, indigestion and as a carminative (reduces intestinal gas).[G3, G4] In addition to these benefits, Ginger is useful here as a circulatory stimulant,[G3, G4] helping to deliver the entire formula throughout the body. Ginger is well known as an antispasmodic.[48,49,50,51] Traditionally, Ginger has also been recognized as having use with painful menstruation [G12] and uterine cramping. [13] Ginger has strong antioxidant properties and is one of the most powerful botanical inhibitors of 5-lipoxygenase,[52] an enzyme responsible for excessive production of pro-inflammatory prostaglandins and thromboxanes. Ginger is used in many traditional Ayurvedic formulas that were traditionally employed in people with arthritis and other inflammatory disorders.[53] Ginger is also valued in traditional Western herbalism for arthritis, rheumatism, muscle aches, migraine, and flatulence.[54]

THERAPEUTIC APPLICATIONS*

Note: The intention of the following information is to represent the traditional use of the individual botanicals found in these formulas and to inform the reader of any evolving scientific inquiry relevant to the formula's ingredients.

SUPPORTED BY TRADITIONAL USE

Increase overall physical performance, and endurance,[55] resistance to disease and stressful influences,[56, 57] circulatory stimulant.[G3, G4]

SCOPE OF RELEVANT SCIENTIFIC INVESTIGATION

<u>Antioxidants with anticancer properties</u>, mediate many of the cancer chemoprotective effects, free radical scavenging activity, stimulation of detoxification systems, inverse association between green tea consumption and cancer risk." [58, 59] anticancer activity by inhibiting cancer's, initiation, promotion and progression,[60, 61] inhibit oxidative damage to DNA, [62, 63] protective effects against several chemical carcinogens,[64] decreases urinary mutagens,[65] inhibits leukotriene formation, platelet aggregation, excessive neutrophil response involved in inflammation.[66]

CAUTIONS, CONTRA-INDICATIONS AND DRUG INTERACTIONS

Please reference Chapter 9. Do not use during pregnancy or lactation.

COMPLIMENTARY HERBS/FORMULAS

Anti-Oxidant Supreme, Vision Enhancement, Cell Wise

REFERENCES

1 Brown MD. Review of green tea's role in cancer prevention. *Alt Med Rev* 1999;4(5):360-70.

2 Katiyar SK, Agarwal R, Mukhtar H. Inhibition of spontaneous and photo-enhanced lipid peroxidation in mouse epidermal microsomes by epicatechin derivatives from green tea. *Cancer Lett* 1994;79:61-66.

3 Imai K, Nakachi K. Cross sectional study of effects of drinking green tea on cardiovascular and liver diseases. *BMJ* 1995;310:693-6.

4 Murray, M. The healing power of herbs-Rocklin, Ca Prima publishing; 1995, 328..

5 Nagabhushan N and Bhide SV: Nonmutagenicity of curcumin and its antimutagenic action versus chili and capsiacin, *Nutr Cancer* 8, 201-210, 1986.

6 Shalini VK and Srinivas L: Lipid peroxide induced DNA damage: Protection by turmeric . *Mol Cell Biochem* 77,3-10,1989.

7 Srivivas L and Shalini VK: DNA damage by smoke; Protection by turmeric and other inhibitors of ROS. *Free Radical Biol Med* 11,277-283, 1991.

8 Boone CW, Steele VE, and Delloff GJ: Screening of chemopreventive (anticarcinogenic) compounds in rodents. *Mutat Res* 267, 251-255,1992.

9 Polasa K, *et al.*: Effect of turmeric on urinary mutagens in smokers. *Mutagenesis* 7, 107-109, 1992.

10 Snow JM. *Curcuma longa* L. (Zingiberaceae). The Protocol Journal of Botanical Medicine. 1995; 1(2):43-46.

11 Wren RC. Potter's New Cyclopaedia of Botanical drugs and preparations. Essex, UK. Saffron Walden;1988.

12 Bartram T. Encyclopedia of Herbal Medicine.Dorset. Grace Publishers;1995.

13 Shama OP: Antioxidant properties of curcumin and related compounds. Biochem Pharmacol 25,1811-18-1825, 1976.

14 Satoskar RR,: Evaluation of anti-inflammatory property of curcumin in patients with postoperative inflammation. *Int J Clin Pharmalcol Ther Toxico* 245, 651-654, 1986.

15 Deodhar SD, Sethi R, and Srimal RC: Preliminary studies on anti-rheumatic activity of curcumin. Indian JH Med Res 71,632-34, 1980.

16 Patacchini R, Maggi CA, and Meli A: Capsaicin-like activity of some natural pungent substances on peripheral ending of visceral primary afferents. Arch Pharmacol 342, 72-77,1990

17 Yan LJ, Droy-Lefaix MT, Packer L. *Ginkgo biloba* extract (EGb 761) protects human low density lipoproteins against oxidative modification mediated by copper. *Biochem Biophys Res Comm* 1995;212:360-6.

18 Haramaki N, Aggarwal S, Kawabata T, *et al.* Effects of natural antioxidant *Ginkgo biloba* extract (EGB 761) on myocardial ischemia-reperfusion injury. *Free Rad Biol Med* 1994;16:780-94.

19 Oken BS, Storzbach DM, Kaye JA. The efficacy of *Ginkgo biloba* on cognitive function in Alzheimer disease. *Arch Neurol* 1998;55:1409-15.

20 Peters H, Kieser M, Hölscher U. Demonstration of the efficacy of *Ginkgo biloba* special extract EGb 761" on intermittent claudication—a placebo controlled, double-blind multicenter trial. *Vasa* 1998;27:106-10 [in German].

21 Marcocci L, Maguire JJ, Droy-Lefaix MT, *et al*. The nitric oxide-scavenging properties of Ginkgo biloba extract EGb 761. *Biochem Biophys Res Commun* 1994;201:748-55.

22 DeFeudis FV (ed.):Ginkgo biloba Extract (Egb 761): Pharmacologivcal Activities and Clinical Applications.. Elsevier, Paris, 1991

23 Funfgeld EW: A natural and broad spectrum nootropic substance for treatment of SDAT-the Ginkgo biloba extract. In:Alzheimer's Disease and Related Disorders(IqbalK, Sisniewske HM, and winblad B, eds.). Alan Liss, New York, 1989, 1247-1260.

24 Murray M. The Healing Power of Herbs - The enlightened persons guide to the wonders of medicinal plants. 2nd ed. Prima publishing. Rocklin, Ca. 1995.

25 Snow JM. *Ginkgo biloba* L. (Ginkgoaceae). *The Protocol Journal Of Botanical Medicine*. 1996; 2(1): 9-15.

26 Tamura Y, Nishikawa T, Yamada K, *et al*. Effects of glycyrrhetinic acid and its derivatives on 4-sulpha- and 5-beta-reductase in rat liver. *Arzneim Forsch* 1979;29:647-9.

27 Yoshikawa M, Matsui Y, Kawamoto H, *et al*. Effects of glycyrrhizin on immune-mediated cytotoxicity. *J Gastroenterol Hepatol* 1997;12:243-8.

28 Van Rossum TGJ, Vulto AG, Hop WCJ, *et al*. Intravenous glycyrrhizin for the treatment of chronic hepatitis C: A double-blind, randomized, placebo-controlled phase I/II trial. *J Gastroenterol Hepatol* 1999;14:1093-9.

29 Suzuki H, Ohta Y, Takino T, *et al*. Effects of glycyrrhizin on biochemical tests in patients with chronic hepatitis. Double blind trial. *Asian Med J* 1983;26:423-38.

30 Arase Y, Ikeda K, Murashima N. The long term efficacy of glycyrrhizin in chronic hepatitis C patients. *Cancer* 1997;79:1494-500.

31 Felter HW. *Eclectic Materia Medica, Pharmacology and Therapeutics*. Sandy, OR: Eclectic Medical Publications, 1922:395.

32 Weiss RF. *Herbal Medicine*. Gothenberg, Sweden: Ab Arcanum and Beaconsfield: Beaconsfield Publishers Ltd, trans. Meuss AR, 1985:59-61.

33 Hoffmann D. *The Complete Illustrated Herbal*. New York: Barnes & Noble Books, 1996:99.

34 Davis EA, Morris DJ. Medicinal uses of licorice through the millennia: The good and plenty of it. *Mol Cell Endocrinol* 1991;78:1-6.

35 Foster S, Yue CX. *Herbal Emissaries: Bringing Chinese Herbs to the West*. Rochester VT: Healing Arts Press, 1992:112-121.

36 Leung A, Foster S. Encyclopedia of Common Natural Ingredients. NY: Wiley;1996.

37 Bradley P (Ed.). British herbal Compendium. Dorset. British Herbal Medical Assoc.; 1992.

38 Ben-Hur E. and Fulder S. Effect of P. ginseng saponins and Eleutherococcus senticosus extract on survival of cultured mammalian cells after ionizing radiation. *Am J Chin Med* 9, 48-56,1981

39 Farnsworth N.R. *et al.*Siberian Ginseng (*Eleutherococcus senticosus*): Current Status as an Adaptogen. In *Economic and Medicinal Plant Research*, Volume 1. London Academic Press 1985. 155-215.

40 Ho CT, Ferraro T, Chen QY, *et al.* Phytochemicals in teas and rosemary and their cancer-preventive properties. In: Ho CT, Osawa T, Huang MT, Rosen RT (eds) *Food Phytochemicals for Cancer Prevention II: Teas, Spices and Herbs.* Washington, DC: American Chemical Society, 1994:2-19.

41 Grieve M. *A Modern Herbal* vol 2. New York: Dover, 1931, 1971:681-3.

42 Leung A, Foster S. Encyclopedia of Common Natural Ingredients. NY: Wiley;1996.492-495.

43 Wang BX. Tianjin Xiyao Zazhi. 1965; 7(338).

44 Brekhman II, Dardymov IV. *Ann Rev Pharmacol.* 1969: 419.

45 Li XY. Bioactivity of neo-lignans from fructus scizandrae. *Mem Inst Oswaldo Cruz.* 1991:31-7.

46 Guyton AC, Hall JE. The major tonic herbs, 18.

47 Panossian AG, *et al.* Effects of heavy physical exercise and adaptogens on nitric oxide content in human saliva. *Phytomedicine* 1999;6(1):17-26.

48 Willard T. Wild Rose Scientific Herbal. Wild rose College of Natural Healing; Alberta; 1991.

49 Bisset NG. Herbal Drugs and Phytopharmaceuticals. Ann Arbor. CRC Press;1994.

50 Schulick P. Ginger, common spice or wonder drug. Herbal Free Press, Vermont. USA.

51 Newmark TM, Schulick P. Beyond Aspirin. Prescott, Az. HOHM Press. 2000. Pg. 244.

52 Srivastava KC. Isolation and effects of some ginger components on platelet aggregation and eicosanoid biosynthesis. *Prostaglandins Leukotrienes Med* 1986;25:187-98.

53 Chopra A, Lavin P, Patwardhan B, Chitre D. Randomized double blind trial of an Ayurvedic plant derived formulation for treatment of rheumatoid arthritis. *J Rheumatol* 2000;27:1365-72.

54 Srivastava CK, Mustafa T. Ginger (*Zingiber officinale*) in rheumatism and musculoskeletal disroders. *Medical Hypoth* 1992;39:342-48.

55 Wang BX. Tianjin Xiyao Zazhi. 1965; 7(338).

56 Leung A, Foster S. Encyclopedia of Common Natural Ingredients. NY: Wiley;1996.

57 Bradley P (Ed.). British herbal Compendium. Dorset. British Herbal Medical Assoc.; 1992.

58 Brown MD. Review of green tea's role in cancer prevention. *Alt Med Rev* 1999;4(5):360-70.

59 Katiyar SK, Agarwal R, Mukhtar H. Inhibition of spontaneous and photo-enhanced lipid peroxidation in mouse epidermal microsomes by epicatechin derivatives from green tea. *Cancer Lett* 1994;79:61-66.

60 Murray, M. The healing power of herbs-Rocklin, Ca Prima publishing; 1995, 328..

61 Nagabhushan N and Bhide SV: Nonmutagenicity of curcumin and its antimutagenic action versus chili and capsaicin, *Nutr Cancer* 8, 201-210, 1986.

62 Shalini VK and Srinivas L: Lipid peroxide induced DNA damage: Protection by turmeric . *Mol Cell Biochem* 77,3-10,1989.

63 Srivas L and Shalini VK: DNA damage by smoke; Protection by turmeric and other inhibitors of ROS. *Free Radical Biol Med* 11,277-283, 1991.

64 Boone CW, Steele VE, and Delloff GJ: Screening of chemopreventive (anticarcinogenic) compounds in rodents. *Mutat Res* 267, 251-255,1992.

65 Polasa K, *et al.*: Effect of turmeric on urinary mutagens in smokers. *Mutagenesis* 7, 107-109, 1992.

66 Satoskar RR,: Evaluation of anti-inflammatory property of curcumin in patients with postoperative inflammation. *Int J Clin Pharmalcol Ther Toxico* 245, 651-654, 1986.

PLANTAIN/BUCHU SUPREME

*Strengthen the Organs of the Urinary Tract and its Functions**

FORMULA

Plantain leaf	(*Plantago lanceolata*)
African Buchu leaf	(*Barosma betulina*)
Corn Silk	(*Zea mays*)
Horsetail Grass	(*Equisitum arvense*)
St. Johns Wort flower buds	(*Hypericum perforatum*)
Arnica flowers	(*Arnica latifolia*)
Thuja leaf	(*Thuja occidentalis*)

Concentration:	1:1 Herb strength ratio
Dosage:	20-30 drops, 3-4 times daily
	Children: 5-15 drops, 3-4 times daily
	for 1-2 months
Duration of use:	2-3 months for best results
Best taken:	Between meals with warm water

DESCRIPTION OF FORMULA

This formula acts to strengthen the musculature and tone of the membranes of the urinary system. The soothing and restorative properties of these herbs relieve irritation and weakness of the urinary tract. This compound is specifically indicated for urinary incontinence in both children and adults. Several of these herbs have traditional descriptions as diuretics, which may seem contradictory to their use for an incontinence formula. These herbs are used in small quantities and together they stimulate circulation to the urinary system and the mucous membranes that line the

urinary tract. These herbs may be used as a restorative tonic to strengthen the muscle walls and functions of the pelvic organs.

Plantain leaf is an astringent and demulcent that is helpful in cystitis.[1] Apigenin and Baicalein are constituents that are anti-inflammatory. Extracts of the plant have been shown to be antimicrobial.[2] Plantain has been reported effective in bedwetting due to its positive effect on tonification of the bladder and the sphincter. Externally applied it is a mild hemostatic for small bleeding surfaces.[3] The extract has proven bacteriostatic and bactericidal effects.[4]

African Buchu contains flavonoids (monoterpene disophenol) and volatile oils[5]. Buchu is a renal tonic suited for chronic conditions of the kidney and bladder. It has mild diuretic and urinary antiseptic properties[6] and is used in cystitis, chronic irritable bladder, urethritis and prostatitis.[7,8]

Corn Silk has flavonoids, rutin, anthocyanidins and phytosterols. It is a urinary demulcent with the effect of soothing inflamed mucous membranes.[9] It is a mild diuretic and may mildly lower blood pressure. In China it has been used for edema and kidney disorders.[10]

Horsetail is used for genitourinary complaints. It has an ability to strengthen the connective tissues due to its significant silicon content.[11] It has been traditionally described to have a hemostatic effect, the ability to slow or stop blood loss in the kidneys or bladder.[G1]

St. John's Wort flower buds have been used as a medicine for more than 2000 years. Beyond its widely reported antidepressant[12] effect, it is utilized here for its affect as a valuable anti-inflammatory and antiviral agent.[13,14] Although such use is seldom mentioned, St. John's Wort has traditionally been used for its positive affect upon digestion and liver function.

Arnica Flowers have been recommended by Eclectic physicians to strengthen the integrity of the urinary tract.

Thuja has a traditional use for the urinary system:

1. Elderly men with enlarged prostate with dribbling of urine.
2. Enuresis of children

3. Elderly women with a weak or relaxed bladder who have urine expulsion on cough or exertion. [15,16]

THERAPEUTIC APPLICATIONS*

Note: The intention of the following information is to represent the traditional use of the individual botanicals found in these formulas and to inform the reader of any evolving scientific inquiry relevant to the formula's ingredients.

SUPPORTED BY TRADITIONAL USE

Cystitis, [18] antimicrobial, [19] bedwetting, [20] chronic irritable bladder, urethritis, prostatitis, [21, 22] urinary demulcent, sooth inflamed mucous membranes, [23] in China used for edema and kidney disorders, [24] enlarged prostate with dribbling of urine, enuresis of children, elderly women with a weak or relaxed bladder who have urine expulsion on cough or exertion. [25, 26]

SCOPE OF RELEVANT SCIENTIFIC INVESTIGATION

Bactericidal effects. [27]

CAUTIONS, CONTRA-INDICATIONS AND DRUG INTERACTIONS

Please reference Chapter 9. Do not use during pregnancy or lactation. Thuja is potentially a hazardous in moderate dosages. It is to be used only in very small, nonirritating doses.

COMPLIMENTARY HERBS/FORMULAS

Calcium Supreme Elixir

REFERENCES

1 Hoffman, D. The Holistic Herbal. Dorset Elements; 1983

2 Wren RC. Potter's New Cyclopaedia of Botanical drugs and preparations. Essex, UK. Saffron Walden;1988.

3 Felter H, Lloyd JU. King's American Dispensatory. Portland. Eclectic medical Publications; 1983.

4 Gruenwald J, Brendler T, Jaenicke C, et al, eds. PDR for Herbal Medicines. Montvale, NJ: Medical Economics, 1998.

5 Wichtl M. Herbal Drugs and Phytopharmaceuticals. CRC Press, 1994, 102-3.

6 Leung A. Encyclopedia of Common Natural Ingredients Used in Food, Drugs and Cosmetics. John Wiley and Sons, 1996, 104-5.

7 Bradley PR, ed. British Herbal Compendium, vol 1. Bournemouth, England: British Herbal Medicine Association, 1992.

8 Mitchell, W., Naturopathic Applications of the Botanical remedies, 1983

9 Bradley PR, ed. British Herbal Compendium, vol 1. Bournemouth, England: British Herbal Medicine Association, 1992, 43-5.

10 Leung A, Foster S. Encyclopedia of Common Natural Ingredients. NY: Wiley;1996. pg 195, Jiangsu reference

11 Bradley P (Ed.). British Herbal Compendium. Dorset. British Herbal Medical Assoc.; 1992. page 93-3

12 Wren RC. Potter's New Cyclopaedia of Botanical drugs and preparations. Essex, UK. Saffron Walden;1988, pg 149

12 Leung A, Foster S. Encyclopedia of Common Natural Ingredients. NY: Wiley;1996.

13 Wren RC. Potter's New Cyclopaedia of Botanical drugs and preparations. Essex, UK. Saffron

14 Walden;1988.Leung A, Foster S. Encyclopedia of Common Natural Ingredients. NY: Wiley;1996.

15 Felter H, Lloyd JU. King's American Dispensatory. Portland. Eclectic Medical Publications; 1983 pg. 1936.

17 Millet Y. Toxicity of some Essential plant oils, Clin Toxicol, 1981 Dec:18:1485-98

18 Hoffman, D. The Holistic Herbal. Dorset Elements; 1983

19 Wren RC. Potter's New Cyclopaedia of Botanical drugs and preparations. Essex, UK. Saffron Walden;1988.

20 Felter H, Lloyd JU. King's American Dispensatory. Portland. Eclectic medical Publications; 1983.

21 Bradley PR, ed. British Herbal Compendium, vol 1. Bournemouth, England: British Herbal Medicine Association, 1992.

22 Mitchell, W., Naturopathic Applications of the Botanical remedies, 1983

23 Bradley PR, ed. British Herbal Compendium, vol 1. Bournemouth, England: British Herbal Medicine Association, 1992, 43-5.

24 Leung A, Foster S. Encyclopedia of Common Natural Ingredients. NY: Wiley;1996. pg 195, Jiangsu reference

25 Felter H, Lloyd JU. King's American Dispensatory. Portland. Eclectic Medical Publications; 1983 pg. 1936.

27 Gruenwald J, Brendler T, Jaenicke C, et al, eds. PDR for Herbal Medicines. Montvale, NJ: Medical Economics, 1998.

RED CLOVER SUPREME

*A Blood and Lymphatic Alterative**
FORMULA

Red Clover Blossoms	(*Trifolium pratense*)
Stinging Nettle Leaf	(*Urtica dioica*)
Cleavers	(*Galium aparine*)
Yellow Dock Root	(*Rumex crispus*)
Burdock Root	(*Arctium lappa*)
Yarrow Flowers	(*Achillea millefolium*)
Plantain Leaf & Corm	(*Plantago lanceolata*)
Licorice Root	(*Glycyrrhiza glabra*)
Prickly Ash Bark	(*Xanthoxylum clava-herculis*)

Concentration:	1:1 Herb strength ratio
Dosage:	30-40 drops, 3-4 times daily
Duration of use:	2-4 months
Best taken:	Between meals with warm water

DESCRIPTION OF FORMULA

This formula contains blood and lymphatic alteratives that improve metabolism and the elimination of catabolic wastes at the cellular level. The functions of the liver, adrenals and skin are assisted, improving the function and restoring their vitality with an improved delivery of nutrients. Excessive toxins from the gut that are absorbed into the circulatory fluids often times are the source of metabolic changes in tissues. The herbs in Red Clover Supreme have beneficial effects on these endotoxins and cleanse the blood and liver improving the function and appearance of the skin. Red Clover has been used for eczema, psoriasis, lymphatic stagnation, lymphatic edema, swollen lymph glands and fatigue. This formula may be used as a spring tonic to promote detoxification and improved metabolism.

Red Clover blossoms have traditionally been used for conditions where the eliminative properties of a diuretic and alterative would be of benefit, including bronchitis, skin sores and ulcers, and whooping cough. [1,2] This common weed has also been used extensively with cancer. [3] In addition, it is reported that Red Clover reduces platelet aggregation (blood stickiness) and angiogenesis (development of tumor vascular-networks), inhibits leukotriene production (a pro-inflammatory and induces cellular proliferation), [4] and contains compounds that may impede tumor development by blocking estrogen receptors. [5,6] Topoisomerase 2 inhibition has also been reported. [7]

Stinging Nettle leaf & seed are able to exert numerous effects on the signals sent by the immune system that provoke chronic inflammation. Studies have shown that nettle can block formation of pro-inflammatory cytokines [8] and prostaglandins. [9] It may even be able to convert some T cells, cells that control the rest of the immune system, into forms that inhibit rather than promote inflammatory reactions. [10] Nettle has been shown to help maintain a healthy urine flow. [11,12] Nettle leaf and seed were widely used in traditional medicine to relieve arthritis pain, help fight bladder infections, and for gout, chronic skin diseases such as eczema, autoimmune diseases such as lupus and rheumatoid arthritis, bleeding, diarrhea, kidney inflammations, wounds, and sciatica. [13]

Cleavers has been traditionally known as one of the best tonics to the lymphatic system and is used for swollen glands and skin conditions. It has a long tradition of use with tumors which is why it is used in this formula as an alterative and for lymphatic drainage. [14]

Yellow Dock Root is a gentle herb that is used as an alterative effecting the skin, gastrointestinal tract and the liver. [15] It is considered a tonic alterative with mild laxative action. [16,17] Native Americans and eclectic physicians of the last century used the Yellow Dock for the treatment of skin conditions. [18] The Eclectic physicians noted that it was particularly useful where lymphatic congestion was present. Yellow Dock improves digestion and reduces liver congestion, [8] making it particularly useful in this formula.

Burdock root is an alterative that is similar in action to Yellow Dock. [19,20,21] It has long been used for rheumatism, skin disorders, and to stimulate urination. [10] It is also well known for its ability to stimulate liver/bile related functions.[22] Traditional cancer research reports that is has some anti-tumor activity.[11,23]

Plantain leaf is an astringent and demulcent.[24] Apigenin and Baicalein are constituents that are anti-inflammatory. Extracts of the plant have been shown to be antimicrobial.[25] Externally applied it is a mild hemostatic for small bleeding surfaces.[26]

Licorice root is one of the most widely researched herbs. Licorice root blocks the breakdown of the body's own cortisol,[27] thus acting as an indirect anti-inflammatory throughout the body. Studies suggest that part of the benefit of licorice in people with hepatitis is mediated by the effects of this herb on the immune system.[28] Licorice has been used in traditional Western herbalism as a demulcent and expectorant for coughs,[29] to heal stomach ulcers,[30] to relieve Addison's disease (low adrenal function),[31] and for people with asthma, diabetes, urinary tract infections, tumors, and pain.[32] In traditional Chinese herbalism, licorice was widely used, including liver problems, asthma, coughs, abdominal problems including ulcers, and to make other herbs work together well in a formula.[33]

Prickly Ash bark is a circulatory stimulant[34,35, 36] and as such, appears in this formula to help drive the other botanicals throughout the body. The Eclectic physicians used this plant to 'stimulate the nerve centers', and to 'sustain the vital forces through any crisis that occurs'.[37] It is a potent alterative and has a long history of use with "chronic muscular rheumatism," lumbar back pain and myalgia. Dr. Felter gave it high marks when the nerve force is low and neural irritation is present but where recuperation is possible.[38]

THERAPEUTIC APPLICATIONS*

Note: The intention of this information is to represent the traditional use of the individual botanicals found in these formulas and to inform the reader of any evolving scientific inquiry relevant to the formula's ingredients.

SUPPORTED BY TRADITIONAL USE

Skin sores, ulcers,[39, 40] arthritis pain, bladder infections, gout, chronic skin diseases, eczema, autoimmune diseases, lupus, rheumatoid arthritis, wounds, kidney inflammations,[41] used as an alterative, with tumors, and for lymphatic drainage,[42] cancer,[43] liver problems, asthma,[44] chronic muscular rheumatism, when the nerve force is low and neural irritation is present.[45]

SCOPE OF RELEVANT SCIENTIFIC INVESTIGATION

Reduces platelet aggregation, angiogenesis, inhibits leukotriene production reduces cellular proliferation,[46] contains compounds that may impede tumor development by blocking estrogen receptors,[47, 48] topoisomerase-2 inhibition,[49] block formation of pro-inflammatory cytokines,[50, 51] and slows the breakdown of the body's own cortisol.[52]

CAUTIONS, CONTRA-INDICATIONS AND DRUG INTERACTIONS

Please reference Chapter 9. Do not use during pregnancy or lactation.

COMPLIMENTARY HERBS/FORMULAS

Supreme Cleanse, Rejuve-Powder, Juniper Berry Supreme, Daily Detox

REFERENCES

1 Felter H, Lloyd JU. King's American Dispensatory. Portland. Eclectic medical Publications; 1983.

2 Wren RC. Potter's New Cyclopaedia of Botanical drugs and preparations. Essex, UK. Saffron Walden;1988.

3 Leung A, Foster S. Encyclopedia of Common Natural Ingredients. NY: Wiley;1996.

4 Beckstrom-Sternberg and Duke Phytochemical Database: http://www.ars-grin.gov/~ngrlsb.

5 Hartwell JL. Plants used against cancer: A survey. Lloydia. 1967-1971, 30.

6 Budavari, S, et al. The Merck Index: An Encyclopedia of Chemicals, Drugs, and Biologicals, 11th ed.

7 Messina M, Barnes S. The role of soy products in reducing risk of cancer. J Natl Cancer Inst. 1991; 83: 541-546.

8 Obertreis B, Ruttkowski T, Teucher T, et al. Ex-vivo in-vitro inhibition of lipopolysaccharide stimulated tumor necrosis factor-_ and interleukin-1_ secretion in human whole blood by extractum Urticae dioicae foliorum. Arzneim Forsch 1996;46:389-94.

9 Obertreis B, Giller K, et al. (1996) Antiphlogistic effects of Urtica dioica folia extract in comparison to caffeic malic acid. Arzneim Forsch 1996;46:52-6 [in German].

10 Klingelhoefer S, Obertreis B, Quast S, Behnke B. Antirheumatic effect of IDS 23, a stinging nettle leaf extract, on in vitro expression of T helper cytokines. J Rheumatol 1999;26:2517-22.

11 Kirchhoff HW. Urtica juice as a diuretic. Z Phytother 1983;4:621-6 [in German].

12 Blumenthal M, et al. Ed. The Complete German Commission E Monographs. Austin, TX: American Botanical Council. 1998.

13 Yarnell E. Stinging nettle: A modern view of an ancient healing plant. Altern Complem Ther 1998;4:180-6.

14 Clymer RS. Natures Healing Agents. Philadelphia. Dorrance and Company. 1963.

15 Hoffman D. *The Herbal Handbook: A User's Guide to Medical Herbalism.* Rochester, VT: Healing Arts Press, 1988,40.

16 Felter H, Lloyd JU. King's American Dispensatory. Portland, Oregon: Eclectic Medical Publications. 1983.

17 Culbreth D. A manual of materia medica and pharmacology. Philadelphia. Lea & Febiger; 1927.

18 Willard T. Wild Rose Scientific Herbal. Wild rose College of Natural Healing; Alberta; 1991.

19 Boik J. Cancer and Natural Medicine: A Textbook of Basic Science and Clinical Research. Oregon   Medical Press, Princeton, MN.1996.

20 Ellingwood F. American Materia Medica, Therapeutics and Pharmacognosy. Portland. Eclectic Medical Publications;1985.

21 Witchl M. (Bisset NG, Ed.) Herbal Drugs and Phytopharmaceuticals. Medpharm, CRC Press: Boca Raton. 1994.

22 Bradley P (Ed.). British herbal Compendium. Dorset. British Herbal Medical Assoc.; 1992.

23 Leung A, Foster S. Encyclopedia of Common Natural Ingredients. NY: Wiley;1996.

24 Hoffman, D. The Holistic Herbal. Dorset Elements; 1983

25 Wren RC. Potter's New Cyclopaedia of Botanical drugs and preparations. Essex, UK. Saffron Walden;1988.

26 Felter H, Lloyd JU. King's American Dispensatory. Portland. Eclectic medical Publications; 1983.

27 Tamura Y, Nishikawa T, Yamada K, *et al.* Effects of glycyrrhetinic acid and its derivatives on 4-sulpha- and 5-beta-reductase in rat liver. *Arzneim Forsch* 1979;29:647-9.

28 Yoshikawa M, Matsui Y, Kawamoto H, *et al.* Effects of glycyrrhizin on immune-mediated cytotoxicity. *J Gastroenterol Hepatol* 1997;12:243-8.

29 Felter HW. *Eclectic Materia Medica, Pharmacology and Therapeutics.* Sandy, OR: Eclectic Medical Publications, 1922:395.

30 Weiss RF. *Herbal Medicine.* Gothenberg, Sweden: Ab Arcanum and Beaconsfield: Beaconsfield Publishers Ltd, trans. Meuss AR, 1985:59-61.

31 Hoffmann D. *The Complete Illustrated Herbal.* New York: Barnes & Noble Books, 1996;:99.

32 Davis EA, Morris DJ. Medicinal uses of licorice through the millennia: The good and plenty of it. *Mol Cell Endocrinol* 1991;78:1-6.

33 Foster S, Yue CX. *Herbal Emissaries: Bringing Chinese Herbs to the West.* Rochester VT: Healing Arts Press, 1992:112-121.

34 Wren RC. Potter's New Cyclopaedia of Botanical drugs and preparations. Essex, UK. Saffron Walden;1988

35 Leung A, Foster S. Encyclopedia of Common Natural Ingredients. NY: Wiley;1996.

36 Bradley P (Ed.). British herbal Compendium. Dorset. British Herbal Medical Assoc.; 1992.

37 Ellingwood F. American Materia Medica, Therapeutics and Pharmacognosy. Portland. Eclectic Medical Publications;1985.

38 Felter HW. The Eclectic Materia Medica, Pharmacology and Therapeutics. Portland, Oregon: Eclectic Medical publications. 1985.697-8

39 Felter H, Lloyd JU. King's American Dispensatory. Portland. Eclectic medical Publications; 1983.

40 Wren RC. Potter's New Cyclopaedia of Botanical drugs and preparations. Essex, UK. Saffron Walden;1988.

41 Yarnell E. Stinging nettle: A modern view of an ancient healing plant. *Altern Complem Ther* 1998;4:180-6.

42 Clymer RS. Natures Healing Agents. Philadelphia. Dorrance and Company. 1963.

43 Leung A, Foster S. Encyclopedia of Common Natural Ingredients. NY: Wiley;1996.

44 Foster S, Yue CX. *Herbal Emissaries: Bringing Chinese Herbs to the West.* Rochester VT: Healing Arts Press, 1992:112-121.

45 Felter HW. The Eclectic Materia Medica, Pharmacology and Therapeutics. Portland, Oregon: Eclectic Medical publications. 1985.697-8

46 Beckstrom-Sternberg and Duke Phytochemical Database: http://www.ars-grin.gov/~ngrlsb.

47 Hartwell JL. Plants used against cancer: A survey. *Lloydia.* 1967-1971, 30.

48 Budavari, S, *et al.* The Merck Index: An Encyclopedia of Chemicals, Drugs, and Biologicals, 11th ed.

49 Messina M, Barnes S. The role of soy products in reducing risk of cancer. *J Natl Cancer Inst.* 1991; 83: 541-546.

50 Obertreis B, Ruttkowski T, Teucher T, *et al.* Ex-vivo in-vitro inhibition of lipopolysaccharide stimulated tumor necrosis factor-_ and interleukin-1_ secretion in human whole blood by extractum Urticae dioicae foliorum. *Arzneim Forsch* 1996;46:389-94.

51 Obertreis B, Giller K, *et al.* (1996) Antiphlogistic effects of *Urtica dioica* folia extract in comparison to caffeic malic acid. *Arzneim Forsch* 1996;46:52-6 [in German].

52 Tamura Y, Nishikawa T, Yamada K, *et al.* Effects of glycyrrhetinic acid and its derivatives on 4-sulpha- and 5-beta-reductase in rat liver. *Arzneim Forsch* 1979;29:647-9.

REISHI/BUPLEURUM SUPREME

An Anti Retro-Viral, Immune and Liver Enhancing Formula*

FORMULA

Reishi Mushroom	(*Ganoderma lucidum*)
Chinese Bupleurum Root	(*Bupleurum falcatum*)
Astragalus Root	(*Astragalus membranaceus*)
St. John's Wort Floral Buds	(*Hypericum perforatum*)
Chinese Skullcap Root	(*Scutellaria baicalensis*)
Lomatium Root	(*Lomatium dissectum*)
Red Root	(*Ceanothus americanus*)
Licorice Root	(*Glycyrrhiza glabra*)
Thuja Leaf	(*Thuja occidentalis*)
Prickly Ash Bark	(*Xanthoxylum clava-herculis*)

Concentration:	1:1 Herb strength ratio
Dosage:	40-60 drops, 4 times daily
Duration of use:	2-3 months for best results
Best taken:	Between meals with warm water

DESCRIPTION OF FORMULA

This is a formula for compromised immune systems with liver involvement. It encourages the immune cells (lymphocytes) to become more immunologically competent. Research has indicated that these herbs inhibit retro-viruses. This formula supports the foundation of the immune system, the production of immune cells from the bone marrow.

Reishi Mushroom helps modulate the immune system, eliminate free radicals, and protects normal liver function.[1,2] Among the active constituents are four polysaccharides including Beta-D-Glucan with promising immunostimulating actions.[3] One lab study showed (in vitro) human macrophages exposed to polysaccharide found in Reishi produced a twenty-nine fold increase in Interleukin-6 and a nine fold increase in tumor necrosis factor, and T-lymphocytes production greatly increased amounts of interferon.[4] It has been used for millennia in China as a longevity promoting tonic. Numerous studies have confirmed its uses in traditional Chinese medicine for cancer, hypertension, heart disease, infections, diabetes, and liver disease.[5]

Chinese Bupleurum Root has polysaccharides with a wide spectrum of immunologic effects. It has been researched as part of a traditional Chinese formula known as sho-saiko-to (which contains about 20% bupleurum). Sho-saiko-to has been shown to foster normal liver function in people with hepatitis C, hepatitis B, and other situations in which the liver is compromised.[6, 7, 8] Chinese Bupleurum appears to protect the liver by decreasing inflammation, calming the immune system, and possibly by directly supporting protein synthesis in the liver.[9, 10, 11] Preliminary research also suggests that bupleurum may help to block fibrosis of the liver.[12] Bupleurum is highly regarded in traditional Chinese herbal medicine where it is considered helpful for infections, fever, liver problems, chest pain, and hemorrhoids.[13]

Astragalus Root restores normal functions to the immune system and protects the liver from harm.[14, 15] Natural killer cell activity was markedly enhanced when treated with Astragalus extract in human umbilical cord.[16] Astragalus has a long history of use in traditional Chinese medicine for fatigue, loss of appetite, edema, debility, weakness, chronic ulcers, and wasting. Consistent with its traditional indications as a restorative tonic, Astragalus has been shown to effect immune system function. [17]

St. John's Wort has been used as a medicine for more than 2000 years. Two components, hypericin and psuedohypericin have been shown to inhibit a variety of encapsulated viruses including Herpes simplex, para-influenza virus and cytomegalovirus.[18, 19] It is an effective antidepressant. In several recent studies when compared to standard antidepressant drugs it proves as effective, better tolerated and has much fewer side effects.[20] St. John's Wort has been shown to be effective in Seasonal Affective Disorder(SAD).[21] In addition to its antidepressant effect, it also is a valuable anti-inflammatory.[22] It accelerates wound healing in burns, incisions and wounds.[23,24]

Chinese Skullcap Root provides potent antioxidant and anti-inflammatory defenses.[25] It is considered useful for people with viral hepatitis in China.[26] In traditional Chinese medicine it was recommended for all manner of "hot" (inflammatory) conditions and infections including dysentery, hepatitis, meningitis, jaundice, allergies, and hypertension.[27]

Lomatium Root is useful as a viricide has been attributed to the coumarin glycosides.[28] It has been used by Native Americans for centuries as a lung medicine. Herbalist, Michael Moore attributes antimicrobial action to Lomatium, saying that it is of particular assistance with "limiting the severity and number of respiratory infections", especially when so-called "slow viruses" are involved.[29] One Canadian study appears to offer some support for this clinical observation, reporting that an extract of Lomatium completely inhibited rotavirus.[30]

Red Root is indicated where there is need to stimulate the spleen, liver and stomach if the liver and/or spleen is inflamed, enlarged or painful. It is astringent, sedative and antispasmodic.[31] M. Moore describes it as a lymphatic remedy, stimulating lymph and interstitial fluid circulation in tonsillitis, sore throats, enlarged lymph nodes and for shrinking nonfibrous cysts.[32]

Licorice Root is one of the most widely researched herbs. Licorice root blocks the breakdown of the body's own cortisol,[33] thus acting as an indirect anti-inflammatory throughout the body. The presence of higher amounts of natural cortisol would also tend to act as a break on excessive immune reactions. In particular it has been shown to support normal liver function in people with hepatitis C as well as other forms of viral hepatitis.[34, 35] It has been shown to prevent long-term problems in people with hepatitis C.[36] Licorice has been used in traditional Western herbalism as a demulcent and expectorant for coughs,[37] to heal stomach ulcers,[38] to relieve Addison's disease (low adrenal function),[39] and for people with asthma, diabetes, urinary tract infections, tumors, and pain.[40] In traditional Chinese herbalism, licorice was widely used, including liver problems, asthma, coughs, and to make other herbs work together well in a formula.[41]

Thuja has a traditional use as an antiviral. It is used topically and internally as a homeopathic tincture for the treatment of warts. Other traditional uses are for the urinary system[1] elderly men with enlarged prostate with dribbling of urine,[2] enuresis of children,[3] elderly women with a weak or relaxed bladder who have urine expulsion on cough or exertion.[42] Thuja is potentially hazardous in moderate dosages. It is to be used only in very small, nonirritating doses.[43]

Prickly Ash Bark is considered an ideal gastric stimulant when poor digestion needs assistance or constipation is present. It is a potent alterative and has a long history of use with chronic muscular rheumatism, lumbar back pain, and myalgia. Dr. Felter gave it high marks when the nerve force is low and neural irritation is present but where recuperation is possible.[44] Prickly Ash bark is considered a circulatory stimulant and nerve tonic in traditional herbal medicine.[45]

THERAPEUTIC APPLICATIONS*
Note: The intention of the following information is to represent the traditional use of the individual botanicals found in these formulas and to inform the reader of any evolving scientific inquiry relevant to the formula's ingredients.

SUPPORTED BY TRADITIONAL USE

Longevity promoting tonic, <u>cancer</u>, hypertension, heart disease, <u>infections</u>, diabetes, and liver disease,[46, 47, 48] fibrosis of the liver,[49] fever, chest pain, hemorrhoids,[50] decreasing inflammation, supports protein synthesis in the liver,[51, 52, 53] fatigue, loss of appetite, edema, debility, weakness, chronic ulcers, and wasting.[54]

SCOPE OF RELEVANT SCIENTIFIC INVESTIGATION

Increase Interleukin-6, tumor necrosis factor, T-lymphocytes produce increased interferon,[55] viricide,[56] <u>viral hepatitis</u>,[57 58]

CAUTIONS, CONTRA-INDICATIONS AND DRUG INTERACTIONS

Please reference Chapter 9. Do not use during pregnancy or lactation. Thuja is potentially hazardous in moderate dosages. It is to be used only in very small, nonirritating doses.[59]

COMPLIMENTARY HERBS/FORMULAS

Cell Wise, Daily Detox, Astragalus Supreme, Hep C

REFERENCES

1 Shiao MS, Lee KR, Lin LJ, Wang CT. Natural products and biological activities of the Chinese medicinal fungus Ganoderma lucidum. In: Ho CT, Osawa T, Huang MT, Rosen RT (eds) Food Phytochemicals for Cancer Prevention II: Teas, Spices and Herbs. Washington, DC: American Chemical Society, 1994: 342-54.

2 Lin JM, Lin CC, Chen MF, *et al.* Radical scavenger and antihepatotoxic activity of Ganoderma formosanum, Ganoderma lucidum and Ganoderma neo-japonicum. J Ethnopharmacol 1995;47:33-41.

3 Hobbs C. Medicinal Mushrooms, Interweave Press, Loveland, Co, 1996, 96-107.

4 Wang, S.Y. *et al.* The antitumor effect of Ganoderma lucidum is mediated by cytokines released from activated macrophages and T lymphocytes. International Journal of Cancer 70:699-705

5 Jones K. Reishi mushroom: Ancient medicine in modern times. Alt Compl Ther 1998;4(4):256-67.

6 Gibo Y, Nakamura Y, Takahashi N, *et al.* Clinical study of sho-saiko-to therapy for Japanese patients with chronic hepatitis C (CH-C). Prog Med 1994;14:217-9.

7 Oka H, Yamamoto S, Kuroki T, *et al.* Prospective study of chemoprevention of hepatocellular carcinoma with sho-saiko-to (TJ-9). Cancer 1995;76:743-9.

8 Reichert R. Phytotherapeutic alternatives for chronic active hepatitis. Q Rev Natural Med 1997;summer:103-8.

9 Werbach M, Murray M. Botanical Influences on Illness. Tarzana, CA: Third Line Press, 1994:176-83

10 Mizoguchi Y, Sakagami Y, Okura Y, *et al.* Effects of sho-saiko-to (TJ-9) in hepatitis patients and on the metabolism of arachidonic acid. In: Hoyosa E, Yamamura Y (eds) Recent Advances in the Pharmacology of Kampo (Japanese Herbal) Medicines. Amsterdam: Excerpta Medica, 1988:396-404.

11 Yamamoto M, Kumagai A, Yamamura Y. Structure and actions of saikosaponins isolated from Bupleurum falcatum L. I. Anti-inflammatory action of saikosaponins. Arzneim Forsch 1975;25:1021-3.

12 Shimizu I, Ma YR, Mizobuchi Y, *et al.* Effects of sho-saiko-to, a Japanese herbal medicine, on hepatic fibrosis in rats. Hepatology 1999;29:149-60.

13 Bensky D, Gamble A, Kaptchuk T. Chinese Herbal Medicine Materia Medica, Revised Edition. Seattle: Eastland Press, 1993: 49-50.

14 Zhang ZL, Wen QZ, Liu CX. Hepatoprotective effects of astragalus root. J Ethnopharmacol 1990;30:145-9.

15 Murray M, Pizzorno P. An Encyclopedia of Natural Medicine. Rocklin, CA: Prima Publishing, 1991:230.

16 Jing JP, Lim WF,Preliminary study on effects of mechanism of juman umbilical cord blood derived interferon-x and of astragalus membranaceus on neutral killer toxicity. 1983, 3:293-6.

17 Bensky D, Gamble A, Kaptchuk T. Chinese Herbal Medicine Materia Medica, Revised Edition. Seattle: Eastland Press, 1993:318-20.

18 Yip L *et al.* Antiviral, activity of a derivative of the photosensitive compound hypericin. 1996, Phytomedicine 3:185-90.

19 Leung A, Foster S. Encyclopedia of Common Natural Ingredients. NY: Wiley;1996, 310-312.

20 Linde, K., Ramirez, G., Mulrow, C.D. *et al.* (1996). St. John's Wort for depression-an overview and meta analysis of randomized clinical trials. British Medical Journal 313:253-258.

21 Wheatley D. Hypericum in seasonal affective disorder (SAD). Curr Med Res Opin 1999; 15:33-37

22 Wren RC. Potter's New Cyclopaedia of Botanical drugs and preparations. Essex, UK. Saffron Walden;1988.

23 Rao S.G. *et al.*Calendula and Hypericum two homeopathic drugs promoting wound healing in rats. Fitoterapia 6:508-510.

24 Hobbs C:St. John's Wort, Hypericum perforatum L. Herbalgram 18/19, 24-33, 1989.

25 van Loon IM. The golden root: Clinical applications of Scutellaria baicalensis Georgi flavonoids as modulators of the inflammatory response. Alt Med Rev 1997;2:472-80.

26 Huang CK. The Pharmacology of Chinese Herbs. 290-1.

27 van Loon IM. The golden root: Clinical applications of Scutellaria baicalensis Georgi flavonoids as modulators of the inflammatory response. Alt Med Rev 1997;2:472-80.

28 Alstat E, Lomatium Dissectum: and herbal virucide?, Complement. Med.,May/June 1987,32-4.

29 Moore M. Medicinal Plants of the Pacific West. Red Crane Books. Santa Fe, NM. 1995.

30 McCutcheon Ar, *et al.* Antiviral screening of British Columbian medicinal plants. J Ethnopharmacol. 1995;49(2):101-10.

31 Felter H, Lloyd JU. King's American Dispensatory. Portland, Oregon: Eclectic Medical Publications. 1983.472-3.

32 Moore M. Medicinal Plants of the Pacific West, Santa Fe, Red Crane Books,1989, 140-1.

33 Tamura Y, Nishikawa T, Yamada K, *et al.* Effects of glycyrrhetinic acid and its derivatives on 4-sulpha- and 5-beta-reductase in rat liver. Arzneim Forsch 1979;29:647-9.

34 Van Rossum TGJ, Vulto AG, Hop WCJ, *et al.* Intravenous glycyrrhizin for the treatment of chronic hepatitis C: A double-blind, randomized, placebo-controlled phase I/II trial. J Gastroenterol Hepatol 1999;14:1093-9.

35 Suzuki H, Ohta Y, Takino T, *et al.* Effects of glycyrrhizin on biochemical tests in patients with chronic hepatitis. Double blind trial. Asian Med J 1983;26:423-38.

36 Arase Y, Ikeda K, Murashima N. The long term efficacy of glycyrrhizin in chronic hepatitis C patients. Cancer 1997;79:1494-500.

37 Felter HW. Eclectic Materia Medica, Pharmacology and Therapeutics. Sandy, OR: Eclectic Medical Publications, 1922:395.

38 Weiss RF. Herbal Medicine. Gothenberg, Sweden: Ab Arcanum and Beaconsfield: Beaconsfield Publishers Ltd, trans. Meuss AR, 1985:59-61.

39 Hoffmann D. The Complete Illustrated Herbal. New York: Barnes & Noble Books, 1996;:99.

40 Davis EA, Morris DJ. Medicinal uses of licorice through the millennia: The good and plenty of it. Mol Cell Endocrinol 1991;78:1-6.

41 Foster S, Yue CX. Herbal Emissaries: Bringing Chinese Herbs to the West. Rochester VT: Healing Arts Press, 1992:112-121.

42 Felter H, Lloyd JU. King's American Dispensatory. Portland. Eclectic Medical Publications; 1983 pg. 1936.

43 Millet Y. Toxicity of some Essential plant oils, Clin Toxicol, 1981 Dec:18:1485-98

44 Felter HW. The Eclectic Materia Medica, Pharmacology and Therapeutics. Portland, Oregon: Eclectic Medical publications. 1985.697-8

45 Ellingwood F. American Materia Medica, Pharmacognosy and Therapeutics 11th ed. Sandy, OR: Eclectic Medical Publications, 1919:165-6.

46 Jones K. Reishi mushroom: Ancient medicine in modern times. Alt Compl Ther 1998;4(4):256-67.

47 Zhang ZL, Wen QZ, Liu CX. Hepatoprotective effects of astragalus root. J Ethnopharmacol 1990;30:145-9.

48 Murray M, Pizzorno P. An Encyclopedia of Natural Medicine. Rocklin, CA: Prima Publishing, 1991:230.

49 Shimizu I, Ma YR, Mizobuchi Y, *et al.* Effects of sho-saiko-to, a Japanese herbal medicine, on hepatic fibrosis in rats. Hepatology 1999;29:149-60.

50 Bensky D, Gamble A, Kaptchuk T. Chinese Herbal Medicine Materia Medica, Revised Edition. Seattle: Eastland Press, 1993: 49-50.

51 Werbach M, Murray M. Botanical Influences on Illness. Tarzana, CA: Third Line Press, 1994:176-83

52 Mizoguchi Y, Sakagami Y, Okura Y, *et al.* Effects of sho-saiko-to (TJ-9) in hepatitis patients and on the metabolism of arachidonic acid. In: Hoyosa E, Yamamura Y (eds) Recent Advances in the Pharmacology of Kampo (Japanese Herbal) Medicines. Amsterdam: Excerpta Medica, 1988:396-404.

53 Yamamoto M, Kumagai A, Yamamura Y. Structure and actions of saikosaponins isolated from Bupleurum falcatum L. I. Anti-inflammatory action of saikosaponins. Arzneim Forsch 1975;25:1021-3.

54 Bensky D, Gamble A, Kaptchuk T. Chinese Herbal Medicine Materia Medica, Revised Edition. Seattle: Eastland Press, 1993:318-20.

55 Wang, S.Y. *et al.* The antitumor effect of Ganoderma lucidum is mediated by cytokines released from activated macrophages and T lymphocytes. International Journal of Cancer 70:699-705

56 Alstat E, Lomatium Dissectum: and herbal virucide?, Complement. Med.,May/June 1987,32-4.

57 Van Rossum TGJ, Vulto AG, Hop WCJ, *et al.* Intravenous glycyrrhizin for the treatment of chronic hepatitis C: A double-blind, randomized, placebo-controlled phase I/II trial. J Gastroenterol Hepatol 1999;14:1093-9.

58 Suzuki H, Ohta Y, Takino T, *et al.* Effects of glycyrrhizin on biochemical tests in patients with chronic hepatitis. Double blind trial. Asian Med J 1983;26:423-38.

59 Millet Y. Toxicity of some Essential plant oils, Clin Toxicol, 1981 Dec:18:1485-98

REJUVE - POWDER SUPREME

A Digestive/Internal Cleansing Formula *
FORMULA

Psyllium Husks	(*Plantago ovata*)
Triphala Powder	(*Ayurvedic blend of Emblica officinalis, Terminalia bellerica, and Terminalia chebula*)
Marshmallow Root	(*Althaea officinalis*)
DGL Licorice Root	(*Glycyrrhiza glabra*)
Ginger Root	(*Zingiber officinale*)

Concentration:	All Powders
Dosage:	Use 1 heaping teaspoon in 8-10 ounces warm water. Shake well and take 2 times daily
Duration of use:	2-4 weeks each season for best results
Best taken:	In the morning before breakfast and 1 hour before bedtime with warm water

DESCRIPTION OF FORMULA

This formula revitalizes digestion and absorption of nutrients while enhancing elimination. The herbs promote a soothing bulk to the bowels and stool. Can be used each season for a GI cleanse and detox.

Psyllium Husk is a colon bulking fiber that is effective for constipation and diarrhea. It has 25% mucilage content that increases the fecal bacterial population of the colon and the fiber increases the weight and water content of the stool. Bowel transit time decreases which increases frequency of BM's. Helpful for irritable bowel syndrome[1] and can lower total cholesterol levels.[2]

Triphala Powder, according to Ayurvedic principles, enhances the functions of digestion and assimilation while revitalizing the entire metabolic process. Composed of equal parts of 3 herbs it is a mild laxative used for dyspepsia, constipation, hemorrhoids, enlarged liver and headaches.[3]

Emblica officinalis or Indian Gooseberry is a diuretic, laxative and stomactic and has spasmolytic activity.[3]

Terminalia bellerica is an astringent, tonic rejuvenative and laxative. Its traditional uses are chronic diarrhea, dysentery, parasites, bronchitis, sore throat and cough.[4]

Terminalia chebula is one of the most important herbs in Ayurvedic medicine. It is rejuvinative; it feeds the nerves and the brain. Indicated for malabsorbtion, abdominal distention, skin diseases and nervous disorders.[5]

Marshmallow root is soothing to inflamed and painful mucous membranes due to its high content of mucilage.[6,7] It has traditionally been used with gastrointestinal irritation and inflammation[8], painful urinary disorders, such as cystitis (kidney inflammation),[9,10] and bladder irritation. Marshmallow is also reported to possess immunostimulating properties.[11]

Deglycyrrhizinated Licorice (DGL) is one of the most widely researched herbs. DGL has had the Glycyrrhizin removed that can have the effect of increasing blood pressure in sensitive individuals. DGL is very effective for treating duodenal ulcers,[12] canker sores[13] and gastric ulcers for both short term treatment and maintenance therapy.[14] Licorice has been used in traditional Western herbalism as a demulcent and expectorant for coughs,[15] and in asthma, diabetes and urinary tract infections.[16]

Ginger is used in traditional medicine to stimulate the appetite, treat stomachaches, nausea,[17] diarrhea, and cholera. Ginger has strong antioxidant properties, and is a digestive stimulant.[18] Ginger is one of the most powerful botanical inhibitors of 5-lipoxygenase,[19, 20, 21] an enzyme responsible for excessive production of pro-inflammatory prostaglandins and thromboxanes. Ginger is used in many traditional Ayurvedic formulas that were traditionally employed in people with arthritis and other inflammatory disorders.[22] Ginger is also valued in traditional Western herbalism for arthritis, rheumatism, muscle aches, migraine, and flatulence.[23]

THERAPEUTIC APPLICATIONS*

Note: The intention of the following information is to represent the traditional use of the individual botanicals found in these formulas and to inform the reader of any evolving scientific inquiry relevant to the formula's ingredients.

SUPPORTED BY TRADITIONAL USE

Enhances the functions of digestion and assimilation while revitalizing the entire metabolic process, mild laxative, dyspepsia, constipation, hemorrhoids, enlarged liver, headaches,[24] irritable bowel syndrome,[25] lower total cholesterol levels,[26] chronic diarrhea, dysentery, parasites, bronchitis, sore throat, cough,[27] gastrointestinal irritation and inflammation[28], painful urinary disorders, such as cystitis,[29, 30] immunostimulating properties, duodenal ulcers,[31] canker sores[32] and gastric ulcers[33]

SCOPE OF RELEVANT SCIENTIFIC INVESTIGATION

Inhibitors of 5-lipoxygenase an enzyme responsible for excessive production of pro-inflammatory prostaglandins and thromboxanes,[34, 35, 36] arthritis, rheumatism, muscle aches, migraine.[37]

CAUTIONS, CONTRA-INDICATIONS AND DRUG INTERACTIONS

Please reference Chapter 9. Do not use during pregnancy or lactation.

COMPLIMENTARY HERBS/FORMULAS

Daily Detox, Sweetish Bitters

REFERENCES

1 Bradley P (Ed.). British Herbal Compendium. Dorset. British Herbal Medical Assoc. 1992.136-7.

2 Davidson MH, et al.a psyllium-enriched cereal for the treatment of hypercholesterolemia in children: a controlled, double blind study. Am J Clin Nutr 1996;63(1):96-102.

3 Kapoor LD. CRC Handbook of Ayurvedic Medicinal Plants. CRC Press Boca Raton. 1990,175.

4 Lad V, Frawley D. The Yoga of Herbs, An Ayurvedic Guide to Herbal Medicine. Lotus Press: New Mexico. 1986,164.

5 Lad V. Ibid pg174.

6 Ellingwood F. American Materia Medica, Therapeutics and Pharmacognosy. Portland. Eclectic Medical Publications;1985.

7 Tang W, Eisenbrand G. Chinese Drugs of Plant Origin. New York. Springer-Verlag;1992.

8 Felter H. *The Eclectic Materia Medica, Pharmacology, and Therapeutics*, John K. Scudder, Cincinnati, Ohio, 1922, 177-8

9 Witchl M. (Bisset NG, Ed.) Herbal Drugs and Phytopharmaceuticals.

Medpharm, CRC Press: Boca Raton. 1994.

10 Coon N. Using plants for healing. Philadelphia, Pa. Rodale Press. 1979.

11 Blumenthal M, et al. Ed. *The Complete German Commission E Monographs.*Austin, TX: American Botanical Council; 1998.

12 Rewari SN,Wilson AK. Deglycyrrhizinated licorice in duodenal ulcer. Practitioner 210,,820-825, 1972

13 Murray M. The healing power of herbs - The enlightened persons guide to the wonders of medicinal plants. Rocklin, Ca. Prima publishing;1995.236.

14 Weiss RF. *Herbal Medicine.* Gothenberg, Sweden: Ab Arcanum and Beaconsfield: Beaconsfield Publishers Ltd, trans. Meuss AR, 1985:59-61.

15 Felter HW. *Eclectic Materia Medica, Pharmacology and Therapeutics.* Sandy, OR: Eclectic Medical Publications, 1922:395.

16 Davis EA, Morris DJ. Medicinal uses of licorice through the millennia: The good and plenty of it. *Mol Cell Endocrinol* 1991;78:1-6.

17 Bone ME, Wilkinson DJ, Young JR, et al. Ginger root—a new antiemetic: The effect of ginger root on postoperative nausea and vomiting after major gynaecological surgery. *Anaesthesia* 1990;45:669-71.

18 Leung A, Foster S. Encyclopedia of Common Natural Ingredients. NY: Wiley;1996.272-3.

19 Srivastava KC. Isolation and effects of some ginger components on platelet aggregation and eicosanoid biosynthesis. *Prostaglandins Leukotrienes* Med 1986;25:187-98.

20 Kawakishi S, Morimitsu Y, Osawa T. Chemistry of ginger components and inhibitory factors of the arachidonic acid cascade. In: Ho CT, Osawa T, Huang MT, Rosen RT (eds) *Food Phytochemicals for Cancer Prevention vol 2: Tea, Spices and Herbs.* Washington, DC: American Chemical Society, 1994:244-50.

21 Kiuchi F, Iwakami S, Shibuya M, et al. Inhibition of prostaglandin and leukotriene biosynthesis by gingerols and diarylheptanoids. *Chem Pharm Bull* 1992;40:387-91.

22 Chopra A, Lavin P, Patwardhan B, Chitre D. Randomized double blind trial of an Ayurvedic plant derived formulation for treatment of rheumatoid arthritis. *J Rheumatol* 2000;27:1365-72.

23 Srivastava CK, Mustafa T. Ginger (*Zingiber officinale*) in rheumatism and musculoskeletal disroders. *Medical Hypoth* 1992;39:342-48.

24 Kapoor LD. CRC Handbook of Ayurvedic Medicinal Plants. CRC Press Boca Raton. 1990,175.

25 Bradley P (Ed.). British Herbal Compendium. Dorset. British Herbal Medical Assoc. 1992.136-7.

26 Davidson MH, et al.a psyllium-enriched cereal for the treatment of hypercholesterolemia in children: a controlled, double blind study. Am J Clin Nutr 1996;63(1):96-102.

27 Lad V, Frawley D. The Yoga of Herbs, An Ayurvedic Guide to Herbal Medicine. Lotus Press: New Mexico. 1986,164.

28 Felter H. *The Eclectic Materia Medica, Pharmacology, and Therapeutics,* John K. Scudder, Cincinnati, Ohio, 1922, 177-8

29 Witchl M. (Bisset NG, Ed.) Herbal Drugs and Phytopharmaceuticals. Medpharm, CRC Press: Boca Raton. 1994.

30 Coon N. Using plants for healing. Philadelphia, Pa. Rodale Press. 1979.

31 Rewari SN,Wilson AK. Deglycyrrhizinated licorice in duodenal ulcer. Practitioner 210,,820-825, 1972

32 Murray M. The healing power of herbs - The enlightened persons guide to the wonders of medicinal plants. Rocklin, Ca. Prima publishing;1995.236.

33 Blumenthal M, *et al.* Ed. *The Complete German Commission E Monographs.*Austin, TX: American Botanical Council; 1998.

34 Srivastava KC. Isolation and effects of some ginger components on platelet aggregation and eicosanoid biosynthesis. *Prostaglandins Leukotrienes Med* 1986;25:187-98.

35 Kawakishi S, Morimitsu Y, Osawa T. Chemistry of ginger components and inhibitory factors of the arachidonic acid cascade. In: Ho CT, Osawa T, Huang MT, Rosen RT (eds) *Food Phytochemicals for Cancer Prevention vol 2: Tea, Spices and Herbs.* Washington, DC: American Chemical Society, 1994:244-50.

36 Kiuchi F, Iwakami S, Shibuya M, *et al.* Inhibition of prostaglandin and leukotriene biosynthesis by gingerols and diarylheptanoids. *Chem Pharm Bull* 1992;40:387-91.

37 Srivastava CK, Mustafa T. Ginger (*Zingiber officinale*) in rheumatism and musculoskeletal disroders. *Medical Hypoth* 1992;39:342-48.

ROBERT'S FORMULA

*Enhances and Strengthens Digestive Function**

FORMULA

Goldenseal Root	(*Hydrastis canadensis*)
Marshmallow Root	(*Althaea officinalis*)
Echinacea Root	(*Echinacea angustifolia and purpurea*)
Geranium Root	(*Geranium maculatum*)
Slippery Elm Bark	(*Ulmus rubra*)
Poke Root	(*Phytolacca americana*)

Concentration:	1:1 Herb strength ratio
Dosage:	30-50 drops, 3-4 times daily
Duration of use:	1-2 months for best results
Best taken:	Between meals with warm water

DESCRIPTION OF FORMULA

This is a traditional naturopathic herbal formula used for digestive disorders. It targets the lining of the gastrointestinal tract and corrects enteric bacterial imbalances and functional disturbances of the intestinal tract. Useful in the treatment of acidic stomach, gastric irritation, gastric ulcerations, irritable bowel syndrome, spastic colon, bacterial imbalances of the colon, toxemia and digestive metabolic disorders.

Goldenseal Root is a important herbal medicine for gastric and intestinal conditions and was used extensively by the Eclectic physicians and native americans.[1] It contains the isoquinoline alkaloids, hydrastine and berberine among others. The active ingredients have potent antibiotic activity against candida, bacteria, fungi and protazoa [2,3] including *Entamoeba histolytica, Giardia* and *Tricomonas vaginalis*.[4] Berberine makes it difficult for streptococci bacteria to adhere to GI cells resulting in the unwanted organism passing through the GI system instead of infecting it. Berberine does this at dosages lower than those required for its antibacterial action.[5] This combination of immune stimulation, antibiotic action and prevention of the adherence of infective organisms creates a dynamic therapeutic action.

Marshmallow root is soothing to inflamed and painful mucous membranes due to its high content of mucilage.[6,7] It has traditionally found use with gastrointestinal irritation and inflammation[8], painful urinary disorders, such as cystitis [9,10] and bladder irritation. Marshmallow is also reported to possess immunostimulating properties.[11]

Echinacea is included in this formula as an immuno-stimulant, that has anti-inflammatory, antibacterial, and antiviral properties.[14] It is well known for its benefits with various chronic catarrhal (congestive) conditions.[12] Today, science is supporting much of its established traditional use, by showing that extracts of Echinacea spp. have the ability to increase antibody production systemically providing resistance to various infections.[3]

Geranium Root is used to treat duodenal or gastric ulcers, dysentery, diarrhea and hemorrhoids, and has an astringent effect.[13]

Poke Root acts on the lymphatic tissues and the mucous lining of the digestive tract.[14] It is specific for pallid (pale) mucous membranes with ulcerations. [15]

Slippery Elm Bark contains abundant mucilage made up of polysaccharides, that are demulcent and emollient and are readily digestible.[16] It is soothing to inflammations and ulcerations of the digestive tract.[17] The polysaccharides may absorb endotoxins in the gut providing relief in dysbiosis (author).

THERAPEUTIC APPLICATIONS*

Note: The intention of the following information is to represent the traditional use of the individual botanicals found in these formulas and to inform the reader of any evolving scientific inquiry relevant to the formula's ingredients.

SUPPORTED BY TRADITIONAL USE

Gastric and intestinal conditions,[18] inflamed and painful mucous membranes,[19, 20] lymphatic tissues and the mucous lining of the digestive tract,[21] gastrointestinal irritation and inflammation[22], painful urinary disorders, cystitis,[23, 24] duodenal or gastric ulcers, dysentery, diarrhea and hemorrhoids,[25] benefits various chronic catarrhal (congestive) conditions.[26]

SCOPE OF RELEVANT SCIENTIFIC INVESTIGATION

Active ingredients have antibiotic activity against candida, bacteria, fungi and protazoa[27, 28] including *Entamoeba histolytica, Giardia* and *Tricomonas vaginalis*.[29] Berberine prevents adherance of streptococci bacteria.[30]

CAUTIONS, CONTRA-INDICATIONS AND DRUG INTERACTIONS

Please reference Chapter 9. Do not use during pregnancy or lactation.

COMPLIMENTARY HERBS/FORMULAS

Friendly bacterial probiotics, DGL-Deglycyrrhizinated Licorice Powder, Rejuve-Powder

REFERENCES

1 Felter H, Lloyd JU. King's American Dispensatory. Portland. Eclectic Medical Publications;1983. 1025-8.

2 Murray M. The healing power of herbs - The enlightened persons guide to the wonders of medicinal plants. Rocklin, Ca. Prima publishing;1995. 169-172

3 Hahn FE and Ciak J: Berberine. *Antibiotics* 3, 577-588, 1976

4 Kaneda Y, *et al.*: In vitro effects of berberine sulfate on the growth of *Entamoeba histolytica, Giardia lamblia and Tricomonas vaginalis. Ann Trop Med Parasiol* 85, 417-425, 1991

5 Sun D. et al, Berberine sulfate blocks adherence of *Streptococcus pyogenes* to epithelial cells, fibronectin, and hexsadecane. Antimicrob Agents Chemother 32, 1370-1374, 1988

6 Ellingwood F. American Materia Medica, Therapeutics and Pharmacognosy. Portland. Eclectic Medical Publications;1985.

7 Tang W, Eisenbrand G. Chinese Drugs of Plant Origin. New York. Springer-Verlag;1992.

8 Felter H. *The Eclectic Materia Medica, Pharmacology, and Therapeutics*, John K. Scudder, Cincinnati, Ohio, 1922, 177-8

9 Witchl M. (Bisset NG, Ed.) Herbal Drugs and Phytopharmaceuticals. Medpharm, CRC Press: Boca Raton. 1994.

10 Coon N. Using plants for healing. Philadelphia, Pa. Rodale Press. 1979.

11 Blumenthal M, *et al*. Ed. *The Complete German Commission E Monographs.*Austin, TX: American Botanical Council; 1998.

12 Felter H, Lloyd JU. King's American Dispensatory. Portland. Eclectic medical Publications; 1983.

13 Felter H, Lloyd JU. King's American Dispensatory. Portland. Eclectic Medical Publications; 1983. 928-929.

14 Felter H, Lloyd JU. King's American Dispensatory. Portland. Eclectic Medical Publications; 1983. 1473-4.

15 Felter H. *The Eclectic Materia Medica, Pharmacology, and Therapeutics*, John K. Scudder, Cincinnati, Ohio, 1922, 536-7

16 Beverage R.J., Some Structural Features of Mucilage from Ulmus fulva. Carbohyd.Res.1969,9,429-39

17 Bradley P (Ed.). British herbal Compendium. Dorset. British Herbal Medical Assoc.; 1992.202

18 Felter H, Lloyd JU. King's American Dispensatory. Portland. Eclectic Medical Publications;1983. 1025-8.

19 Ellingwood F. American Materia Medica, Therapeutics and Pharmacognosy. Portland. Eclectic Medical Publications;1985.

20 Tang W, Eisenbrand G. Chinese Drugs of Plant Origin. New York. Springer-Verlag;1992.

21 Felter H, Lloyd JU. King's American Dispensatory. Portland. Eclectic Medical Publications; 1983. 1473-4.

22 Felter H. *The Eclectic Materia Medica, Pharmacology, and Therapeutics*, John K. Scudder, Cincinnati, Ohio, 1922, 177-8

23 Witchl M. (Bisset NG, Ed.) Herbal Drugs and Phytopharmaceuticals. Medpharm, CRC Press: Boca Raton. 1994.

24 Coon N. Using plants for healing. Philadelphia, Pa. Rodale Press. 1979.

25 Felter H, Lloyd JU. King's American Dispensatory. Portland. Eclectic Medical Publications; 1983. 928-929.

26 Felter H, Lloyd JU. King's American Dispensatory. Portland. Eclectic medical Publications; 1983.

27 Murray M. The healing power of herbs - The enlightened persons guide to the wonders of medicinal plants. Rocklin, Ca. Prima publishing;1995. 169-172

28 Hahn FE and Ciak J: Berberine. *Antibiotics* 3, 577-588, 1976

29 Kaneda Y, *et al*.: In vitro effects of berberine sulfate on the growth of *Entamoeba histolytica, Giardia lamblia and Tricomonas vaginalis. Ann Trop Med Parasiol* 85, 417-425, 1991

30 Sun D. et al, Berberine sulfate blocks adherence of *Streptococcus pyogenes* to epithelial cells, fibronectin, and hexsadecane. Antimicrob Agents Chemother 32, 1370-1374, 1988

SAW PALMETTO SUPREME

A Formula to Promote Healthy Prostate Function *
FORMULA

Saw Palmetto Berry	(*Serenoa repens*)
Echinacea Supreme	(*E. angustifolia and Purpurea roots*)
Stinging Nettle Root	(*Urtica dioica*)
Poplar Buds	(*Populus tremuloides*)
Pipsissewa Herb	(*Chimaphila umbellata*)
Thuja leaf	(*Thuja occidentalis*)

Concentration:	1:1 Herb strength ratio
Dosage:	30-50 drops, 3-4 times daily
Duration of use:	2-3 months for best results
Best taken:	Between meals with warm water

DESCRIPTION OF FORMULA

This formula targets the functions of the prostate gland with a specific focus on benign prostatic hypertrophy. The researched herbs are combined with lower dosages of traditionally used herbs to produce a restorative tonic to strengthen the prostate and decrease the symptoms of BPH.

Saw Palmetto has been demonstrated in multiple studies to be effective in the treatment of BPH, benign prostatic hypertrophy. [1,2,3] Saw palmetto contains fatty acids and sterols that have the effect of inhibiting the conversion of testosterone to a stronger form, DHT (dihydrotestosterone), which stimulates the prostate cells to multiply and the gland to enlarge. [4] Saw palmetto has also been shown to have an anti-estrogenic effect that results in improvement of benign prostatic hypertrophy. Nighttime urination has been shown to decrease in 73% of patients. [5] There have been multiple double blind placebo controlled studies that have compared Saw Palmetto to the drug Finasteride or Proscar and shown improved symptom reduction in a decreased time.[6,7]

Echinacea is included in this formula as an immuno-stimulant, anti-inflammatory, antibacterial, and antiviral.[8,9] Traditionally, Echinacea has been used by Native Americans to treat colds, coughs, sore throats.[10] The Eclectic medical doctors, from the first half of the last century, also praised Echinacea for its benefits with various chronic catarrhal (congestive) conditions of the respiratory tract.[11] Today, science is supporting much of its established traditional use, by showing that extracts of Echinacea spp. have the ability to increase antibody production, along with resistance to various infections.[12,13] Research has further shown that extracts of Echinacea significantly enhance natural killer cell function, and have phagocytic, metabolic and bactericidal influence on macrophages,[14,15] that adds therapeutic value to this prostate formula.[16]

Stinging Nettle Root contains polysaccharides and lectins[17] that have been shown in double blind studies to be useful in benign prostatic hypertrophy.[18] This effect is through decreasing the protein carrier molecules of the sex hormones testosterone and estrogen.[19]

Poplar Buds and Leaf contain salicylates and flavonoids that have an anti-inflammatory action with beneficial effects in complaints following prostate hypertrophy.[20] Poplar has a long tradition of use in remedies for urinary complaints.[21]

Pipsissewa contains arbutin and other flavonoids that have urinary antiseptic properties. Pipsissewa also has tonic and astringent properties.[22] Dr. Felter described its specific uses in "atonic and debilitated states of the urinary tract...chronic irritation of the prostate and urethra..."[23]

Thuja has the traditional indication for use on the urinary system of elderly men with enlarged prostate with dribbling of urine, enuresis of children and elderly women with a weak or relaxed bladder who have urine expulsion on cough or exertion.[24] Thuja is potentially hazardous in moderate dosages. It is to be used only in very small, nonirritating doses.[25]

THERAPEUTIC APPLICATIONS*

Note: The intention of the following information is to represent the traditional use of the individual botanicals found in these formulas and to inform the reader of any evolving scientific inquiry relevant to the formula's ingredients.

SUPPORTED BY TRADITIONAL USE

Prostate enlargement and inflammation,[26] anti-inflammatory, antibacterial, antiviral,[27, 28] chronic irritation of the prostate and urethra.[29]

SCOPE OF RELEVANT SCIENTIFIC INVESTIGATION

Benign prostatic hypertrophy, [30, 31, 32] Fatty acids and sterols inhibit conversion of testosterone to dihydrotestosterone,[33] anti-estrogenic effect, nighttime urination decrease in 73% of patients.[34]

CAUTIONS, CONTRA-INDICATIONS AND DRUG INTERACTIONS

Please reference Chapter 9. Do not use during pregnancy or lactation. Thuja is potentially a hazardous in moderate dosages. It is to be used here in very small, nonirritating doses.

COMPLIMENTARY HERBS/FORMULAS

Juniper Berry Supreme, Pygeum Bark, Saw Palmetto Liquid Phyto-Cap, Male Libido

REFERENCES

1 Braeckman J, Bruhwyler J, Vandekerckhove K, Géczy J. Efficacy and safety of the extract of Serenoa repens in the treatment of benign prostatic hyperplasia: Therapeutic equivalence between twice and once daily dosage forms. Phytotherapy Res 1997;11:558-63.

2 Redecker KD, Hölscher U. Extractum Sabal fructus in benign prostatic hyperplasia (BPH)-clinical trial in BPH stages I and II according to Alken. Extracta Urologica 1998;21:23-5.

3 Ziegler, K, Hölscher U. Efficacy of special extract WS 1473 from saw palmetto fruit in patients with BPH (stage I and II according to Alken). Jatros Uro 1998;3:36-43.

4 Di Silverio F, Monti S, Sciarra A, et al. Effects of long-term treatment with Serenoa repens (Permixon(r)) on the concentrations and regional distribution of androgens and epidermal growth factor in benign prostatic hyperplasia. Prostate 1998;37:77-83.

5 Bach D, Ebeling L. Long-term drug treatment of benign prostatic hyperplasia-results of a prospective 3-year multicenter study using Sabal extract IDS 89. Phytomedicine 1996;3:105-11 (originally published in Urologe [B] 1995;35:178-83).

6 Braeckman J. The extract of Serenoa repens in the treatment of benign prostatic hyperplasia: multicenter open study. Curr Ther Res 1994;55:776-85.

7 Carraro JC, Raynaud JP, Koch G, *et al.* Comparison of phytotherapy (Permixon(r)) with finasteride in the treatment of benign prostate hyperplasia: A randomized international study of 1,098 patients. Prostate 1996;29:231-40

8 Wren RC. Potter's New Cyclopaedia of Botanical drugs and preparations. Essex, UK. Saffron Walden;1988.

9 Bradley P (Ed.). British herbal Compendium. Dorset. British Herbal Medical Assoc.; 1992.

10 Snow JM. Echinacea (Moench) Spp. Asteraceae. The Protocol Journal of Botanical Medicine. 1997; 2 (2): 18-24.

11 Felter H, Lloyd JU. King's American Dispensatory. Portland. Eclectic medical Publications; 1983.

12 Snow JM. Echinacea (Moench) Spp. Asteraceae. The Protocol Journal of Botanical Medicine. 1997; 2 (2): 18-24.

13 Bauer R, Wagner H. Echinacea species as potential immunostimulatory drugs. Economic and Medicinal Plant Research. San Diego: Academic press Ltd.; 1991.

14 Schranner I, Wurdinger M, *et al.* Modification of avian humeral immunoreactions by Influx and Echinacea angustifolia extract. Zentralbl Veterinarmed (B) 1989; 36.

15 Bukovsky M, Kostalova D, Magnusova R, Vaverkova S. Testing for immunomodulating effects of ethanol-water extracts of the above ground parts of the plants Echinaceae and Rudbeckia. Cesk Farm. 1993; 42.

16 Witchl M. (Bisset NG, Ed.) Herbal Drugs and Phytopharmaceuticals. Medpharm, CRC Press: Boca Raton. 1994.

17 Hirano T, Homma M, Oka K. Effects of stinging nettle root extracts and their steroidal components on the Na+,K+-ATPase of the benign prostatic hyperplasia. Planta Med 1994; 60:30-3.

18 Vontobel H, Herzog R, Rutishauser G, Kres H. Results of a double-blind study on the effectiveness of ERU (extractum radicis urticae) capsules in conservative treatment of benign prostatic hyperplasia. Urologe 1985;24(1):49-51 [in German].

19 Blumenthal M, Busse WR, Goldberg A, et al, eds. The Complete Commission E Monographs: Therapeutic Guide to Herbal Medicines. Boston, MA: Integrative Medicine Communications, 1998, 216-7.

20 Gruenwald J. PDR for Herbal Medicines, Medical Economics Company. Montvale, New Jersey. 1998.1059-61.

21 Wren RC. Potter's New Cyclopaedia of Botanical drugs and preparations. Essex, UK. Saffron Walden;1988.222-223

22 Leung A, Foster S. Encyclopedia of Common Natural Ingredients. NY: Wiley;1996.421-22

23 Felter H, Lloyd JU. King's American Dispensatory. Portland. Eclectic Medical Publications; 1983. 495-97

24 Felter H, Lloyd JU. King's American Dispensatory. Portland. Eclectic Medical Publications; 1983 pg. 1936.

25 Millet Y. Toxicity of some Essential plant oils, Clin Toxicol, 1981 Dec:18:1485-98

26 Leung A, Foster S. Encyclopedia of Common Natural Ingredients. NY: Wiley;1996.

27 Wren RC. Potter's New Cyclopaedia of Botanical drugs and preparations. Essex, UK. Saffron Walden;1988.

28 Bradley P (Ed.). British herbal Compendium. Dorset. British Herbal Medical Assoc.; 1992.

29 Felter H, Lloyd JU. King's American Dispensatory. Portland. Eclectic Medical Publications; 1983. 495-97

30 Braeckman J, Bruhwyler J, Vandekerckhove K, Géczy J. Efficacy and safety of the extract of Serenoa repens in the treatment of benign prostatic hyperplasia: Therapeutic equivalence between twice and once daily dosage forms. Phytotherapy Res 1997;11:558-63.

31 Redecker KD, Hölscher U. Extractum Sabal fructus in benign prostatic hyperplasia (BPH)-clinical trial in BPH stages I and II according to Alken. Extracta Urologica 1998;21:23-5.

32 Ziegler, K, Hölscher U. Efficacy of special extract WS 1473 from saw palmetto fruit in patients with BPH (stage I and II according to Alken). Jatros Uro 1998;3:36-43.

33 Di Silverio F, Monti S, Sciarra A, et al. Effects of long-term treatment with Serenoa repens (Permixon(r)) on the concentrations and regional distribution of androgens and epidermal growth factor in benign prostatic hyperplasia. Prostate 1998;37:77-83.

34 Bach D, Ebeling L. Long-term drug treatment of benign prostatic hyperplasia-results of a prospective 3-year multicenter study using Sabal extract IDS 89. Phytomedicine 1996;3:105-11 (originally published in Urologe [B] 1995;35:178-83).

SCUDDER'S ALTERATIVE
*A Deep Tissue Alterative for Detoxification**
FORMULA

Corydalis tubers	(*Dicentra canadensis*)
Black alder bark	(*Alnus serrulata*)
Mayapple root	(*Podophyllum peltatum*)
Figwort	(*Scrophularia nodosa*)
Yellowdock root	(*Rumex crispus*)

Concentration:	1:1 Herb strength ratio
Dosage:	30-40 drops, 3 times daily
Duration of use:	3-4 months
Best taken:	Between meals, with warm water

DESCRIPTION OF FORMULA

Originally compounded by Dr. John Scudder, MD, this alterative formula increases the removal of cellular wastes and promotes correct nutrition. When this balance of basic cellular function is normalized, we remove the 'obstacles to cure', and allow the healing force within the body to overcome disorder. This type of formula represents the most profound, yet basic, principle underlying Naturopathic Botanical Medicine. This Detox formula is of value where the use of tissue repair is required.

Corydalis tubers were held in high regard by the Physiomedicalists and the Eclectic physicians of the last century. [G15, 1, 3] It is said that "all the excretive avenues of the body are more or less emptied of injurious and impure contents"[1] and that "its efficacy is not equaled by any other agent as an alterative tonic".[G12] It is also of value in this formula for its ability to improve digestion.[G15]

Black alder bark has a long history of use as a pain-relieving alterative. [G12] Dr. John Scudder, the medical doctor who created this formula, said that the Black alder is simply the ideal alterative, due to the fact that "it exerts a specific influence upon the processes of waste and nutrition, increasing one and stimulating the other". [2] It is reported to have particular effect where indigestion, [G12, G15] or lymphatic congestion is present. [G12] Dr. Scudder also noted its use with conditions of the skin and mucous membranes. [2]

Mayapple root is another example of a highly respected alterative. [G12, 1, 3] Scudder discovered that if Mayapple is extracted in hot water, that the alterative compounds within the plant are extracted and the laxative compounds in the plant are left behind. The hot water extracted Mayapple is used here. Its reported affinity for improving weakened digestion, [G12] along with its established use with liver disorders, [G12, 3] make it of particular benefit in this formula.

Figwort joins this formula of noted alteratives. It has been described as a "mild and gently stimulating alterative", [1] "probably as certain in its action as any of the vegetable alteratives". [2] It is particularly respected for its influence with conditions of the skin. [1, 2]

Yellow Dock root is considered a tonic alterative with mild laxative action. [G12, 3] It is interesting that Native Americans and the eclectic physicians of the last century used the Yellowdock for its mild laxative quality, and for the treatment of skin conditions. [G12, 4] The Eclectic physicians noted that it was particularly useful where lymphatic congestion was present. [G12] Yellowdock is also noted to improve digestion and reduce liver congestion. [3]

THERAPEUTIC APPLICATIONS*

Note: The intention of the following information is to represent the traditional use of the individual botanicals found in these formulas and to inform the reader of any evolving scientific inquiry relevant to the formula's ingredients.

SUPPORTED BY TRADITIONAL USE

<u>Alterative,</u> [G12, G15, 1, 2, 3] Improves digestion, [G12, G15, 3] <u>Lymphatic congestion,</u> [G12] Skin conditions, [G12, 1, 2, 4] Liver disorders, [G12, 3]

SCOPE OF RELEVANT SCIENTIFIC INVESTIGATION

None relevant

CAUTIONS, CONTRA-INDICATIONS AND DRUG INTERACTIONS

Please reference Chapter 9. Do not use during pregnancy or lactation.

COMPLIMENTARY HERBS/FORMULAS

Daily Detox, Cell Wise, Red Clover Supreme,
Sheep Sorrel/ Burdock Supreme

REFERENCES

1. Lyle TJ. Physiomedical Therapeutics, Materia Medica and Pharmacy. London. National Association of Medical Herbalists; 1897.
2. Scudder JM. Specific Medication. Eclectic Medical Publications. 1985.
3. Culbreth D. A manual of materia medica and pharmacology. Philadelphia. Lea & Febiger; 1927.
4. Willard T. Wild Rose Scientific Herbal. Wild rose College of Natural Healing; Alberta; 1991.

SHEEP SORREL/BURDOCK SUPREME

*An Alterative Formula for Degenerative Processes**

FORMULA

Sheep Sorrel	(*Rumex acetosella*)
Burdock Root	(*Arctium lappa*)
Slippery Elm Bark	(*Ulmus rubra*)
Turkey Rhubarb Root	(*Rhuem palmatum*)

Concentration:	1:1 Herb strength ratio
Dosage:	30-50 drops, 3-4 times daily
Duration of use:	2-3 months for best results
Best taken:	Between meals with warm water

DESCRIPTION OF FORMULA

This formula is a replication of Renee Caisse's traditional formula used for a wide variety of degenerative disorders. It contains herbs for the liver, a laxative, a soothing demulcent and an herb for chronic catarrh (mucous). The formula was described as "breaking down catabolic (diseased) tissue and promoting the development of healthy new tissue."[1]

Sheep Sorrel is used for acute and chronic inflammation of the nasal passages and respiratory tract. It has a mild antibacterial effect. [2] Sheep Sorrel has long been described as a remedy for cancer. Dr. Scudder described its use in the 1800's as "a remedy where there is a tendency to degeneration of tissue, whether in syphilis, scrofula (tuberculosis) or cancer the indication for its use is the replacement of tissue with lower organization."[3]

Burdock root is an alterative that is similar in action to Yellow Dock.[4,5,6] It has long been used for rheumatism, skin disorders, and to stimulate urination.[10] It is also well known for its ability to stimulate liver/bile related functions.[7] Traditional cancer research reports that is has some anti-tumor activity, along with the ability to induce cell differentiation.[8]

Slippery Elm Bark contains abundant mucilage made up of polysaccharides, that are demulcent and emollient and are readily digestible.[9] It is soothing to inflammations and ulcerations of the digestive tract.[10] The polysaccharides may absorb endotoxins in the gut providing relief in dysbiosis (author).

Turkey Rhubarb Root has a laxative effect and is analgesic and anti-inflammatory. This combination of properties makes a good addition to this "rejuvinative formula" in order to stimulate excretion and elimination via the bowels. It has a high tannin content so that it is also astringent toning up the mucous membranes of the colon as it exits.[11] In low doses it acts as an appetite stimulant and increases gastric secretions.[12]

THERAPEUTIC APPLICATIONS*

Note: The intention of the following information is to represent the traditional use of the individual botanicals found in these formulas and to inform the reader of any evolving scientific inquiry relevant to the formula's ingredients.

SUPPORTED BY TRADITIONAL USE

Acute and chronic inflammation of the nasal passages and respiratory tract, mild antibacterial effect,[13] rheumatism, skin disorders,[10] stimulates liver and bile functions,[14] soothing to inflammations and ulcerations of the digestive tract,[15] appetite stimulant and increases gastric secretions.[16]

SCOPE OF RELEVANT SCIENTIFIC INVESTIGATION

Some anti-tumor activity, ability to induce cell differentiation.[11,17]

CAUTIONS, CONTRA-INDICATIONS AND DRUG INTERACTIONS

Please reference Chapter 9. Do not use during pregnancy or lactation.

COMPLIMENTARY HERBS/FORMULAS

Red Clover Supreme, Daily Detox, Cell Wise

REFERENCES

1 Scudder, Specific Medication.

2 PDR for Herbal Medicines, Medical Economics Company. Montvale, New Jersey. 1998. 1105-6

3 See Scudder, Specific Medication.

4 Boik J. Cancer and Natural Medicine: A Textbook of Basic Science and Clinical Research. Oregon Medical Press, Princeton, MN.1996.

5 Ellingwood F. American Materia Medica, Therapeutics and Pharmacognosy. Portland. Eclectic Medical Publications; 1985.

6 Witchl M. (Bisset NG, Ed.) Herbal Drugs and Phytopharmaceuticals. Medpharm, CRC Press: Boca Raton. 1994.

7 Bradley P (Ed.). British herbal Compendium. Dorset. British Herbal Medical Assoc.; 1992.

8 Leung A, Foster S. Encyclopedia of Common Natural Ingredients. NY: Wiley; 1996.

9 Beverage R.J., Some Structural Features of Mucilage from Ulmus fulva. Carbohyd.Res.1969,9,429-39

10 Bradley P (Ed.). British herbal Compendium. Dorset. British Herbal Medical Assoc.; 1992.202

11 Bradley P (Ed.). British herbal Compendium. Dorset. British Herbal Medical Assoc. 1992. 188-9

12 Wren RC. Potter's New Cyclopaedia of Botanical drugs and preparations. Essex, UK. Saffron Walden;1988.23

13 PDR for Herbal Medicines, Medical Economics Company. Montvale, New Jersey. 1998. 1105-6

14 Bradley P (Ed.). British herbal Compendium. Dorset. British Herbal Medical Assoc.; 1992.

15 Bradley P (Ed.). British herbal Compendium. Dorset. British Herbal Medical Assoc.; 1992.202

16 Wren RC. Potter's New Cyclopaedia of Botanical drugs and preparations. Essex, UK. Saffron Walden;1988.23

17 Leung A, Foster S. Encyclopedia of Common Natural Ingredients. NY: Wiley; 1996.

SKULLCAP/ST. JOHN'S WORT SUPREME

Nervous System Tonic, Trauma and Sleep formula*

FORMULA

Skullcap Herb	(*Scutellaria laterifolia*)
St. John's Wort Flower Buds	(*Hypericum perforatum*)
Chamomile Flowers	(*Matricaria recutita*)
Calendula Flowers	(*Calendula officialis*)
California Poppy	(*Eschscholzia californica*)
Wild Oats	(*Avena sativa*)
Valerian Root	(*Valeriana officinalis*)

Concentration:	1:1 Herb strength ratio
Dosage:	30-40 drops, 3-4 times daily
Duration of use:	2-6 weeks
Best taken:	Between meals with warm water

DESCRIPTION OF FORMULA

This formula is formulated as a nerve restorative, antispasmodic and soothing anodyne. The specific herbs in this formula soothe nervous agitation and exert a mild sedative and calming action. These herbs are helpful in promoting sleep.

Skullcap is a tonic to the nerves and has a long and trusted use as an antispasmodic. It is used in restlessness, insomnia and nervous excitability.[1] It is helpful for physical or mental over-work, or nervous exhaustion following acute illness. Skullcap is reported to act on the cerebrospinal centers of the brain and may have a beneficial effect on epilepsy and heart symptoms of a nervous origin.[2] Skullcap has been used in teething, neuralgia and headache.[3] For insomnia it calms nervous irritability.[4]

St. John's Wort has been used as a medicine for more than 2000 years. It is an effective antidepressant. In several recent studies when compared to standard antidepressant drugs it proves as effective, better tolerated and has much fewer side effects.[5] St. John's Wort has been shown to be effective in Seasonal Affective Disorder(SAD).[6] It has also been shown to increase libido in contrast to conventional medications. In addition to its antidepressant effect, it also is a valuable anti-inflammatory[7], wound healing[8] and antiviral agent. [9]

Chamomile is an excellent and reliable nervine that relaxes and is tonic to the nervous system. It produces a calming action for infants, children and adults who are restless, discontented and impatient.[10] It is a traditional remedy for nervous apprehension that is out of proportion to the actual pain suffered. Chamomile is soothing to the GI tract and is effective for a simple bellyache, diarrhea or constipation.[11,12] Its volatile oils have fungicidal and bactericidal properties.[13]

Calendula used internally has a traditional use as an antiphlogistic (anti-inflammatory) in colitis, gastritis, bladder infections, gall bladder pain,[14] gastric and duodenal ulcers.[15] It is a valued herb as an external application for cuts, wounds and burns as an anti-inflammatory and to speed healing.[16,17]

California Poppy has anti-anxiety and sedative effects as well as mild analgesic effects at higher doses. It been reported useful in quieting "hyperactive bright eyed children who can't fall asleep"[18] It has pain relieving and antispasmodic influence in stomach cramps and muscle aches.[19] Its main alkaloid is cryptopine which has been shown to have antispasmotic properties.[20]

Wild Oats is indicated in assisting convalescence for nervous exhaustion and debility in chronic conditions and cardiac weakness. An acute indication for use is for a headache from over work. "It is not a remedy of great power...probably its chief value as a medicine is to energize in nervous exhaustion", Harvey W. Felter, MD.[21]

Valerian root is a nerve tonic that reduces symptoms of anxiety, helping people to deal with stress more effectively[22] without the negative effects of a narcotic. [23] It has proven effective for insomnia by reducing sleep latency, improve sleep quality, and decrease nighttime waking.[24] The mechanism for these actions appears to be by valerian binding to GABA receptors in the brain creating the sedative effect.[25] These have been common uses for valerian for many centuries.

THERAPEUTIC APPLICATIONS*

Note: The intention of this information is to represent the traditional use of the individual botanicals found in these formulas and to inform the reader of any evolving scientific inquiry relevant to the formula's ingredients.

SUPPORTED BY TRADITIONAL USE

Antispasmodic, restlessness, insomnia[26], teething, neuralgia headache[27], heart symptoms of a nervous origin[28], useful in quieting "hyperactive bright eyed children who can't fall asleep"[29] pain relieving, antispasmodic in stomach cramps and muscle aches.[30]

SCOPE OF RELEVANT SCIENTIFIC INVESTIGATION

Effective antidepressant, better tolerated and fewer side effects,[31] effective in Seasonal Affective Disorder(SAD).[32] Its main alkaloid is cryptopine has antispasmodic properties.[33] Helps insomnia by reducing sleep latency, improve sleep quality, and decrease nighttime waking,[34] binding to GABA receptors in the brain creating the sedative effect.[35]

CAUTIONS, CONTRA-INDICATIONS AND DRUG INTERACTIONS

Please reference Chapter 9. Do not use during pregnancy or lactation.

COMPLIMENTARY HERBS/FORMULAS

Serenity with Kava, Calcium Supreme, Valerian Root

REFERENCES

1 Hoffman D. *The Herbal Handbook: A User's Guide to Medical Herbalism.* Rochester, VT: Healing Arts Press, 1988, 77.

2 Felter H, Lloyd JU. King's American Dispensatory. Portland, Oregon: Eclectic Medical Publications. 1983, 17339-41.

3 Grieve M. A Modern Herbal, Dover Publications NY.1971,725.

4 Ellingwood F. American Materia Medica, Therapeutics and Pharmacognosy. Portland, Oregon: Eclectic Medical Publications. 1985, 625.

5 Linde, K., Ramirez, G., Mulrow, C.D. *et al.* (1996). St. John's Wort for depression-an overview and meta analysis of randomized clinical trials. British Medical Journal 313:253-258.

6 Wheatley D. Hypericum in seasonal affective disorder (SAD). Curr Med Res Opin 1999; 15:33-37

7 Wren RC. Potter's New Cyclopaedia of Botanical drugs and preparations. Essex, UK. Saffron Walden;1988.

8 Hobbs C:St. John's Wort, *Hypericum perforatum L. Herbalgram* 18/19, 24-33, 1989.

9 Leung A, Foster S. Encyclopedia of Common Natural Ingredients. NY: Wiley;1996, 310-312.

10 Felter HW. The Eclectic Materia Medica, Pharmacology and Therapeutics. Portland, Oregon: Eclectic Medical publications. 1985.475-6.

11 Bisset N. Herbal Drugs and Phytopharmaceuticals, Medpharm Scientific Publishers, Stuttgart, 1994, 322-25.

12 Hoffman D. *The Holistic Herbal.* Moray. The Findhorn Press; 1984.185

13 Leung A, Foster S. Encyclopedia of Common Natural Ingredients. NY: Wiley;1996, 145-48.

14 Bisset N. Herbal Drugs and Phytopharmaceuticals, Medpharm Scientific Publishers, Stuttgart, 1994, 118-120.

15 Wren RC. Potter's New Cyclopaedia of Botanical drugs and preparations. Essex, UK. Saffron Walden;1988.184-5.

16 Felter HW. The Eclectic Materia Medica, Pharmacology and Therapeutics. Portland, Oregon: Eclectic Medical publications. 1985.262-3.

17 Wren RC. Potter's New Cyclopaedia of Botanical drugs and preparations. Essex, UK. Saffron Walden;1988,184-185.

18 Moore M. *Medicinal Plants of the Pacific West*, Santa Fe, Red Crane Books, 110-112.

19 Hoffman D. *The Holistic Herbal.* Moray. The Findhorn Press; 1984.177.

20 Blumenthal M, *et al.* Ed. *The Complete German Commission E Monographs.* Austin, TX: American Botanical Council. 1998, 389.

21 Felter HW. The Eclectic Materia Medica, Pharmacology and Therapeutics. Portland, Oregon: Eclectic Medical publications. 1985.235.

22 Kohnen R, The effectsof valerian, propranolol and their combination on activationperformance and mood of healthy volunteers under social stress conditions. Pharmacopsychiatry 1988;21:447-8.

23 Coon N. Using plants for healing. Philadelphia, Pa. Rodale Press. 1979.

24 Leatherwood P, *et al.*: Aqueous extract of valerian root improves sleep quality in man. *Pharmacol Biochem Behav* n 17,65-71.

25 Mennini T, Bernasconi P, *et al.* In vitro study on the interaction of extracts and pure compounds from *Valeriana officinalis* roots with GABA, benzodiazepine and barbiturate receptors. *Fitoterapia* 1993;64:291-300.

26 Hoffman D. *The Herbal Handbook: A User's Guide to Medical Herbalism.* Rochester, VT: Healing Arts Press, 1988, 77.

27 Grieve M. A Modern Herbal, Dover Publications NY.1971,725.

28 Felter H, Lloyd JU. King's American Dispensatory. Portland, Oregon: Eclectic Medical Publications. 1983, 17339-41.

29 Moore M. *Medicinal Plants of the Pacific West*, Santa Fe, Red Crane Books, 110-112.

30 Hoffman D. The Holistic Herbal. Moray. The Findhorn Press; 1984.177.

31 Linde, K., Ramirez, G., Mulrow, C.D. *et al.* (1996). St. John's Wort for depression-an overview and meta analysis of randomized clinical trials. British Medical Journal 313:253-258.

32 Wheatley D. Hypericum in seasonal affective disorder (SAD). Curr Med Res Opin 1999; 15:33-37

33 Blumenthal M, *et al.* Ed. *The Complete German Commission E Monographs.* Austin, TX: American Botanical Council. 1998, 389.

34 Leatherwood P, *et al.*: Aqueous extract of valerian root improves sleep quality in man. *Pharmacol Biochem Behav* n 17,65-71.

35 Mennini T, Bernasconi P, *et al.* In vitro study on the interaction of extracts and pure compounds from *Valeriana officinalis* roots with GABA, benzodiazepine and barbiturate receptors. *Fitoterapia* 1993;64:291-300.

SMILAX/DAMIANA SUPREME

*A Male/Female Virility Formula**
FORMULA

Sarsaparilla Root	(*Smilax officinalis*)
Damiana	(*Turnera diffusa*)
American ginseng	(*Panax quinquifolium*)
Ashwagandha	(*Withinia somnifera*)
Shatavari Root	(*Asparagus racemosus*)
Wild Oats	(*Avena sativa*)
Licorice Root	(*Glycyrrhiza glabra*)
Hawthorn Berry	(*Crataegus oxyacantha*)
Prickly Ash Bark	(*Xanthoxylum clava-herculis*)

Concentration:	1:1 Herb strength ratio
Dosage:	30-40 Drops 3-4 times daily
Duration of use:	3-4 months for best results
Best taken:	Between meals with warm water

DESCRIPTION OF FORMULA

This formula is a restorative for men and women desiring more stamina and virility. It is a useful adjunct to a fitness or body building program. The herbs contain natural phytosterols that target the same receptors as endogenous hormones, while hormonal imbalances and liver dysfunction are also addressed.

Sarsaparilla is an alterative that is known for its anti-inflammatory affect with conditions such as psoriasis, rheumatism, and rheumatoid arthritis. Liver protective action is also noted. It is included in this virility formula for its tonifying influence combined with its ability to restore correct metabolism. Contains steroidal saponins and phytosterols.[1][2][3]

Damiana has a long history of use as a trophorestorative (builds nervous reserve) and an even longer history as an aphrodisiac.[4][5][6] In fact, Damiana was once referred to by the latin, *Damiana* *aphrodisiaca* because of this reputation. The physicians of the physio-medicalist school referred to Damiana as a stimulating nervous system tonic and trophorestorative.[7]

American Ginseng belongs to a genus (a sub-group of a family) named Panax, which is derived from the word panacea, meaning 'cure-all'. The common name also distinguishes this highly regarded herb, as Ginseng means 'wonder of the world'.[8] American Ginseng is said, energetically speaking, to be cooler than Asian Ginseng.[9] Traditionally used as a yin tonic, it is used to build condensed energy which nourishes the body fluids and 'essence', in the most debilitated of conditions. Western medicine has also held this plant in high regard, as it was used in medical practice, here in the U.S. as a mild sedative and a tonic to the nerve centers, which was said to improve their tone with its use.[10] Ginseng was also in the United States Pharmacopoeia from 1842 to 1882, as a stimulant and a digestive aid.[11] This plant is the tonic *par excellence*.

Ashwaghanda is considered the Ginseng of India in Ayurvedic medicine. It is adaptogenic and strengthens the body's power of resistance. It is a general tonic to enhance virility and vitality.[12]

Shatavari Root is described as an aphrodisiac but is probably described better as a nutritive tonic.[13]

Wild Oats are present here for its influence with nervous exhaustion. [G12] Often used with complaints of the digestive system where there is also physical weakness and fatigue. [13] Wild Oats may be used during convalescence from chronic disease, [G12] or from nicotine abuse.[13] This plant also combines well with Saw Palmetto where nervous exhaustion leads to impotence. [G6]

Licorice root blocks the breakdown of the body's own cortisol,[14] thus acting as an indirect anti-inflammatory throughout the body. Licorice has been used in traditional Western herbalism as a demulcent and expectorant for coughs,[16] to heal stomach ulcers,[17] to relieve Addison's disease (low adrenal function),[18] and for people with asthma, diabetes, urinary tract infections, tumors, and pain.[19] In traditional Chinese herbalism, licorice was widely used to make other herbs work together well in a formula.[20]

Hawthorn berry has long been used as a tonic for the cardiovascular system. Hawthorn berry has been shown to reduce free-radical damage to cellular phospholipids,[21] and to inhibit the initial release of compounds such as prostaglandins, leukotrienes, etc. which are highly pro-inflammatory. Hawthorns ability to reduce free-radical damage to collagen is the proposed process by which it is able to stabilize connective tissue. [22, 23]

Prickly Ash bark is a circulatory stimulant[24, 25, 26] and as such, appears in this formula to help drive the other botanicals throughout the body. The Eclectic physicians used this plant to 'stimulate the nerve centers', and to 'sustain the vital forces through any crisis that occurs'.[27] It is a potent alterative and has a long history of use with "chronic muscular rheumatism," lumbar back pain and myalgia. Dr. Felter gave it high marks when the nerve force is low and neural irritation is present but where recuperation is possible.[28]

THERAPEUTIC APPLICATIONS*
Note: The intention of the following information is to represent the traditional use of the individual botanicals found in these formulas and to inform the reader of any evolving scientific inquiry relevant to the formula's ingredients.

SUPPORTED BY TRADITIONAL USE
Sexual restorative, nervous exhaustion,[29, 30] aphrodisiac.[31, 32, 33] Tonic,[34] Physical weakness and fatigue,[13] Anti-inflammatory.[35] nervous system tonic and trophorestorative.[36]

SCOPE OF RELEVANT SCIENTIFIC INVESTIGATION
None found.

CAUTIONS, CONTRA-INDICATIONS AND DRUG INTERACTIONS
Please reference Chapter 9. Do not use during pregnancy or lactation.

COMPLIMENTARY HERBS/FORMULAS
Energy & Vitality, Siberian Ginseng Tonic, Male Libido, Woman's Libido

REFERENCES

1 Leung A, Foster S. Encyclopedia of Common Natural Ingredients. NY: Wiley;1996.

2 Bradley P (Ed.). British herbal Compendium. Dorset. British Herbal Medical Assoc.; 1992.

3 Newall CA, *et al.* Herbal Medicines: A Guide for Health-Care

Professionals.London: Pharmaceutical Press;1996.

4 Bradley P (Ed.). British herbal Compendium. Dorset. British Herbal Medical Assoc.; 1992.

5 Leung A, Foster S. Encyclopedia of Common Natural Ingredients. NY: Wiley;1996.204.

6 Wren RC. Potter's New Cyclopaedia of Botanical drugs and preparations. Essex, UK. Saffron Walden;1988,100.

7 Priest AW, Priest LR. Herbal medication. A clinical dispensary handbook. 1982

8 Coon N. Using plants for healing. Philadelphia, Pa. Rodale Press. 1979.

9 Leung A, Foster S. Encyclopedia of Common Natural Ingredients. NY: Wiley;1996.Bradley P (Ed.). British herbal Compendium. Dorset. British Herbal Medical Assoc.; 1992.

10 Ellingwood F. American Materia Medica, Therapeutics and Pharmacognosy. Portland. Eclectic Medical Publications;1985.

11 Coon N. Ibid

12 Naturopathic handbook of Herbal Formulas, Herbal Research Publications, Ayer, Massachusetts, 1995,91.

13 Kapoor LD. CRC Handbook of Ayurvedic Medicinal Plants. CRC Press Boca Raton. 1990,56.

14 Tamura Y, Nishikawa T, Yamada K, et al. Effects of glycyrrhetinic acid and its derivatives on 4-sulpha- and 5-beta-reductase in rat liver. Arzneim Forsch 1979;29:647-9.

15 Yoshikawa M, Matsui Y, Kawamoto H, et al. Effects of glycyrrhizin on immune-mediated cytotoxicity. J Gastroenterol Hepatol 1997;12:243-8.

16 Felter HW. Eclectic Materia Medica, Pharmacology and Therapeutics. Sandy, OR: Eclectic Medical Publications, 1922:395.

17 Weiss RF. Herbal Medicine. Gothenberg, Sweden: Ab Arcanum and Beaconsfield: Beaconsfield Publishers Ltd, trans. Meuss AR, 1985:59-61.

18 Hoffmann D. The Complete Illustrated Herbal. New York: Barnes & Noble Books, 1996;:99.

19 Davis EA, Morris DJ. Medicinal uses of licorice through the millennia: The good and plenty of it. Mol Cell Endocrinol 1991;78:1-6.

20 Foster S, Yue CX. Herbal Emissaries: Bringing Chinese Herbs to the West. Rochester VT: Healing Arts Press, 1992:112-121.

21 Bensky D, Gamble A. Chinese Herbal Medicine: Materia Medica. Seattle: Eastland, 1986.

22 Djumlija LC. Crataegus oxycantha. The Australian Journal of Medical Herbalism. 1994; 6(2): 37-42.

23 Snow JM. Ginkgo biloba L. (Ginkgoaceae). The Protocol Journal of Botanical Medicine. 1996; 2(1): 9-15.

24 Wren RC. Potter's New Cyclopaedia of Botanical drugs and preparations. Essex, UK. Saffron Walden;1988

25 Leung A, Foster S. Encyclopedia of Common Natural Ingredients. NY: Wiley;1996.

26 Bradley P (Ed.). British herbal Compendium. Dorset. British Herbal Medical Assoc.; 1992.

27 Ellingwood F. American Materia Medica, Therapeutics and Pharmacognosy. Portland. Eclectic Medical Publications;1985.

28 Felter HW. The Eclectic Materia Medica, Pharmacology and Therapeutics. Portland, Oregon: Eclectic Medical publications. 1985.697-8

29 Ellingwood F. American Materia Medica, Therapeutics and Pharmacognosy.

Portland. Eclectic Medical Publications;1985.

30 Felter H, Lloyd JU. King's American Dispensatory. Portland. Eclectic medical Publications; 1983.

31 Bradley P (Ed.). British herbal Compendium. Dorset. British Herbal Medical Assoc.; 1992.

32 Leung A, Foster S. Encyclopedia of Common Natural Ingredients. NY: Wiley;1996.204.

33 Wren RC. Potter's New Cyclopaedia of Botanical drugs and preparations. Essex, UK. Saffron Walden;1988,100.

34 Bensky D, Gamble A. Chinese Herbal Medicine: Materia Medica. Seattle: Eastland, 1986.

35 Newall CA, *et al. Herbal Medicines: A Guide for Health-Care Professionals.*London: Pharmaceutical Press;1996.

36 Priest AW, Priest LR. Herbal medication. A clinical dispensary handbook. 1982

SPILANTHES SUPREME
*Anti-Yeast and Anti-Fungal Formula**
FORMULA

Spilanthes Flowering tops and Root	(*Spilanthes acmella*)
Oregon Grape root	(*Berberis aquifolium*)
Juniper Berry	(*Juniperus communis*)
Usnea Lichen	(*Usnea spp.*)
Myrrh Gum	(*Commiphora molmol*)

Concentration:	1:1 Herb strength ratio
Dosage:	30-50 drops, 3-4 times daily
Duration of use:	3-4 months for best results
Best taken:	Between meals with warm water

DESCRIPTION OF FORMULA

These herbs are natural anti-fungal, anti-yeast and anti-bacterial.

Spilanthes Flowering tops and Root has enjoyed a long history of indigenous use for numerous disorders, including the removal of intestinal worms. This plant is immunotonic, anti-inflammatory, anti-bacterial, anti-fungal, anti-viral and anti-malarial. As a mouthwash it heals herpes sores and keeps gingiva healthy.[1] The Eclectic physicians of North America considered it to be a useful digestive stimulant.[2]

Oregon Grape root has a history of traditional use closely resembling that of Goldenseal due to the berberine alkaloids shared by each. Berberine has been shown to effect *Giardia lambria, Tricomonas vaginalis, and Entameba histolytica-candida.*[5] Oregon Grape root has a therapeutic effect with skin conditions, such as psoriasis, eczema, and acne.[6]

Juniper Berry is a soothing diuretic suited to chronic disorders of the kidneys.[7,1] It is used to restore normal action and function of the kidneys following acute, irritating[1] disorders.[8] This remedy is useful for indigestion,[2, 3] bronchitis (using steam inhalation), various gastrointestinal disorders,[2] snakebites, and as a carminative to treat intestinal flatulence and colic.[9, 10, 11] Pharmacological research reports that the oil from Juniper possesses an antispasmodic influence over smooth muscle.[8]

Usnea is a lichen that contains usneic acid, which has strong antibacterial and anti-fungal activity. It is used in many European anti-bacterial and anti-fungal creams.[12]

Myrrh Gum is used as an antiseptic and astringent for mucous membranes in sore throats, cough and gingivitis. It has been used traditionally for wounds, bleeding and pain.[13]

THERAPEUTIC APPLICATIONS*

Note: The intention of the following information is to represent the traditional use of the individual botanicals found in these formulas and to inform the reader of any evolving scientific inquiry relevant to the formula's ingredients.

SUPPORTED BY TRADITIONAL USE

Anti-fungal,[14] anti-viral, anti-malarial, mouthwash heals herpes sores, keeps gingiva healthy.[15] Intestinal worms, digestive stimulant,[16] carminative to treat intestinal flatulence and colic.[17 18 19]

SCOPE OF RELEVANT SCIENTIFIC INVESTIGATION

Effective against *Giardia lambria, Tricomonas vaginalis, and Entameba histolytica-candida.*[20]

CAUTIONS, CONTRA-INDICATIONS AND DRUG INTERACTIONS

Please reference Chapter 9. Do not use during pregnancy or lactation.

COMPLIMENTARY HERBS/FORMULAS

Candida Supreme Vital Cleanse, Sweetish Bitters

REFERENCES

1 Agricultural Research Service. Dr. Duke's Phytochemical and Ethnobotanical Databases: Ethnobotanical uses *Maytenus ilicifolia*. Online. Internet. [8/30/00]. Available WWW: http://www.ars-grin.gov/cgi-bin/duke/ethnobot.pl

2 Felter H, Lloyd JU. King's American Dispensatory. Portland. Eclectic Medical Publications; 1983.1808.

3 Wagner H, Breu W, *et al.* In vitro Inhibition of Arachidonate Metabolism by some Alkamides and Prenylated phenols. *Planta Medica.* 1989;55:566-567.

4 Fabry W, *et al.* Activity of East African medicinal plants against *Heliobacter pylori. Chemotherapy.* 1996;42(5):315-317.

5 Kaneda Y, *et al.*: In vitro effects of berberine sulfate on the growth of Entamoeba histolytica, Giardia lamblia and Tricomonas vaginalis. Ann Tpp Med Parasitol 85, 417-425, 1991.

6 Murray M. The healing power of herbs - The enlightened persons guide to the wonders of medicinal plants. Rocklin, Ca. Prima publishing; 1995.

7 Wren RC. Potter's New Cyclopaedia of Botanical drugs and preparations. Essex, UK. Saffron Walden;1988.

8 Ellingwood F. American Materia Medica, Therapeutics and Pharmacognosy. Portland. Eclectic Medical Publications;1985.

9 Witchl M. (Bisset NG, Ed.) Herbal Drugs and Phytopharmaceuticals. Medpharm, CRC Press: Boca Raton. 1994.

10 Grieve M, Mrs. A Modern Herbal. New York. Dover; 1982.

11 Leung A, Foster S. Encyclopedia of Common Natural Ingredients. NY: Wiley;1996.

12 Hobbs C. Usnea: The herbal Antibiotic, Interweave Press, Loveland, Co, 1996, 96-107.

13 Leung A, Foster S. Encyclopedia of Common Natural Ingredients. NY: Wiley;1996, 382-3.

14 Hobbs C. Usnea: The herbal Antibiotic, Interweave Press, Loveland, Co, 1996, 96-107.

15 Agricultural Research Service. Dr. Duke's Phytochemical and Ethnobotanical Databases: Ethnobotanical uses *Maytenus ilicifolia.* Online. Internet. [8/30/00]. Available WWW: http://www.ars-grin.gov/cgi-bin/duke/ethnobot.pl

16 Felter H, Lloyd JU. King's American Dispensatory. Portland. Eclectic Medical Publications; 1983.1808.

17 Witchl M. (Bisset NG, Ed.) Herbal Drugs and Phytopharmaceuticals. Medpharm, CRC Press: Boca Raton. 1994. Grieve M, Mrs. A Modern Herbal. New York. Dover; 1982.

18 Grieve M, Mrs. A Modern Herbal. New York. Dover; 1982.

19 Leung A, Foster S. Encyclopedia of Common Natural Ingredients. NY: Wiley;1996.

20 Kaneda Y, *et al.*: In vitro effects of berberine sulfate on the growth of Entamoeba histolytica, Giardia lamblia and Tricomonas vaginalis. Ann Tpp Med Parasitol 85, 417-425, 1991.

TURMERIC/CATECHU SUPREME

*An Immediate Hypersensitivity, Allergy, and Anti-Inflammatory Formula**

FORMULA

Turmeric Root	(*Curcuma longa*)
Black Catechu	(*Catechu nigra*)
Grindelia Floral Buds	(*Grindelia robusta*)
Licorice Root	(*Glycyrrhiza glabra*)
Rose Hips	(*Rosa rugosa*)
Chinese Skullcap	(*Scutellaria baicalensis*)
Ginkgo Leaf	(*Ginkgo biloba*)
Devil's Claw Root	(*Harpagophytum procumbens*)
Yarrow Flowers	(*Achillea millefolium*)
Lobelia Herb & Seed	(*Lobelia inflata*)

Concentration:	1:1 Herb strength ratio
Dosage:	30-40 drops, 4-5 times daily
Duration of use:	3-4 months
Best taken:	Between meals with warm water

DESCRIPTION OF FORMULA

The herbs in this formula contain active constituents that act as anti-inflammatory, antihistamine, bronchial dilators, respiratory antispasmodics and enhance mucous membrane integrity. These herbs are powerful anti-hepatotoxic agents; they protect the liver from circulating antigens and allergens. This compound is formulated to provide adrenal support when it is needed by the body to compensate for the excess anti-inflammatory responses generated from the chronic presence of allergens. The specific action in this formula is to stabilize mast cells of the respiratory system, mucous membranes and epidermal skin tissue.

Turmeric Root has been shown to possess antioxidant,[1] anti-inflammatory, and liver protective effects.[2][3] The volatile oils and curcumin are the most active components. Curcumin is a potent antioxidant and combats free radicals better than vitamin E.[4] The anticancer effects of curcumin act in several ways inhibiting cancer's formation, initiation, promotion and progression.[5,6] The anti-inflammatory effects of curcumin have been demonstrated in animal studies. They are as effective as cortisone in acute inflammation[7] and half as effective in chronic models studied but without toxicity.[8] In one clinical trial patients with rheumatoid arthritis using curcumin were compared with those using tophenlybutazone. The improvements in activities of daily living were comparable, but without the side-effects.[9] Curcumin is an effective analgesic as it depletes the nerve endings of substance P, the neurotransmitter of pain receptors.[10] Turmeric inhibits leukotriene formation, platelet aggregation, and excessive neu-trophil response involved in the inflammation process by stabiliz-ing the cell membranes.[11] It also supports the functioning of the adrenal corticosteroids. Curcumin protects the liver through its antioxidant, anti-inflammatory and choleric effects. Turmeric also protects against ulcer formation from stress, alcohol and some toxins.

Black Catechu contains 2-12% catechins with a tannin content of 20-60% making it a potent astringent, antiseptic and antioxi-dant. It is used for gingivitis, colitis and pharyngitis.[12,13]

Grindelia floral buds have traditionally been used as an effec-tive treatment for congested respiratory disorders including asth-ma.[14] They have also been used to treat eczema, inflammatory disorders, and to restore digestion particularly when it is associ-ated with sluggish liver function.[15] Hoffman reports that Grindelia produces it results by relaxing the smooth muscles of the chest and the heart.[16]

Licorice Root has been used medicinally for over 3000 years.[17] It has anti-inflammatory and anti-allergy properties. Licorice enhances the immune response and has antiviral properties by stimulating the body to produce interferon.[18] It is used for cough and bronchitis because of its expectorant qualities especially in the area of the trachea.[19,20] Its historical use in asthma is now being 'rediscovered' by modern scientific research.[21] Like Schizandra, it also increases intracellular cyclic AMP and has the ability of to protect against the damage caused by free-radicals to liver cells.[22]

Chinese Skullcap has a long history of traditional applications including use as a detoxifying herb and an anti-inflammatory.[23] Modern science confirms its anti-inflammatory influence by selectively inhibiting COX-2 enzymes. [24,25] The COX-2 inhibitory action results in reduced inflammation, without the highly destructive gastric side-effects of the class of pharmaceutical drugs known as Non-Steroidal Anti-inflammatory Drugs (NSAID's). [26] Similar to the other ingredients of this formula, Chinese Skullcap provides further support for the reduction of the inflammation-induced free-radical stress that is generated at times of chemical challenge from a external or internal toxin.

Rosehip solid extract is used in this formula for its nutritive value as one of the best sources of natural vitamin C and bioflavonoids.[27] It is an excellent tonic for 'general debility and exhaustion'.[28]

Ginkgo leaf activites pathways that reduce the tissue damage caused by excess inflammation. Ginkgo decreases platelet aggregation and inhibits platelet adhesion and the release of inflammatory mediators from injured cells.[29] This decreases damage to the circulatory system secondary to allergic reactions and trauma. Fragile cell membranes are susceptible to damage by inflammation and lipid peroxidation by free radicals. Ginkgo's anti-oxidant properties neutralize this damage.[30] Ginkgo leaf has an affinity for the circulatory system of the brain. It has been shown to reduce symptoms related to Cerebral Vascular Insufficiency (CVI), including impaired mental performance, dizziness, headache, depression, ringing in the ears, and short-term memory loss.[31,32]

Devil's Claw Root is a plant from southern Africa long valued by the native peoples there as an anti-inflammatory, for migraines, wounds, labor pains, and as a digestive tonic.[33] It is still not known how devil's claw works, though it does not work like nonsteroidal anti-inflammatory drugs (NSAIDs like ibuprofen).[34] Thus it does not damage the stomach like these drugs do. In fact, it may even help maintain healthy digestion.[35] Regardless of how it works, devil's claw is well established to maintain normal joint function and back mobility.[36, 37]

Yarrow is a highly aromatic flower containing eucalyptol, camphor, and a variety of aromatics called sesquiterpene lactones.[38] It has a traditional use as a tea for fevers and colds to stimulate perspiration and is helpful in relieving fevers, stimulating digestion, and useful for bladder infections. Animal studies have shown yarrow to have the effect of reducing muscle spasms though the inhibition of cyclooxygenase 5-lipoxygenase[39] which might further explain its usefulness gastrointestinal conditions. The volatile oil, gives yarrow its anti-inflammatory activity.[40] The alkaloid obtained from yarrow, known as achilletin, reportedly stops bleeding in animals. [41]

Lobelia is a powerful herb popularized by the Thomsonian herbalists in the 1800's. It is used as an antispasmodic and expectorant in respiratory conditions including asthma, bronchitis and whooping cough.[42] Lobelia stimulates the release of hormones from the adrenal gland that relaxes the smooth muscle of the bronchioles to relax.[43] In larger doses it stimulates vomiting.

Licorice Root has been used medicinally for over 3000 years. It has anti-inflammatory and anti-allergy properties. Licorice enhances the immune response and has antiviral properties by stimulating the body to produce interferon.[44] It is used for cough and bronchitis because of its expectorant qualities especially in the area of the trachea.[45,46]

THERAPEUTIC APPLICATIONS*

Note: The intention of the following information is to represent the traditional use of the individual botanicals found in these formulas and to inform the reader of any evolving scientific inquiry relevant to the formula's ingredients.

SUPPORTED BY TRADITIONAL USE

Antioxidant,[47] anti-inflammatory, and liver protective effects.[48][49] Antispasmodic and expectorant in respiratory conditions including asthma, bronchitis and whooping cough.[50]

SCOPE OF RELEVANT SCIENTIFIC INVESTIGATION

Inhibits leukotriene formation, platelet aggregation, and excessive neutrophil response involved in the inflammation process by stabilizing the cell membranes.[51] Combats free radicals better than vitamin E,[52] anti-inflammatory effects in animal studies as effective as cortisone in acute inflammation,[53] reduces muscle spasms through the inhibition of cyclooxygenase 5-lipoxygenase[54]

CAUTIONS, CONTRA-INDICATIONS AND DRUG INTERACTIONS

Please reference Chapter 9. Do not use during pregnancy or lactation. Moderate doses of lobelia (larger that present in this formula) may cause nausea and vomiting. Large doses can be toxic causing mental confusion, and collapse.

COMPLIMENTARY HERBS/FORMULAS

Nettle Leaf, Infla-Profen, Migra-Profen, Devil's Claw/Chaparral Supreme

REFERENCES

1 Snow JM. *Curcuma longa* L. (Zingiberaceae). The Protocol Journal of Botanical Medicine. 1995; 1(2):43-46.

2 Wren RC. Potter's New Cyclopaedia of Botanical drugs and preparations. Essex, UK. Saffron Walden;1988.

3 Bartram T. Encyclopedia of Herbal Medicine.Dorset. Grace Publishers;1995.

4 Shama OP: Antioxidant properties of curcumin and related compounds. Biochem Pharmacol 25,1811-18-1825, 1976.

5 Nagabhushan N and Bhide SV: Nonmutagenicity of curcumin and its antimutagenic action versus chili and capsiacin, Nutr Cancer 8, 201-210, 1986.

6 Shalini VK and Srinivas L: Lipid peroxide induced DNA damage: Protection by turmeric . *Mol Cell Biochem* 77,3-10,1989.

7 Arora R, *et al.*:Anti-inflamitory studies on *Curcuma Longa* (turmeric). Indian J Med Res 59,1289-95, 1971

8 Mudhopadhyay A, *et al.*:Anti-inflamitory and irritant activities of curcumin analogues in rats. Agents Actions 12,508-515, 1982

9 Deodhar SD, Sethi R, and Srimal RC: Preliminary studies on anti-rheumatic activity of curcumin. Indian JH Med Res 71,632-34, 1980.

10 Patacchini R, Maggi CA, and Meli A: Capsaicin-like activity of some natural pungent substances on peripheral ending of visceral primary afferents. Arch Pharmacol 342, 72-77,1990

11 Satoskar RR,: Evaluation of anti-inflammatory property of curcumin in patients with postoperative inflammation. *Int J Clin Pharmalcol Ther Toxico* 245, 651-654, 1986.

12 Grieve M. A Modern Herbal, Dover Publications NY.1971.

13 Leung A, Foster S. Encyclopedia of Common Natural Ingredients. NY: Wiley;1996.

14 Wren RC. Potter's New Cyclopaedia of Botanical drugs and preparations. Essex, UK. Saffron Walden;1988.

15 Felter H, Lloyd JU. King's American Dispensatory. Portland. Eclectic medical Publications; 1983.

16 Hoffman D. The Herbal Handbook. Rochester, Vt. Healing Arts Press. 1988.

17 Davis E, Morris DJ. Medicinal uses of Licorice through the millennia: The good and plenty of it. *Molecular and Cellular Endocrinology.* 1991; 78:1-6.

18 Murray M. The healing power of herbs - The enlightened persons guide to the wonders of medicinal plants. Rocklin, Ca. Prima publishing;1995. 230-234.

19 Bradley P (Ed.). British herbal Compendium. Dorset. British Herbal Medical Assoc.; 1992.145-7

20 Hikano H. Economic and Medicinal Plant Research, Volume 1, London, Academic Press. 1985,53-85.

21 Kent C. Licorice - More than just candy. *Journal of the Australian Traditional Medicine Society.* 1994; Autumn: 9-14

22 Pizzorno J, Murray M. Textbook of Natural medicine. New York. Churchill Livingstone; 1999.

23 Detoxification Profile. GSDL Education Monograph. Great Smokies Diagnostic Lab (GSDL). Asheville, NC. 1998.

24 Leung A, Foster S. Encyclopedia of Common Natural Ingredients. NY: Wiley;1996.

25 Huang KC. The Pharmacology of Chinese Herbs. Ann Arbor. CRC Press;1993.

26 Newmark TM, Schulick P. Beyond Aspirin. Prescott, Az. HOHM Press. 2000.

27 Coon N. Using plants for healing. Philadelphia, Pa. Rodale Press. 1979.

28 Hoffman D. The Holistic Herbal. Moray, Scotland. The Findhorn Press. 1984.

29 Kleijnen J and Knipschild P: *Ginkgo biloba. Lancet* 340, 1136-9, 1992

30 DeFeudis FV: *Ginkgo biloba extract; Pharmacological Activities and Clinical Applications.* Elsevier, Paris. 1991.

31 Le Poncin, *et al.*: Effect of *Ginkgo biloba* on changes induced by quantitative cerebral microembolization in rats. *Arch Int Pharmacodyn Ther* 243, 236-244, 1980

32 Murray M. IBID Pg 143-160.

33 Mills S, Bone K. *Principles and Practice of Phytotherapy: Modern Herbal Medicine.* Edinburgh: Churchill Livingstone, 2000:345-9.

34 Moussard C, Alber D, Toubin MM, *et al.* A drug used in traditional medicine, *Harpagophytum procumbens:* No evidence for NSAID-like effect on whole blood eicosanoid production in human. *Prostagland Leukotr Essential Fatty Acids* 1992;46:283-6.

35 Blumenthal M, Busse WR, Goldberg A, *et al.* (eds). *The Complete German Commission E Monographs: Therapeutic Guide to Herbal Medicines.* Austin: American Botanical Council and Boston: Integrative Medicine Communications, 1998:120-1.

36 Chantre P, Cappelaere A, Leblan D, *et al.* Efficacy and tolerance of *Harpagophytum procumbens* versus diacerhein in the treatment of osteoarthritis. *Phytomedicine* 2000;7:177-83

37 Chrubasik S, Junck H, Breitschwerdt H, *et al.* Effectiveness of *Harpagophytum* extract WS 1531 in the treatment of exacerbation of low back pain: A randomized placebo-controlled double-blind study. *Eur J Anaesthesiol* 1999;16:118-29.

38 Zitterl-Eglseer K, Sesquiterpene lactones of Achillea setacea with antiphlogistic activity. Planta Med 1991;57(5)444-6

39 Muller-Jakic B, Breu W, Probstle A, *et al.* In vitro inhibition of cyclooxygenase and 5-lipoxygenase by alkamides from Echinacea and Achillea species. Planta Med 1994;60(1):37-40.

40 Tewari JP, Srivastava MC, Bajpai JL. Pharmacologic studies of Achillea millefolium Linn.Indian J Med Sci 1994;28(8):331-6.

41 Duke JA. CRC Handbook of Medicinal Herbs. Boca Raton, FL: CRC Press, 1985, 10-1.

42 McGuffin M, Hobbs C, Upton R, Goldberg A. American Herbal Products Association'sBotanical Safety Handbook. Boca Raton, FL: CRC Press, 1997, 71

43 Ellingwood F. American Materia Medica, Therapeutics and Pharmacognosy, 11th ed. Sandy, OR: Eclectic Medical Publications, 1919, 1998, 235-42.

44 Murray M. IBID pg. 230-234.

45 Bradley P (Ed.). British herbal Compendium. Dorset. British Herbal Medical Assoc.; 1992.145-7

46 Hikano H. Economic and Medicinal Plant Research, Volume 1, London, Academic Press. 1985,53-85.

47 Snow JM. *Curcuma longa* L. (Zingiberaceae). The Protocol Journal of Botanical Medicine. 1995; 1(2):43-46.

48 Wren RC. Potter's New Cyclopaedia of Botanical drugs and preparations. Essex, UK. Saffron Walden;1988.

49 Bartram T. Encyclopedia of Herbal Medicine.Dorset. Grace Publishers;1995.

50 McGuffin M, Hobbs C, Upton R, Goldberg A. American Herbal Products Association's Botanical Safety Handbook. Boca Raton, FL: CRC Press, 1997, 71

51 Satoskar RR,: Evaluation of anti-inflammatory property of curcumin in patients with postoperative inflammation. *Int J Clin Pharmalcol Ther Toxico* 245, 651-654, 1986.

52 Shama OP: Antioxidant properties of curcumin and related compounds. Biochem Pharmacol 25,1811-18-1825, 1976.

53 Arora R, *et al.*:Anti-inflamitory studies on *Curcuma Longa* (turmeric). Indian J Med Res 59,1289-95, 1971

54 Muller-Jakic B, Breu W, Probstle A, *et al.* In vitro inhibition of cyclooxygenase and 5-lipoxygenase by alkamides from Echinacea and Achillea species. Planta Med 1994;60(1):37-40.

USNEA/UVA URSI SUPREME

*For Support of Healthy Urinary Function**
FORMULA

Usnea Lichen	(*Usnea spp.*)
Uva Ursi Leaf	(*Arctostaphylos uva ursi*)
Pipsissewa leaf	(*Chimaphilia umbellata*)
Echinacea Root	(*Echinacea spp.*)

Concentration:	1:1 Herb strength ratio
Dosage:	Acute use: 40-60 drops every 2-4 hours
Duration of use:	5-7 days
Best taken:	Between meals, with warm water

DESCRIPTION OF FORMULA

This formula has antibacterial compounds that target the urinary tract including bladder and kidney.

Usnea is a lichen that contains usneic acid, which has strong urinary antiseptic and antibacterial activity. It is also used topically in many European anti-bacterial and anti-fungal creams.[1]

Uva Ursi Leaf contains arbutin that is a urinary antiseptic effective against E.coli and Proteus bacteria. The high tannin content causes an astringent action. Its effect as a diuretic has been frequently reported but contradicted in at least one study.[2][3] Arbutin is converted to hydroxyquinone in the urine with a toxicity that may occur at doses higher than in this formula, equivalent to 1/2 ounce of fresh leaf. [4]

Pipsissewa contains arbutin and other flavonoids that have urinary antiseptic properties. Pipsissewa also has tonic and astringent properties. [5] Dr. Felter described its specific uses in "atonic and debilitated states of the urinary tract...chronic irritation of the prostate and urethra..."[6]

Echinacea is an immune-stimulant, whose anti-inflammatory, antibacterial, antiviral, and wound healing properties have been widely reported.[7][8] Extracts of Echinacea spp. have the ability to increase antibody production, along with resistance to various infections.[9, 10] Research has further shown that alcohol/water extracts of Echinacea significantly enhance natural killer cell function, and have phagocytic, metabolic and bactericidal influence on macrophages.[11, 12]

THERAPEUTIC APPLICATIONS*

Note: The intention of the following information is to represent the traditional use of the individual botanicals found in these formulas and to inform the reader of any evolving scientific inquiry relevant to the formula's ingredients.

SUPPORTED BY TRADITIONAL USE

Urinary antiseptic and urinary antibiotic,[14] has tonic and astringent properties.[15] "Atonic and debilitated states of the urinary tract...chronic irritation of the prostate and urethra..."[16]

SCOPE OF RELEVANT SCIENTIFIC INVESTIGATION

Arbutin is a urinary antiseptic effective against *E.coli and Proteus bacteria.*[17 18] Anti-inflammatory, antibacterial, antiviral, and wound healing properties have been widely reported.[19 20]

CAUTIONS, CONTRA-INDICATIONS AND DRUG INTERACTIONS

Please reference Chapter 9. Do not use during pregnancy or lactation. Arbutin in Uva Ursi is converted to hydroxyquinone in the urine with a toxicity that may occur at doses equivalent to 1/2 ounce of fresh leaf.[21]

A kidney infection is a serious condition that requires medical supervision and should not be treated with this formula alone.

COMPLIMENTARY HERBS/FORMULAS

Uva Ursi solid extract, Echinacea Supreme

REFERENCES

1 Hobbs C. Usnea: The herbal Antibiotic, Interweave Press, Loveland, Co, 1996, 96-107.

2 Leung A, Foster S. Encyclopedia of Common Natural Ingredients. NY: Wiley;1996.505-6.

3 Bradley P (Ed.). British herbal Compendium. Dorset. British Herbal Medical Assoc.; 1992.211.

4 Merck Index, 10th ed. Merck &Co. Rahway,NJ,1983, 796-7.

5 Leung A, Foster S. Encyclopedia of Common Natural Ingredients. NY: Wiley;1996.421-22

6 Felter H, Lloyd JU. King's American Dispensatory. Portland. Eclectic Medical

Publications; 1983. 495-97

7 Wren RC. Potter's New Cyclopaedia of Botanical drugs and preparations. Essex, UK. Saffron Walden;1988.

8 Bradley P (Ed.). British herbal Compendium. Dorset. British Herbal Medical Assoc.; 1992.

9 Snow JM. Echinacea (Moench) Spp. Asteraceae. The Protocol Journal of Botanical Medicine. 1997; 2 (2): 18-24.

10 Bauer R, Wagner H. Echinacea species as potential immunostimulatory drugs. Economic and Medicinal Plant Research. San Diego: Academic press Ltd.; 1991.

11 Schranner I, Wurdinger M, *et al.* Modification of avian humeral immunoreactions by Influx and Echinacea angustifolia extract. Zentralbl Veterinarmed (B) 1989; 36.

12 Bukovsky M, Kostalova D, Magnusova R, Vaverkova S. Testing for immunomodulating effects of ethanol-water extracts of the above ground parts of the plants Echinaceae and Rudbeckia. Cesk Farm. 1993; 42.

13 Witchl M. (Bisset NG, Ed.) Herbal Drugs and Phytopharmaceuticals. Medpharm, CRC Press: Boca Raton. 1994.

14 Hobbs C. Usnea: The herbal Antibiotic, Interweave Press, Loveland, Co, 1996, 96-107.

15 Leung A, Foster S. Encyclopedia of Common Natural Ingredients. NY: Wiley;1996.421-22

16 Felter H, Lloyd JU. King's American Dispensatory. Portland. Eclectic Medical Publications; 1983. 495-97

17 Leung A, Foster S. Encyclopedia of Common Natural Ingredients. NY: Wiley;1996.505-6.

18 Bradley P (Ed.). British herbal Compendium. Dorset. British Herbal Medical Assoc.; 1992.211.

19 Wren RC. Potter's New Cyclopaedia of Botanical drugs and preparations. Essex, UK. Saffron Walden;1988.

20 Bradley P (Ed.). British herbal Compendium. Dorset. British Herbal Medical Assoc.; 1992.

21 Merck Index, 10th ed. Merck &Co. Rahway,NJ,1983, 796-7.

VALERIAN/POPPY SUPREME

*Herbal Insomnia Formula**
FORMULA

Valerian Root	(*Valeriana officinalis*)
California Poppy	(*Eschscholzia californica*)
Skullcap Herb	(*Scutellaria lateriflora*)
Kava Kava Root	(*Piper methysticum*)
Passionflower Vine	(*Passiflora incarnata*)
Chamomile Flowers	(*Matricaria recutita*)
Mugwort Herb	(*Artemesia vulgaris*)

Concentration:	1:1 Herb strength ratio
Dosage:	40-60 drops every 20 minutes beginning one hour before bedtime (3 doses maximum)
Duration of use:	As needed
Best taken:	Before bed

DESCRIPTION OF FORMULA

This formula is used for insomnia, anxiety and stress.

The therapeutic actions of this formula are sedative, anxiolytic and restorative to the nerves.

Valerian root has reportedly been used to induce sleep. [1] German Commission E notes its use for restlessness and nervous disturbances of sleep.[2, 3] The World Health Organization (WHO) also suggests its use as a sleep-promoting herb, stating that it is often used a possible substitute for stronger synthetic sedatives in the treatment of nervous excitement and disturbances of sleep, when associated with anxiety. [4, 5]

California poppy has received acknowledgement from a number of respected clinicians for use as a sleep aid. [6, 7, 8] Dr. Weiss from Europe states that California poppy is "altogether gentle, more in the direction of establishing equilibrium, and not narcotic".[9] One report states "useful in quieting hyperactive, bright eyed children who can't fall asleep"[10]

Skullcap was used extensively by the early Eclectic physicians of the last century as a tonic, nervine, and as an antispasmodic. It was said to be especially useful for nervous afflictions, particularly those manifesting "excitability, restlessness, or wakefulness". Skullcap is used for nervousness from mental or physical exhaustion.[11, 12] Skullcap has been used in teething, neuralgia and headache.[13]

Kava Kava is well known for its relaxing affect. Numerous clinical trials have supported the use of kava for the treatment of nervous anxiety.[15] German Commission E approves Kava for 'conditions of nervous anxiety, stress and restlessness'.[16] Kava is used here to remove the stress and anxiety that can often prevent someone from obtaining deep, restful sleep. Antispasmodic activity has been noted.[17, 18]

Passionflower is another example of a medicinal plant that has traditionally been reported to induce sleep by its simple calming or quieting influence, and not by any narcotic affect. It has also traditionally been used to treat nervous disorders,[19] as an antispasmodic, and for its influence with pain relief.[20] Passionflower has been approved by the European Scientific Co-Operative on Phytotherapy (ESCOP) for "tenseness, restlessness and irritability with difficulty in falling asleep".[21]

A flavonoid, vitexin, acts as a anti-inflammatory and lowers blood pressure.[22]

Chamomile flowers are considered antispasmodic and anti-inflammatory, with specific influence on the gastrointestinal tract.[23] *Matricaria*, a genus of Chamomile comes from the root 'matrix', meaning womb or mother. This reflects the opinion that it is particularly useful with female reproductive disorders.[4] It is used as a sedative in cases of restlessness and irritability, particularly where there is disturbed digestion and flatulence.[24]

Mugwort also receives mention by the German Commission E as a sedative, for use with restlessness, anxiety, and insomnia.[1, 4] Mugwort also stimulates digestion,[4] thereby assisting with an increase overall vitality.

THERAPEUTIC APPLICATIONS*

Note: The intention of the following information is to represent the traditional use of the individual botanicals found in these formulas and to inform the reader of any evolving scientific inquiry relevant to the formula's ingredients.

SUPPORTED BY TRADITIONAL USE

Restlessness and nervous disturbances of sleep,[25][26] sleep aid,[27][28] [29] teething, neuralgia, headache,[30] pain relief.[31]

SCOPE OF RELEVANT SCIENTIFIC INVESTIGATION

Numerous clinical trials have supported the use of these herbs for the treatment of nervous anxiety.[32]

CAUTIONS, CONTRA-INDICATIONS AND DRUG INTERACTIONS

Please reference Chapter 9. Do not use during pregnancy or lactation. Kava may potentiate the effect of alcohol and should not be used with it.

COMPLIMENTARY HERBS/FORMULAS

Sound Sleep, Serenity with Kava Kava

REFERENCES

1 Valpiani C. Valeriana officinalis. Journal of the Australian Traditional Medicine Society. 1995;1(2):57-62.

2 Houghton PJ. The Scientific Basis for the Reputed Activity of Valerian. J. Pharm. Pharmacol. 1999;51:505-512.

3 Blumenthal M, et al. Ed. The Complete German Commission E Monographs.Austin, TX: American Botanical Council; 1998.

4 Brown D. Valerian: Clinical Overview - Phytotherapy Review & Commentary. Townsend Letter for Doctors. 1995:150151.

5 Bisset N. Herbal Drugs and Phytopharmaceuticals, Medpharm Scientific Publishers, Stuttgart, 1994.

6 Newall CA, et al. Herbal Medicines: A Guide for Health-Care Professionals.London: Pharmaceutical Press;1996.

7 Sherman, JA The complete botanical prescriber. Self Published, 1993. Pg. 101.

8 Miller JG, Murray WJ. Herbal Medicinals: A Clinician's Guide. New York: Pharma Prod Press, 1998. Pg. 222.

9 Weiss. Herbal Medicine. Beaconsfield: Beaconsfield Publish, 1998.

10 Moore M. Medicinal Plants of the Pacific West, Santa Fe, Red Crane Books, 110-112.

11 Ellingwood F. American Materia Medica, Therapeutics and Pharmacognosy. Portland. Eclectic Medical Publications;1985.

12 Felter H, Lloyd JU. King's American Dispensatory. Portland. Eclectic medical Publications; 1983.2041-3.

13 Grieve M. A Modern Herbal, Dover Publications NY.1971,725.

14 Harrison T. Savage civilization New York: Alfred A. Knopf; 1937

15 Anonymous. Natural anxiolytics - Kava and L.72 antianxiety formula. *The American Journal of Natural Medicine.* 1994; 1(2): 10-14.

16 Blumenthal M, *et al.* Ed. *The Complete German Commission E Monographs.* Austin, TX: American Botanical Council; 1998.

17 Blumenthal M, *et al.* Ed. *The Complete German Commission E Monographs.* Austin, TX: American Botanical Council; 1998.

18 Lehmann, E., Kinzler, E. and Friedmann, J. Efficacy of a special kava extract, in patients with states of anxiety, tension, and excitedness of non-mental origin, Phytomedicine 1996; 3:113-119.

19 Leung A, Foster S. Encyclopedia of Common Natural Ingredients. NY: Wiley;1996.

20 Felter HW. The Eclectic Materia Medica, Pharmacology and Therapeutics. Portland, Oregon. Eclectic Medical publications;1985, 515.

21 Bartram T. Encyclopedia of Herbal Medicine.Dorset. Grace Publishers;1995.

22 Brinker, Francis ND. *Formulas for Healthful Living.* Sandy, OR: Eclectic Medical Publications;1995.120.

23 Bisset N. Herbal Drugs and Phytopharmaceuticals, Medpharm Scientific Publishers, Stuttgart, 1994, 322-25.

24 Ellingwood F. American Materia Medica, Therapeutics and Pharmacognosy. Portland. Eclectic Medical Publications;1985.

25 Houghton PJ. The Scientific Basis for the Reputed Activity of Valerian. J. Pharm. Pharmacol. 1999;51:505-512.

26 Blumenthal M, *et al.* Ed. The Complete German Commission E Monographs.Austin, TX: American Botanical Council; 1998.

27 Newall CA, *et al.* Herbal Medicines: A Guide for Health-Care Professionals.London: Pharmaceutical Press;1996.

28 Sherman, JA The complete botanical prescriber. Self Published, 1993. Pg. 101.

29 Miller JG, Murray WJ. Herbal Medicinals: A Clinician's Guide. New York: Pharma Prod Press, 1998. Pg. 222.

30 Grieve M. A Modern Herbal, Dover Publications NY.1971,725.

31 Felter HW. The Eclectic Materia Medica, Pharmacology and Therapeutics. Portland, Oregon. Eclectic Medical publications;1985, 515.

32 Anonymous. Natural anxiolytics - Kava and L.72 antianxiety formula. *The American Journal of Natural Medicine.* 1994; 1(2): 10-14.

VITEX/ALFALFA SUPREME

A Menstrual and Menopausal Corrective Formula *

FORMULA

Chaste Tree berry	(*Vitex agnus-castus*)
Alfalfa Solid Extract	(*Medicago sativa*)
Night Blooming Cereus	(*Cactus grandiflorus*)
St. Johns's Wort	(*Hypericum perforatum*)
Sage Leaf	(*Salvia officinalis*)
Wild Oats	(*Avena sativa*)
Motherwort	(*Leonurus cardiaca*)
Essential Oil of Lavender	

Concentration:	1:1 Herb strength ratio
Dosage:	30-40 drops, 3-4 times daily
Duration of use:	3-4 months
Best taken:	Between meals with warm water

DESCRIPTION OF FORMULA

This formula is for menstrual cycle irregularities, premenstrual symptoms and menopausal symptoms. It focuses on the nerve centers and on specific symptoms such as cardiac palpitation, excessive sweating and fluid retention. This formula has phytoestrogen properties.

Vitex or Chaste tree berry has a medicinal history dating back more than 6,000 years.[1,2] It restores normal menstrual flow and regularity by stimulating the corpus luteum to produce an increase in progesterone levels.[3] Vitex stimulates the release of lutenizing hormone and inhibits follicle-stimulating hormone. It decreases the water retention during menstruation. It is used in Europe as an herb to ease the transition off the pill in reestablishing normal menstrual cycle.[4] Vitex influences the pituitary. Clinical trials focusing on the symptoms of PMS have shown it to be of particular benefit in normalizing menstruation (where its dysfunction is due to a deficiency of progesterone and prolactin).[5]

Alfalfa leaf brings several influential benefits to this formula. Its estrogen-like plant compounds are balancing to the system. These phytoestrogens, which are reported to be hundreds of times weaker in their effect than the body's estrogens, exert their reduced influence at receptors where the body's more powerful estrogens would otherwise bind. Thus, the addition of weak estrogen-mimicking compounds may either reduce the overall estrogen signaling in the body (by competing with the powerful estrogens), or increase it by supplying weak estrogens where there is a shortage of the body's more powerful estrogens.[67] Its reputation to be highly nutritive, as well as the reported benefits of its vitamin K_1 content for aiding in the maturing of the body's calcium managing proteins, make this plant a welcome addition to this woman's formula.[8]

Note: Current concerns with Alfalfa inducing a reversible Systemic Lupus Erythematosus (SLE)-like syndrome are based on toxicology studies of canavanine - an alkaloid which is only found in Alfalfa's seeds and sprouts. As canavanine is not found in the mature tops of the plant, this concern is not clinically relevant when using the leaf or blade, as is the case here.

Night Blooming Cereus is indicated by the Eclectic physicians for functional heart condions and disturbances, during the menstrual cycle and menopause, including palpitations and cardiac dyspnea (difficult breathing). It is described as one of the best cardiac tonics.[9] Cactus increases the contractile force of the heart and has been used for angina and edema. It is generally contraindicated for high blood pressure.[10]

St. John's Wort is an effective antidepressant. In several recent studies when compared to standard antidepressant drugs it proves as effective, better tolerated and has much fewer side effects.[11] St. John's Wort has been shown to be effective in Seasonal Affective Disorder(SAD).[12] In addition to its antidepressant effect, it also is a valuable anti-inflammatory.[13] It accelerates wound healing in burns, incisions and wounds.[14,15] Two components, hypericin and psuedohypericin have been shown to inhibit a variety of encapsulated viruses including Herpes simplex, para-influenza virus and cytomegalovirus.[16][17]

Sage Leaf is an antispasmodic and mild antidepressant.[18] It is indicated in menopause symptoms and aids in exhausting sweats.[19]

Wild Oats works in a gentle, subtle manner. An acute indication for use is for a headache from over work. "It is not a remedy of great power...probably its chief value as a medicine is to energize in nervous exhaustion" HarveyW. Felter, MD.[20] Oat is indicated in assisting convalescence for nervous exhaustion and debility in chronic conditions and cardiac weakness. Indicated in menopausal symptoms with depression.[21]

Motherwort herb is present to provide a bitter nervine with specificity for the reproductive tissues. Its bitter principles promote improved digestion while its nervine properties relieve anxiety and emotional unrest associated with cardiac uneasiness. It is an emmenagogue meaning it promotes the normal menstrual flow.[22]

Essential Oil of Lavender is indicated in pelvic and lumbar discomfort and pain. Used for nervous and weak individuals, who faint easily, lavender is a gentle stimulant. [23]

Licorice Root has a small amount of estriol, one of the weakest of the estrogens.[24] Licorice is only used in small quantities so that its aldosterone like effects of retaining fluids are not activated.[25] It has anti-inflammatory and anti-allergy properties.

THERAPEUTIC APPLICATIONS*

Note: The intention of this information is to represent the traditional use of the individual botanicals found in these formulas and to inform the reader of any evolving scientific inquiry relevant to the formula's ingredients.

SUPPORTED BY TRADITIONAL USE

Emmenagogue meaning it promotes the normal menstrual flow.[26] Pelvic and lumbar discomfort and pain. [27] Phytoestrogens are adaptogens that balance the stronger estrogenic effects;[28, 29] restores normal menstrual flow and regularity though its hormonal effects on the pituitary gland and increased progesterone levels;[30] eases the transition off the pill in reestablishing normal menstrual cycle. [31]   Indicated for menstrual symptoms, aids in exhausting sweats.[32] functional heart conditions, palpitations and cardiac dyspnea (difficult breathing).[33]

SCOPE OF RELEVANT SCIENTIFIC INVESTIGATION

It restores normal menstrual flow and regularity by stimulating the corpus luteum to produce an increase in progesterone levels.[34] Normalizing menstruation where it is due to a deficiency of progesterone.[35]

CAUTIONS, CONTRA-INDICATIONS AND DRUG INTERACTIONS

Please reference Chapter 9. Do not use during pregnancy or lactation.

COMPLIMENTARY HERBS/FORMULAS

Phyto-Estrogen, Alfalfa Solid Extract

REFERENCES

1 Snow JM. Vitex agnus-castus L. (Verbenaceae). The Protocol Journal of Botanical Medicine. 1996; Spring: 20-23.

2 Brown D. Vitex agnus-castus Clinical Monograph. The Quarterly Review of Natural Medicine. 1994; Summer: 111-121.

3 Anonymous. Chaste Tree. The Lawrence Review of Natural products. 1994; December.

4 Leung A, Foster S. Encyclopedia of Common Natural Ingredients. NY: Wiley;1996.151-2.

5 Lauritzen CH, *et al*. Treatment of premenstrual tension syndrome with Vitex agnus-castus - Controlled, double-blind study versus pyridoxine. *Phytomedicine*. 1997; 4(3): 183-189.

6 Mitchell W. Plant Medicine. Seattle, Wa: Self-published; 2000. Pg. 14-15.

7 Reilly P. Clinical application Medicago sativa extracts. Journal of Naturopathic Medicine. 1 (1):

8 Boon H, Smith M. The Botanical Pharmacy. Quebec, Canada. Quarry press;1999.

9 Felter HW. The Eclectic Materia Medica, Pharmacology and Therapeutics. Portland, Oregon: Eclectic Medical publications. 1985.253-6.

10 Brinker, Francis ND. *Formulas for Healthful Living*. Sandy, OR: Eclectic Medical Publications;1995.99.

11 Linde, K., Ramirez, G., Mulrow, C.D. *et al*. (1996). St. John's Wort for depression-an overview and meta analysis of randomized clinical trials. British Medical Journal 313:253-258.

12 Wheatley D. Hypericum in seasonal affective disorder (SAD). Curr Med Res Opin 1999; 15:33-37

13 Wren RC. Potter's New Cyclopaedia of Botanical drugs and preparations. Essex, UK. Saffron Walden;1988.

14 Rao S.G. *et al.*Calendula and Hypericum two homeopathic drugs promoting wound healing in rats. Fitoterapia 6:508-510.

15 Hobbs C:St. John's Wort, Hypericum perforatum L. Herbalgram 18/19, 24-33, 1989.

16 Yip L *et al*. Antiviral, activity of a derivative of the photosensitive compound hypericin. 1996, Phytomedicine 3:185-90.

17 Leung A, Foster S. Encyclopedia of Common Natural Ingredients. NY: Wiley;1996, 310-312.

18 Wren RC. Ibid,.240.

19 Felter HW, ibid pg 1705-6.

20 Felter HW. The Eclectic Materia Medica, Pharmacology and Therapeutics. Portland, Oregon: Eclectic Medical publications. 1985.235.

21 Wren RC. Ibid pg 203.

22 Felter HW. The Eclectic Materia Medica, Pharmacology and Therapeutics. Portland, Oregon: Eclectic Medical publications. 1985.443.

23 Felter HW. The Eclectic Materia Medica, Pharmacology and Therapeutics. Portland, Oregon: Eclectic Medical publications. 1985.442-3.

24 Costello CH, Lynn EV, Estrogenic Substances from Plants:I. Glycyrrhiza, J Am Pharm Assoc, 39:177-1950, 80.

25 Brinker, Francis ND. *Formulas for Healthful Living.* Sandy, OR: Eclectic Medical Publications;1995.136.

26 Felter HW. The Eclectic Materia Medica, Pharmacology and Therapeutics. Portland, Oregon: Eclectic Medical publications. 1985.443.

27 Felter HW. The Eclectic Materia Medica, Pharmacology and Therapeutics. Portland, Oregon: Eclectic Medical publications. 1985.442-3.

28 Mitchell W. Plant Medicine. Seattle, Wa: Self-published; 2000. Pg. 14-15.

29 Reilly P. Clinical application Medicago sativa extracts. Journal of Naturopathic Medicine. 1 (1):

30 Anonymous. Chaste Tree. The Lawrence Review of Natural products. 1994; December.

31 Leung A, Foster S. Encyclopedia of Common Natural Ingredients. NY: Wiley;1996.151-2.

32 Felter HW, ibid pg 1705-6.

33 Felter HW. The Eclectic Materia Medica, Pharmacology and Therapeutics. Portland, Oregon: Eclectic Medical publications. 1985.253-6.

34 Anonymous. Chaste Tree. The Lawrence Review of Natural products. 1994; December.

35 Lauritzen CH, *et al.* Treatment of premenstrual tension syndrome with *Vitex agnus-castus* - Controlled, double-blind study versus pyridoxine. *Phytomedicine.* 1997; 4(3): 183-189.

WILD CHERRY SUPREME

An Anti-Coughing Formula*
FORMULA

Wild Cherry Bark	(*Prunus serotina*)
Elecampane Root	(*Inula helenium*)
Yerba Santa Leaf	(*Eriodictyon californicum*)
Red Clover Blossoms	(*Trifolium pratense*)
Licorice Root	(*Glycyrrhiza glabra*)
Butterbur Root	(*Petasites frigida*)

Concentration:	1:1 Herb strength ratio
Dosage:	30-40 drops, 4-6 times daily
Duration of use:	2-4 weeks for acute use
Best taken:	Between meals with warm water

DESCRIPTION OF FORMULA

This formula is used for coughs. It promotes expectoration of mucous and contains respiratory antispasmodic and soothing emollient principles that target the lungs and respiratory membranes.

Wild Cherry Bark is used for irritating coughs with irritation and mucous production. Its main action is to relieve irritation of the mucous membranes.[1] It has been used for bronchitis and whooping cough.[2] It contains cyanogenic glycosides, particularly prunasin which decreases spasms in the smooth muscles lining bronchioles, opening airways and relieving coughs.[3]

Elecampane Root is used in bronchitis, asthma, and whooping cough.[4] The active constituents are 1-4% volatile oils composed of sesquiterpene lactones, inulin (44%) and mucilage.[5] It provides relief by assisting expectoration of mucous. It is used in combination with other remedies when treating chronic lung problems such as asthma.[6]

Yerba Santa Leaf is effective for coughs as an expectorant. It decreases the mucous secretions and inflammation with bronchitis.[7,8]

Red Clover Blossoms have expectorant and antispasmodic effects and are used for coughs, bronchitis and fever.[9]

Licorice Root has been used medicinally for over 3000 years. It has anti-inflammatory and anti-allergy properties. Licorice enhances the immune response and has antiviral properties by stimulating the body to produce interferon.[10] It is used for cough and bronchitis because of its expectorant qualities especially in the area of the trachea.[11,12]

Butterbur Root is used to decrease the spasm and discomfort of a cough. It has an analgesic effect and acts as a "phytotranquilizer" in nervous disturbances of the gastrointestinal tract and in bronchial asthma.[13]

THERAPEUTIC APPLICATIONS*

Note: The intention of this information is to represent the traditional use of the individual botanicals found in these formulas and to inform the reader of any evolving scientific inquiry relevant to the formula's ingredients.

SUPPORTED BY TRADITIONAL USE

Cough, mucous production, relieves irritation of the mucous membranes,[14] bronchitis, whooping cough,[15] bronchitis and fever,[16] expectorant qualities.[17, 18]

SCOPE OF RELEVANT SCIENTIFIC INVESTIGATION

Cyanogenic glycosides decrease spasms in the smooth muscles lining bronchioles, opening airways and relieving coughs.[19]

CAUTIONS, CONTRA-INDICATIONS AND DRUG INTERACTIONS

Please reference Chapter 9. Do not use during pregnancy or lactation.

COMPLIMENTARY HERBS/FORMULAS

Echinacea Supreme, Lobelia, Grindelia, Lomatium/Osha Supreme or Pleurisy Root.

REFERENCES

1 Felter H, Lloyd JU. King's American Dispensatory. Portland, Oregon: Eclectic Medical Publications. 1983.1583-4.

2 Wren RC. Potter's New Cyclopaedia of Botanical drugs and preparations. Essex, UK. Saffron Walden;1988.282.

3 Mills SY. Out of the Earth: The Essential Book of Herbal Medicine. Middlesex, UK: Viking Arkana, 1991, 314.

4 Leung AY, Foster S. Encyclopedia of Common Natural Ingredients Used in Food, Drugs, and Cosmetics. New York: John Wiley & Sons, 1996, 222-4.

5 Wichtl M. Herbal Drugs and Phytopharmaceuticals. Boca Raton, FL: CRC Press, 1994, 254-6.

6 Grieve M. A Modern Herbal, Jonathan Cape, London, 1931. 281

7 MooreM. Medicinal Plants of the Northwest, red Crane Books, Santa Fe, 265-6

8 Felter HW. The Eclectic Materia Medica, Pharmacology and Therapeutics. Portland, Oregon: Eclectic Medical publications. 1985.361.

9 Leung A, Foster S. Encyclopedia of Common Natural Ingredients. NY: Wiley;1996.520.

10 Murray M. The healing power of herbs - The enlightened persons guide to the wonders of medicinal plants. Rocklin, Ca. Prima publishing;1995. 230-234.

11 Bradley P (Ed.). British herbal Compendium. Dorset. British Herbal Medical Assoc.; 1992.145-7

12 Hikano H. Economic and Medicinal Plant Research, Volume 1, London, Academic Press. 1985,53-85.

13 Bisset N. Herbal Drugs and Phytopharmaceuticals, Medpharm Scientific Publishers, Stuttgart, 1994, 367-8.

14 Felter H, Lloyd JU. King's American Dispensatory. Portland, Oregon. Eclectic Medical Publications. 1983.1583-4.

15 Wren RC. Potter's New Cyclopaedia of Botanical drugs and preparations. Essex, UK. Saffron Walden;1988.282.

16 Leung A, Foster S. Encyclopedia of Common Natural Ingredients. NY: Wiley;1996.520.

17 Bradley P (Ed.). British herbal Compendium. Dorset. British Herbal Medical Assoc.; 1992.145-7

18 Hikano H. Economic and Medicinal Plant Research, Volume 1, London, Academic Press. 1985,53-85.

19 Mills SY. Out of the Earth: The Essential Book of Herbal Medicine. Middlesex, UK: Viking Arkana, 1991, 314.

YUCCA/BURDOCK SUPREME

*Anti-Arthritic, Anti-inflammatory Formula**
FORMULA

Yucca root	(*Yucca spp.*)
Echinacea Root	(*Echinacea spp.*)
Burdock Root and Seed	(*Arctium lappa*)
Poke Root	(*Phytolacca americana*)
Celery Seed	(*Apium graveolens*)
Bladderwrack Fronds	(*Fucus vesiculosus*)
Pipsissewa Herb	(*Chimaphilla umbellata*)

Concentration:	1:1 Herb strength ratio
Dosage:	30-40 drops, 3-5 times daily
Duration of use:	3-4 months
Best taken:	Between meals with warm water

DESCRIPTION OF FORMULA

The herbs in this formula have strong anti-inflammatory action for the treatment of arthritis. The formula includes diuretics to promote the excretion of toxins and acids associated with the inflammation of arthritis.

Yucca root is a common desert plant in the southwestern United States. Saponins in yucca root have been shown to help counter chronic joint inflammation, though the mechanisms of action are unknown.[1] Yucca root was and is widely used for arthritis, and prostatitis by traditional herbalists in the desert Southwest.[2] One 15 month study found that yucca saponins extract was effective and well tolerated for the treatment of arthritis.[3]

Echinacea is an immune-stimulant, anti-inflammatory, antibacterial, and antiviral.[4, 5] Traditionally, Echinacea has been used by Native Americans to treat colds, coughs, sore throats, and snakebite.[6] Research has shown that extracts of Echinacea spp. have the ability to increase antibody production, along with resistance to various infections.[7, 8] Research has further shown Echinacea significantly enhances natural killer cell function, phagocytic, metabolic and bactericidal influence on macrophages.[9, 10]

Burdock root & seed have long been used in traditional herbalism for inflammatory conditions including rheumatism and arthritis, gout, and inflammatory skin problems like eczema and psoriasis.[12, 13] Burdock root acts as an antioxidant and interferes with a messenger chemical known as platelet-activating factor that strongly promotes excessive inflammation.[14, 15] It is also well known for its ability to stimulate liver/bile related functions.[16]

Poke Root acts on the lymphatic tissues and the mucous lining of the digestive tract.[17] It is an alterative.[G1, G6, 9] Poke root has been used for rheumatism and skin conditions.[18, 19] It is specific for pallid (pale) mucous membranes with ulcerations.[20] It also has been used traditionally for cancer.[21]

Celery seed has traditionally been used as a remedy for arthritis, gout, rheumatism, bladder infections, congestive heart failure, anxiety, gas, and loss of appetite.[22] It is included because of its anti-inflammatory properties.

Bladderwrack is a seaweed with a long history of use for maintaining thyroid and maintaining a healthy body weight.[23, 24] It was also used in traditional medicine for rheumatism, kidney inflammation, fatty heart, and as a tonic.[25, 26] The complex carbohydrates (alginates) have been extensively studied in the laboratory and clinic and are well known as being useful for helping with heartburn and indigestion, as well as preventing absorption of various radioactive isotopes.[27, 28] Animal studies suggest bladderwrack can help maintain healthy cholesterol levels and can have profound effects on the immune system.[29, 30]

Pipsissewa contains arbutin and other flavonoids that have urinary antiseptic properties. Pipsissewa also has tonic and astringent properties.[31] Dr. Felter described its specific uses in "atonic and debilitated states of the urinary tract...chronic irritation of the prostate and urethra..."[32]

THERAPEUTIC APPLICATIONS*

Note: The intention of this information is to represent the traditional use of the individual botanicals found in these formulas and to inform the reader of any evolving scientific inquiry relevant to the formula's ingredients.

SUPPORTED BY TRADITIONAL USE

Chronic joint inflammation, arthritis, rheumatism, gout, prostatitis and inflammatory skin problems like eczema and psoriasis. [33, 34, 35, 36, 37]

SCOPE OF RELEVANT SCIENTIFIC INVESTIGATION

Increase antibody production, increase resistance to various infections,[38, 39] enhances natural killer cell function, phagocytic, metabolic and bactericidal influence on macrophages.[40, 41] Antioxidant interferes with a messenger chemical known as platelet-activating factor that decreases excessive inflammation.[42, 43]

CAUTIONS, CONTRA-INDICATIONS AND DRUG INTERACTIONS

Please reference Chapter 9. Do not use during pregnancy or lactation.

COMPLIMENTARY HERBS/FORMULAS

Infla-Profen, Devil's Claw/Chaparral Supreme, Turmeric/Catechu Supreme, Nettle Leaf Phyto-Cap

REFERENCES

1 Bingham R, Bellew BA, Bellew JG. Yucca plant saponin in the management of arthritis. *J Appl Nutr* 1975;27:45-50.

2 Moore M. *Medicinal Plants of the Desert and Canyon West.* Santa Fe: Museum of New Mexico Press, 1989:134-5.

3 Anonymous. Feverfew. *The Lawrence Review of Natural products.* 1994; March:1-3.

4 Wren RC. Potter's New Cyclopaedia of Botanical drugs and preparations. Essex, UK. Saffron Walden;1988.

5 Bradley P (Ed.). British herbal Compendium. Dorset. British Herbal Medical Assoc.; 1992.

6 Snow JM. Echinacea (Moench) Spp. Asteraceae. The Protocol Journal of Botanical Medicine. 1997; 2 (2): 18-24.

7 Snow JM. Echinacea (Moench) Spp. Asteraceae. The Protocol Journal of Botanical Medicine. 1997; 2 (2): 18-24.

8 Bauer R, Wagner H. Echinacea species as potential immunostimulatory drugs. Economic and Medicinal Plant Research. San Diego: Academic press Ltd.; 1991.

9 Schranner I, Wurdinger M, *et al.* Modification of avian humeral immunoreactions by Influx and Echinacea angustifolia extract. Zentralbl Veterinarmed (B) 1989; 36.

10 Bukovsky M, Kostalova D, Magnusova R, Vaverkova S. Testing for immunomodulating effects of ethanol-water extracts of the above ground parts of the plants Echinaceae and Rudbeckia. Cesk Farm. 1993; 42.

11 Witchl M. (Bisset NG, Ed.) Herbal Drugs and Phytopharmaceuticals. Medpharm, CRC Press: Boca Raton. 1994.

12 Newall CA, Anderson LA, Phillipson JD. *Herbal Medicines: A Guide for Health-Care Professionals.* London: Pharmaceutical Press, 1996:52-3.

13 Ellingwood F. *American Materia Medica, Pharmacognosy and Therapeutics* 11th ed. Sandy, OR: Eclectic Medical Publications, 1919:378.

14 Lin CC, Lu JM, Yang JJ, *et al.* Anti-inflammatory and radical scavenge effects of Arctium lappa. Am J Chin Med 1996;24:127-37.

15 Iwakami S, Wu J, Ebizuka Y, Sankawa U. Platelet activating factor (PAF) antagonists contained in medicinal plants: Lignans and sesquiterpenes. *Chem Pharm Bull (Tokyo)* 1992;40:1196-8.

16 Bradley P (Ed.). British herbal Compendium. Dorset. British Herbal Medical Assoc.; 1992.

17 17 Felter H, Lloyd JU. King's American Dispensatory. Portland. Eclectic Medical Publications; 1983. 1473-4.

18 Ellingwood F. American Materia Medica, Therapeutics and Pharmacognosy. Portland. Eclectic Medical Publications;1985.

19 Felter HW. The Eclectic Materia Medica, Pharmacology and Therapeutics. Portland, Oregon. Eclectic Medical publications;1985.535-8.

20 Felter H. *The Eclectic Materia Medica, Pharmacology, and Therapeutics*, John K. Scudder, Cincinnati, Ohio, 1922, 536-7

21 Hutchens AR. A handbook of Native American herbs. Shambhalla publications. 1992.

22 Leung AY, Foster S. *Encyclopedia of Common Natural Ingredients Used in Food, Drugs and Cosmetics* 2nd ed. New York: John Wiley & Sons Inc, 1996:141-3.

23 Ellingwood F. *American Materia Medica, Pharmacognosy and Therapeutics* 11th ed. Sandy, OR: Eclectic Medical Publications, 1919:382-3.

24 Mills SY. *Out of the Earth: The Essential Book of Herbal Medicine.* Middlesex, UK: Viking Arkana, 1991:514-6

25 Hoffmann D. *The Complete Illustrated Herbal.* New York: Barnes & Noble Books, 1996:94.

26 Felter HW. *Eclectic Materia Medica, Pharmacology and Therapeutics.* Sandy, OR: Eclectic Medical Publications, 1922:381.

27 Bruneton J. *Pharmacognosy Phytochemistry Medicinal Plants.* Paris: Lavoisier Publishing, 1995:44-47.

28 Schulick P. *Herbal Therapy from the Sea.* 1993.

29 Lamela M, Vázquez-Freire MJ, Calleja JM. Isolation and effects on serum lipid levels of polysaccharide fractions from *Fucus vesiculosus. Phytother Res* 1996;10(suppl):S175-6.

30 Willenborg DO, Parish CR. Inhibition of allergic encephalomyelitis in rats by treatment with sulfated polysaccharides. *J Immunol* 1988;140:3410-5.

31 Leung A, Foster S. Encyclopedia of Common Natural Ingredients. NY: Wiley;1996.421-22

32 Felter H, Lloyd JU. King's American Dispensatory. Portland. Eclectic Medical Publications; 1983. 495-97

33 Bingham R, Bellew BA, Bellew JG. Yucca plant saponin in the management of arthritis. *J Appl Nutr* 1975;27:45-50.

34 Moore M. *Medicinal Plants of the Desert and Canyon West.* Santa Fe: Museum of New Mexico Press, 1989:134-5.

35 Newall CA, Anderson LA, Phillipson JD. *Herbal Medicines: A Guide for Health-Care Professionals.* London: Pharmaceutical Press, 1996:52-3.

36 Ellingwood F. *American Materia Medica, Pharmacognosy and Therapeutics* 11th ed. Sandy, OR: Eclectic Medical Publications, 1919:378.

37 Leung AY, Foster S. *Encyclopedia of Common Natural Ingredients Used in Food, Drugs and Cosmetics* 2nd ed. New York: John Wiley & Sons Inc, 1996:141-3.

38 Snow JM. Echinacea (Moench) Spp. Asteraceae. The Protocol Journal of Botanical Medicine. 1997; 2 (2): 18-24.

39 Bauer R, Wagner H. Echinacea species as potential immunostimulatory drugs. Economic and Medicinal Plant Research. San Diego: Academic press Ltd.; 1991.

40 Schranner I, Wurdinger M, *et al.* Modification of avian humeral immunoreactions by Influx and Echinacea angustifolia extract. Zentralbl Veterinarmed (B) 1989; 36.

41 Bukovsky M, Kostalova D, Magnusova R, Vaverkova S. Testing for immunomodulating effects of ethanol-water extracts of the above ground parts of the plants Echinaceae and Rudbeckia. Cesk Farm. 1993; 42.

42 Lin CC, Lu JM, Yang JJ, *et al.* Anti-inflammatory and radical scavenge effects of *Arctium lappa.* Am J Chin Med 1996;24:127-37.

43 Iwakami S, Wu J, Ebizuka Y, Sankawa U. Platelet activating factor (PAF) antagonists contained in medicinal plants: Lignans and sesquiterpenes. *Chem Pharm Bull (Tokyo)* 1992;40:1196-8.

GENERAL REFERENCES

G1. Wren RC. Potter's New Cyclopaedia of Botanical drugs and preparations. Essex, UK. Saffron Walden;1988.

G2. Bartram T. Encyclopedia of Herbal Medicine.Dorset. Grace Publishers;1995.

G3. Leung A, Foster S. Encyclopedia of Common Natural Ingredients. NY: Wiley;1996.

G4. Bradley P (Ed.). British herbal Compendium. Dorset. British Herbal Medical Assoc.; 1992.

G5. Mills S, Bone K. Principles and practice of Phytotherapy. New York. Churchill Livingstone; 2000.

G6. Ellingwood F. American Materia Medica, Therapeutics and Pharmacognosy. Portland. Eclectic Medical Publications;1985.

G7. Tang W, Eisenbrand G. Chinese Drugs of Plant Origin. New York. Springer-Verlag;1992.

G8. Huang KC. The Pharmacology of Chinese Herbs. Ann Arbor. CRC Press;1993.

G9. McGuffin M, *et al.* Ed. AHPA's Botanical Safety Handbook. Boca Raton: CRC Press, 1997.

G10. Newall CA, *et al. Herbal Medicines: A Guide for Health-Care Professionals.*London: Pharmaceutical Press;1996.

G11. Weiss R. Herbal medicine. Beaconsfield, UK. Beaconsfield Publishers;1985.

G12. Felter H, Lloyd JU. King's American Dispensatory. Portland. Eclectic medical Publications; 1983.

G13. Duke J. Handbook of Medicinal Herbs. Boca Raton. CRC Press;1985.

G14. Hoffman D. The Holistic Herbal. Moray. The Findhorn Press;1984.

G15. Felter HW. The Eclectic materia Medica, Pharmacology and Therapeutics. Portland, Oregon. Eclectic Medical publications;1985.

G16. Boon H, Smith M. The Botanical Pharmacy. Quebec, Canada. Quarry press;1999.

G17. Mills S. The Essential Book of Herbal medicine. London. Penguin;1991.

G18. Brinker, Francis ND. *Herb Contraindications and Drug Interactions.* Sandy, OR: Eclectic Medical Publications;1997.

G19. Miller L. Herbal Medicinals: Selected Clinical Consideration Focusing on Known or Potential Drug-Herb Interactions. *Arch Intern Med.*1998;158: 2200-11.

G20. Newall C, Phillipson JD. "Interactions of Herbs with Other Medicines." Online. Internet. [4/26/00]. Available WWW: http://www.ex.ac.uk/phytonet/phytojournal/

G21. Bensky D, Gamble A. Chinese Herbal Medicine: Materia Medica. Seattle: Eastland, 1986.

G22. DeSmet PAGM. *Adverse Effects of Herbal Drugs.* Berlin: Springer-Verlag. 1993

G23. Bergner P. "Herb-drug Interactions." Medical Herbalism. 1997. Online. Internet. [5/20/99]. Available WWW: http://medherb.com/92DRGHRB.HTM

CHAPTER 8
SPECIFIC INDICATIONS OF
SINGLE HERB REMEDIES

Specific indications are a symptom or clinical occurrence which serves to direct the physician to the treatment of a disease and selection of the most indicated herb.

King's American Dispensatory is a two volume text of 2172 pages. Originally written by Dr. John King its third edition was entirely rewritten by Harvey W. Felter, M.D. and John Uri Lloyd, Phar. M., Ph.D. and published in 1898. It was the cornerstone used by Eclectic physicians in their education and the daily treatment of patients. The third edition of Kings American Dispensatory was reprinted by Eclectic Medical Publications in Sandy, Oregon in 1983.

The following represents excerpts from Kings American Dispensatory on Single Herb Remedies that present Specific Indications. This material indicates how Eclectic physicians differentiated the specific use of these single herbs.

ARNICA FLOWERS   *Arnica latifolia*

King's Disp. Vol 1 p 281

Muscle soreness and pain from strains or over-exertion; advanced stage of disease, with marked enfeeblement, weak circulation, and impaired spinal innervation(the sending out of nerve signals); sleeplessness from impeded respiration, and dull precordial(heart) pain from "heart-strain"; muscular pain and soreness when the limbs are moved; tensive(with spasm)backache, as if bruised or strained; cystitis, with bruised feeling in bladder, or from a fall or blow; headache, with tensive(spasm), bruised feeling and pain on movement; dull aching lumbar pain, or from over-exertion. All cases of debility with enfeebled circulation. Two ounces of tincture has produced death.

Please read Precautions and Contraindications section, use Arnica topically or in very small doses only.

BAYBERRY BARK   *Myrica cerifera*

Kings Disp. Vol 2 pg 1294

Profuse mucous flows; catarrhal states of the gastro-intestinal tract; atonic diarrhea (from weak bowel muscle tone), typhoid dysentery, atony of the cutaneous circulation (weak circulation to the skin); full oppressed pulse. Locally and internally - sore mouth; spongy, flabby, bleeding gums, sore throat of scarlet fever when enfeebled and swollen.

BLACK ALDER BARK   *Alnus serrulata*

King's Disp. Vol 1 page 147

The specific use of this remedy is to improve nutrition and increase waste. It is of particular value in Scrofula (tuberculosis infection in swollen lymph glands of the neck), with feeble vitality, and chronic skin diseases exhibiting scaly or pustular eruptions.

BLACK COHOSH ROOT   *Cimicifuga racemosa*

King's Disp. Vol 1 Page 533

Dr. Scudder gives as the specific indications for this drug: "Muscular pains; uterine pains, with tenderness; false pains; irregular pains; rheumatism (pain and inflammation)of the uterus; dysmenorrhea (difficult or painful menses). As an antirheumatic, when the pain is paroxysmal (sudden and reoccurring)." To these indications may be added a sense of soreness, with dragging pains in the hips and loins (lumbar back), rheumatoid muscular pain; rheumatoid dyspepsia (discomfort and bloating with digestion).

BLACK HAW ROOT & TREE BARK
Viburnum prunifolium

Kings Disp. Vol 2 page 2061

Uterine irritability, and hyperaesthesia (abnormal sensitivity of the skin); threatened abortion; uterine colic; dysmenorrhea (difficult or painful menstruation), with deficient menses; severe lumbar and bearing-down pains; cramp-like, expulsive menstrual pain; intermittent, painful contractions of the pelvic tissues; after-pains and false pains of pregnancy; obstinate hiccough.

BLOODROOT   *Sanguinaria canadensis*

Kings Disp. Vol. 2 page 1713

For its specific indications, Prof. J.M. Scudder gives a "sensation of burning and itching of mucous membrane, especially of fauces(back of mouth and throat), pharynx, Eustachian tubes and ears; less frequently of larynx, trachea, and bronchia, occasionally of stomach and rectum, and rarely of vagina, and urethra. The mucous membrane looks red and irritable. Added to this he gives "nervousness, redness of nose, with acrid discharge, burning and constriction in fauces of pharynx, with irritative cough and difficult respiration. Prof. Locke gives also feeble circulation, with coldness in the extremities.

BLUE FLAG ROOT   *Iris versicolor*

Kings Disp. Vol 2 Page 1713

The specific indications for iris may be stated as fullness of thyroid gland; enlarged spleen; chronic liver complaints with sharp, cutting pain, aggravated by motion; nausea and vomiting of sour liquids, or regurgitation of food, especially after eating rich pastry or fats; with watery, burning bowel discharges; enlarged lymph nodes, soft and yielding; rough, greasy conditions of the skin, disorders of sebaceous follicles; abnormal skin pigmentation; menstrual wrongs, with thyroid fullness; unilateral facial neuralgia; muscular atrophy and other wastings of the tissues; bad blood.

BUCHU LEAVES   *Barosma betulina*

Kings Disp. Vol 1 Page 373

Abnormally acid urine, with constant desire to urinate, with but little relief from it; bladder-renal irritation; copious mucous, or muco-purulent discharges; cystorrhea(bladder pain).

BUGLEWEED   *Lycopus virginica*

Kings Disp. Vol 2 Page 1215

Vascular excitement with inordinately active circulation; frequent pulse, with high temperature; albuminuria (protein in urine); cough, with copious expectoration of mucus, especially debilitating chronic cough; wakefulness and morbid vigilance, and in tubercular deposits.

BURDOCK ROOT

Arctium lappa

Kings Disp. Vol 2 Page 1120

Feeble cutaneous circulation (skin); scaly, dry eruptions; impaired nutrition of skin; urinary irritation; psoriasis.

CALENDULA FLOWERS   *Calendula officinalis*

Kings Disp. Vol 1 page 403

Locally, to <u>wounds</u> and injuries to prevent suppuration and promote rapid healing. Internally, to aid local action, and in chronic suppuration, capillary engorgement, varicose veins, old ulcers, spleen and liver congestion.

CASCARA SAGRADA BARK   *Rhamnus purshiana*

Kings Disp. Vol 2 Page 1656

Constipation, due to neglect or to nervous and muscular atony (weakness) of the intestinal tract; lesser ailments, depending solely upon <u>constipation</u>, with intestinal atony.

CELANDINE TOPS AND ROOTS   *Chelidonium major*

Kings Disp. Vol 1 Page 493

"Full, pale, sallow tongue and mucous membranes; skin pale and sallow, sometimes greenish; "<u>liver congestion</u>; jaundice, due to swollen bile ducts; sluggish hepatic (liver) action; cough, with hepatic pain; fullness, with spasm or throbbing pain in the right hypochondrium(lower rib cage), and pain extending to right shoulder; melancholia, headaches, and gastric disorders, dependent upon faulty action of the liver.

CHAMOMILE FLOWERS, GERMAN
Matricaria recutita

Kings Disp Volume 2 Page 1247

Nervous irritability, with peevishness, fretfulness, discontent, and impatience; sudden fits of temper during the menstrual period; muscular twitching; morbid sensitiveness to pain; head sweats easily; anal discharges, fetid, greenish and watery, and of green mucus with curds of milk, or of yellow and white flocculi (clumps), associated with flatulence, colic, and excoriation of the anal outlet; a remedy particularly fitted for the disorders of teething, and to correct the condition threatening to end in dentition convulsions.

CINNAMON BARK   *Cinnamomum zeylanicum*

Kings Disp. Vol. 1 Page 560

Post-partum (after birth) and other uterine hemorrhages with profuse flow, cold extremities, and pallid surface; hematuria (blood in urine).

CORYDALIS TUBERS *Dicentra canadensis*

Kings Disp. Volume 1 Page 611

Yellow skin with lymphatic enlargements; syphilitic (lymph) nodes. Increases waste (excretion) and improves nutrition.

DAMIANA *Turnera diffusa*

Kings Disp. Volume 1 Page 647

To relieve irritation of the genito-urinary mucous surfaces. Sexual weakness and debility, with nervousness and depression.

DANDELION ROOT AND LEAF
Taraxacum officinalis

Kings Disp. Vol 2 Page 1915

Loss of appetite, <u>weak digestion</u>, hepatic torpor, and constipation.

ECHINACEA ANGUSTIFOLIA ROOT
Echinacea angustifolia

King Disp. Vol 1 Page 671

To correct fluid depravation, "<u>bad blood,</u>" tendency to sepsis and malignancy, as in gangrene, sloughing skin ulcerations, carbuncles (large pus filled inflammation beneath the skin), boils, and various forms of septicemia; foul discharges, with weakness and emaciation; deepened, bluish or purplish coloration of skin or mucous membranes, with a low form of inflammation; dirty-brownish tongue; jet-black tongue; tendency to the formation of multiple abscesses of semi-active character, with marked asthenia(weakness). Of special importance in typhoid, septicemic (bloodborn infection)fevers, and in malignant carbuncle (skin cancer), pulmonary gangrene, cerebro-spinal meningitis and pyosalpinx(kidney infections).

ECHINACEA PURPUREA ROOT
Echinacea purpurea

Kings Disp. Vol 1 Page 677

See Echinacea Angustifolia...

ELDERBERRY　*Sambucus canadensis*

Kings Disp. Volume 2 Page 1708

In skin affections, when the tissues are full, flabby, and edematous(fluid filled swelling); epidermis separates and discharge of serum is abundant, forming crusts; indolent ulcers, with soft edematous borders; mucous patches, with free secretions.

ELECAMPANE ROOT　*Inula helenium*

Kings Disp. Volume 2 Page 1059

Cough, of a teasing, persistent character, accompanied with substernal (under the sternum/chest)pain, and profuse secretion; atony (weakness)of abdominal organs, with engorgement and relaxation; catarrhal (mucous) discharges.

EYEBRIGHT　*Euphrasia officinalis*

Kings Disp. Vol 1 Page 752

Acute catarrhal (mucous secreting) diseases of the eyes, nose, and ears; fluent coryza (headcold with nasal discharge) with copious discharge of watery mucus. "Secretion of acrid mucus from eyes and nose with heat and pain in frontal sinus"

GENTIAN ROOT　*Gentiana lutea*

Kings Disp Volume 2 Page 926

"Sense of depression referred to epigastric (upper stomach) region, and associated with sense of physical and mental weariness" (Scudder).

GERANIUM ROOT　*Geranium maculatum*

Kings Disp. Volume 2 Page 929

Relaxed mucous tissues, with profuse, debilitating discharges; chronic diarrhea, with mucous discharges; chronic dysentery; diarrhea, with constant desire to evacuate the bowels; passive hemorrhages.

GINGER ROOT　*Zingiber officinalis*

Kings Disp. Volume 2 Page 2111

<u>Loss of appetite; flatulence</u>, borborygmus (abdominal noise); spasmodic gastric and intestinal contractions; painful menstruation; acute colds; cool extremities; and cold surface in children's diseases.

GINSENG ROOT   *Panax quinquifolium*

Kings Disp. Volume 2 Page 1432

Intestinal indigestion, with diarrhea of fatty or chylous (partially digested and emulsified) feces, and with flatulence, abdominal pain, nausea, and vomiting; in diseases of mesenteric glands(glands within the small intestine). For temporary effects only.

GRINDELIA FLORAL BUDS   *Grindelia spp.*

Kings Disp. Volume 2 Page 958

Grindelia Robusta: <u>Asthmatic breathing</u>, with soreness and raw feeling in the chest; cough harsh and dry; breathing labored, with a dusky coloration of the face in plethoric individuals(having an excess of blood). Locally, old atonic ulcers; full tissues; rhus poisoning(poison ivy).

Grindella Squarrosa: <u>Spleen congestion</u>, especially when(present with)malarial cachexia(weakness and malnutrition); fullness and dull pain in left hypochondrium (lower chest), with indigestion, pallid, sallow countenance, and general debility; gastric pains associated with spleen congestion.

HELONIAS ROOT   *Chamaelirium luteum*

Kings Disp. Volume 1 Page 490

Mental irritability and despondency; sexual lassitude; <u>atony of the female reproductive organs</u>; gastric debility, with anorexia, nausea, indigestion and mal-assimilation, particularly when due to reflexes of uterine origin; sticky, slimy leucorrhea(milky discharge); atonic urinary tract; dysmenorrhea (difficult or painful menses), with pelvic fullness and heaviness, as if congested, with bearing-down sensation, as if the parts were about to fall out.

HORSETAIL   *Equisetum arvense*

Kings Disp. Volume 1 Page 713

Cystic (bladder) irritation; nocturnal urinary incontinence; (spasmodic)urging to urinate; dropsy, renal calculi.

JAMAICAN DOGWOOD *Piscidia erythrina*

Kings Disp. Volume 2 Page 1511

Insomnia and nervous unrest; to allay spasm, control pain and allay nervous excitability: migraine; neuralgia

KAVA KAVA ROOT *Piper methysticum*

Kings Disp. Volume 2 Page 1507

Neuralgia, particularly of the trigeminal nerve(facial area); toothache; earache; ocular pain; reflex neuralgia; anorexia; dizziness and despondency; gonorrhea; chronic catarrhal inflammations; vesical (bladder)irritation; painful urination.

LIFE ROOT *Senecio aurus*

Kings Disp. Volume 2 Page 1744

Atony of the reproductive organs, with impairment of function; uterine enlargement, with uterine or cervical leucorrhoea; difficult tenesmic micturition(intermittent urination); dragging sensations in the testicles; perineal (genital/anal area)weight and fullness.

LOBELIA HERB & SEED *Lobelia inflata*

Kings Disp. Volume 2 Page 1205

Lobelia is specifically indicated by the full, labored, doughy pulse; the blood moves with difficulty; pain in chest of a heavy, sore, or oppressive character; angina pectoris; cardiac neuralgia; pulmonary apoplexy; mucus accumulation in bronchi; convulsive movements; rigidity of muscular tissues; rigid perineum or vaginal walls; nausea; oppressive sick headache, with nausea. As an emetic when tongue is heavily coated at base.

MILK THISTLE SEED *Silybum marianum*

Kings Disp. Vol 1 Page 448

Splenic, hepatic and renal congestion, face sallow, appetite capricious; nervous irritability; despondency; physical debility; pain in either hypochondrium(lower chest around liver); pelvic tension and weight; congestion of the parts supplied by the celiac nerve(abdominal organs); and non-malarial splenic hypertrophy.

MYRRH GUM   *Commiphora myrrha*

Kings Disp. Volume 2 Page 1300

Chronic bronchitis, with profuse secretion of mucus or muco-pus, with difficult expectoration; membranes lax and pallid, ton-sils enlarged and spongy, throat pale and tumid, soreness and sponginess of the gums; reproductive disorders of women, with weight and dragging in the parts, and leucorrhoea.

NETTLE LEAF   *Urtica dioica*

Kings Disp. Volume 2 Page 2033

Chronic diarrhea and dysentery, with large mucous evacuations; profuse secretion of gastric juice, with eructations (belching)and emesis; choleric discharges (undigested and emulsified stool), summer bowel diseases of children, with copious watery and mucous passages; chronic eczematous eruptions.

NIGHT BLOOMING CEREUS   *Cactus grandiflorus*

Kings Disp. Volume 1 Page 376

Impaired heart-action, whether feeble, violent, or irregular; car-diac disorder, with nervousness, precordial oppression (chest pain or pressure), anxiety, apprehension of danger, or death, hys-teria; tobacco heart; nervous disorders, with heart complications.

OATS, WILD MILKY SEED   *Avena sativa*

Kings Disp.Volume 1 Page 317

Nerve tonic, stimulant, and antispasmodic. Spasmodic and nerv-ous disorders, with exhaustion; cardiac weakness; nervous debili-ty of convalescence; spermatorrhea (involuntary discharge of semen without an orgasm)from the nervous erethism (irritabili-ty)of debility; tensive articular swellings.

OREGON GRAPE ROOT   *Berberis aquifolium*

Kings Disp. Volume 1 Page 348

Syphilitic dyscrasia (disease with debility), constitutional syphilis, with periosteal(bone) or muscular pains; chronic skin affections, with blood dyscrasia; profusely secreting, tumid mucous tissues; indigestion, with hepatic torpor(liver sluggishness); yellow skin, with marked weakness and emaciation.

PASSIONFLOWER   *Passiflora incarnata*

Kings Disp. Volume 2 Page 1441

Irritation of brain and nervous system with atony; <u>sleeplessness</u> from overwork, worry or from febrile excitement, and in the young and aged; neuralgic pains with debility; exhaustion from cerebral fullness, or from excitement; convulsive movements; infantile nervous irritation; nervous headache; tetanus; hysteria; oppressed breathing; cardiac palpitation from excitement or shock.

PEPPERMINT LEAF   *Mentha piperita*

Kings Disp, Vol 2 Page 1255

<u>Gastrodynia(stomach pain)</u>, flatulent colic, and difficult digestion.

PIPSISSEWA   *Chimaphila umbelatta*

Kings Disp. Vol 1 Page 497

<u>Atonic and debilitated states of the urinary organs</u>, giving rise to lingering disorders, with scanty urine, but excessive voiding of mucus, muco-pus, or bloody muco-pus, offensive or non-offensive in character; smarting or burning pain with dysuria(difficult or painful urination); chronic irritation of the urethra and prostate; chronic relaxation of the bladder walls; chronic prostatitis, with vesical catarrh(mucous discharge from bladder).

POKE ROOT   *Phytolaccca americana*

Kings Disp. Volume 2 Page 1475

Pallid mucous membranes with ulceration; sore mouth with small blisters on tongue and mucous membrane of cheeks; sore lips, blanched, with separation of the epidermis; hard, painful, enlarged glands; <u>mastitis, orchitis</u> (infected/swollen testicles); <u>parotitis</u> (infected/swollen parotid gland,ie. mumps), aphthae (oral ulcers on tongue, gums or cheeks); soreness of mammary glands, with impaired respiration; faucial(throat), tonsillar, or pharyngeal ulceration; pallid sore throat, with cough or respiratory difficulty, secretions of mouth give a white glaze to surface of mouth, especially in children; white pultaceous (porridge-like) sloughs at corners of mouth or in the cheek.

POPLAR BARK   *Populus tremuloides*

Kings Disp. Volume 2 Page 1538

Marked debility with impairment of digestion; tenesmic vesical (bladder spasm) irritation; tenesmus after micturition(spasm after urination).

PRICKLY ASH BARK   *Xanthoxylum clava-herculis*

Kings Disp. Volume 2 Page 2091

Xanthoxylum is specifically indicated (in the smaller doses) in hypersecretion from debility and relaxation of mucous tissues; atonicity of the nervous system (larger doses); in capillary engorgement in the exanthemata, sluggish circulation, tympanites (distension of abdomen from gas) in bowel complaints, intestinal and gastric torpor (weak digestion with deficient secretion), dryness of the mucous membrane of mouth and fauces (with glazed, glossy surfaces), flatulent colic, Asiatic cholera, uterine cramps, and neuralgia. For the painful bowel disorders, the preparations of the berries are to be preferred.

RED CLOVER BLOSSOMS   *Trifolium pratense*

Kings Disp. Volume 2 Page 1996

Some forms of whooping-cough; irritation of the larnygo-pulmonic (throat and bronchi) passages; provoking spasmodic cough; cough of measles; cancerous diathesis (susceptibility).

RED ROOT   *Ceanothus americanus*

Kings Disp. Volume 1 Page 473

Enlarged spleen; sallow, doughy skin; expressionless countenance; non-inflammatory, catarrhal states, with profuse secretion.

SAGE LEAF   *Salvia officinalis*

Kings Disp. Volume 2 Page 1706

Skin soft and relaxed, extremities cold, circulation enfeebled; excessive sweating; and urine of low specific gravity.

SAW PALMETTO BERRY   *Serenoa repens*

Kings Disp. Volume 2 Page 1752

Relaxation of parts, with copious catarrhal discharges; lack of development, or wasting away of testicles, ovaries, or breasts; prostatic irritation, with painful urination, and dribbling or urine, particularly in the aged; tenderness of the glands, and other parts concerned in reproduction.

SKULLCAP HERB   *Scutellaria lateriflora*

Kings Disp. Volume 2 Page 1740

<u>Nervousness</u>, attending or following acute or chronic diseases, or from mental or physical exhaustion, teething, etc; nervousness manifesting itself in muscular action; tremors, subsultus(twitching), etc; hysteria, with inability to control the voluntary muscles; functional cardiac disorders of a purely nervous type, with intermittent pulse.

ST. JOHN'S WORT FLOWER BUDS
Hypericum perforatum

Kings Disp. Volume 2 Page 1039

Spinal injuries, shocks, or concussions; throbbing of the whole body without fever; spinal irritation, eliciting tenderness and burning pain upon slight pressure; <u>spinal injuries</u>, and lacerated and punctured wounds of the extremities, with excruciating pain; hysteria; locally to wounds, contusions, etc.

STILLINGIA ROOT   *Stillingia sylvatica*

Kings Disp. Volume 2 Page 1837

Feeble tissues, with tardy removal of broken-down material, and slow renewal of the parts; mucous membranes, tumid, red, and glistening, with scanty secretion; skin affections, with irritation and watery discharge; laryngeal irritation, with paroxysmal, hoarse, croupous cough; irritation of the superior pharynx just behind the fauces, with cough; winter-cough of irritation; periosteal (bone)pain and tendency to form nodes.

THUJA LEAF   *Thuja occidentalis*

Kings Disp Volume 2 Page 1936

<u>Enlarged prostate</u>, with dribbling of urine in the aged, urine easily expelled upon coughing or slight muscular exertion; vesical (bladder)irritation and atony; enuresis of children; verrueous (wartlike) vegetations; trachoma; chancroid (nonsyphilitic venereal ulcer with lymphatic enlargement)

UVA URSI LEAF   *Arctostaphylos uva ursi*

Kings Disp. Volume 2, Page 2039

Relaxation of the urinary tract, with pain and mucous or bloody secretions; feeling of weight and dragging in the loins and per-ineum, when not due to prostatic enlargement; chronic vesical irritation, with pain, spasm, and catarrhal discharges.

VALERIAN ROOT   *Valeriana officinalis*

Kings Disp. Volume 2 Page 2043

A cerebral stimulant. Hysteria, chorea, hemicrania (one sided pain), all with mental depression and despondency; cerebral ane-mia; mild spasmodic movements

WILD INDIGO ROOT   *Baptisia tinctoria*

Kings Disp. Volume 1, Page 326

The indications will be found to be fullness of tissue, with dusky, leaden, purplish, or livid discoloration; tendency to ulceration and decay; sepsis; typhoid conditions; enfeebled capillary circula-tion; color of skin effaced by pressure and returns slowly; patient's face swollen and bluish, appearing like one having been frozen, or long exposed to cold, fetid discharges, with atony, and gangrene.

WILD YAM ROOT   *Dioscorea villosa*

Kings Disp. Volume One Page 661

Bilious colic; other forms of colic with spasmodic contractions; yellow skin and conjunctiva, with nausea and colicky pains; tongue coated, paroxysmal abdominal pain, and stomach deranged; frequent small, flatulent, alvine (stool) passages; colic, with tenderness on pressure; sharp abdominal pain, made worse by motion.

WILLOW BARK   *Salix nigra*

Kings Disp. Volume 2 Page 1703

Black Willow Bark - To moderate sexual erethism (extreme sen-sitivity), irritability, and passion; lascivious dreams; libidinous thoughts; nocturnal emissions; cystitis, urethral irritation, prosta-titis, cystitis, ovaritis, and other sexual disorders arising from sex-ual abuse or excesses.

YARROW FLOWERS   *Achillea millefloium*

Kings Disp. Volume 1 Page 20

To relieve urinary irritation, strangury(difficult and painful passage of urine), urinary suppression; relieves irritation in incipient Bright's disease, capillary relaxation, leucorrhoea with relaxed and irritated vaginal walls, hematuria, gastric and intestinal atony, atonic amenorrhoea, menorrhagia (painful menses)

YELLOW DOCK ROOT   *Rumex crispus*

Kings Disp. Volume 2 Page 1685

Bad blood with chronic skin diseases, bubonic swellings; low deposits in glands and cellular tissues, and tendency to indolent ulcers; feeble recuperative power; irritative, dry laryngo-trachael cough; stubborn, dry, summer cough, chronic sore throat with glandular enlargements and hypersecretion; nervous dyspepsia, with epigastric fullness and pain extending through left half of chest; cough, with dyspnea (difficult breathing)and sense of precordial (chest)fullness

YERBA SANTA LEAF   *Eriodictyon californicum*

Kings Disp. Volume 1 page 729

Chronic asthma with cough, profuse expectoration, thickening of the bronchial mucous membrane, loss of appetite, abundant and easy expectoration.

CHAPTER 9
HERBAL MEDICINE
CAUTIONS, CONTRAINDICATIONS
AND DRUG INTERACTIONS

We are using the terms Cautions, Contraindications and Drug Interactions to describe the side effects and warnings appropriate to the utilization of herbs. The herbal literature referenced here contains a wide variety of scientific articles and herbal reference books. We have principally relied on current herbal pharmacology resources such as the PDR of Herbal Medicine, second edition, German Commission E monographs, several eclectic and English reference works and the writings of Brinker, Brown, Bone and Blumenthal.

Some of these herbs are gentle, some are not. There are several herbs that are described here as Toxic (Ex: Arnica, Poke, and Phytolacca) and we have inserted descriptions of Overdose Symptoms. The use of these herbs as single herb products is never recommended in this book. These potent and powerful herbs are included in a few herbal formulas in a small and safe dosage. This makes the use of these herbs safe. We are advocates of formulas because it is the synergy of the herbs in lower doses that stimulate different metabolic pathways which effects change and healing within a person.

Another category of caution is for plants that contain chemicals having toxic effects over a longer period of usage (Ex: Comfrey, Coltsfoot, Chaparral, Chionanthus). When using these plants it is important to alternate formulas with different herbs but with a similar therapeutic focus.

Throughout this chapter, citations of cautions, contraindications and drug interactions are made on the basis of a single constituent within the herb. Warnings are thus made solely due to the presence of this single constituent within the formula. The reader should be aware that "objectionable" constituents are found in every food that we consume. This does not necessarily make that food harmful. Thus please read this chapter with this frame of reference.

In chronic illness it is essential and necessary to evolve the herbal prescription consistent with the changes in the individuals current "symptom picture" towards the goal of a healthier person. The ability to make a clinical judgement about how to change the formula requires experience and knowledge. It requires an understanding of the physiology of the body and how it speaks to us using the signs and symptoms that it demonstrates physically on an ever-changing basis. Good clinical judgement also requires an understanding of when to use a single herb for a specific focus or a general herbal tonic. In evolving your herbal program and dealing with the concerns associated with these cautions, contraindications and drug interactions, the assistance of a healthcare professional knowledgeable about healing with herbal medicine can be a valuable and essential counselor.

DESCRIPTION OF TERMS

Cautions: Describes a concern or a potential concern for safety. These may be discuss specific side effects, the size of the dose and useful information.

EXAMPLE:

Green Tea-*Camellia sinensis*

No health hazards known with proper use. [67]
Cautions: Nervous system stimulant may irritate sensitive stomachs due to tannin (addition of milk will bind tannin and reduce symptoms). [3]

Contraindication: A contraindication in conventional pharmaceuticals is a specific documented problem with the drug (Ex: Valium) and another medication or a contraindication for use in a specific disease or health condition (such as diabetes or pregnancy). We use the same definition of contraindication here but in addition we include contains less urgent or specific "concerns and potential contraindications." **Regarding the frequent use of C/I in pregnancy and lactation;** many herbs have not been proven safe in pregnancy so the default recommendation is that in pregnancy and in breast feeding their use is a contraindication.

Editors Note: In this section the abbreviation C/I indicates 'contraindication' or the grammatically appropriate form of contraindication (e.g. contraindicated).

EXAMPLE:

Green Tea-*Camellia sinensis*

Contraindications: Caution with use in kidney disorders, due to increased urinary output. Caution with use in duodenal ulcers because of increased gastric acid secretion. Caution with use in tachycardia and heart arrhythmias due to increased heart rate. Caution with use in anxiety, is a nervous system stimulant. [6] Pregnant women and children should limit intake to maximum of 250 mg a day (3 cups).

Drug Interactions: This section describes the biochemical interactions of herbal medicines with specific prescription drugs and other herbs. This section also contains statements that are generalizations about the interactions of drug categories (antidepressants) with herbal categories (sedatives).

EXAMPLE:

Green Tea-*Camellia sinensis*

Drug Interactions
High in tannins and thus may decrease absorption of iron, codeine, ephedrine, pseudoephedrine, theophylline, aminophylline and atropine. [9, 11, 13] If taken with ephedrine can increase thermogenesis and weight loss plus cause agitation, tremors, and insomnia. [6] Excessive amounts combined with MAO Inhibitors could cause a hypertensive crisis. [6] May decrease absorption of tricyclic antidepressants and thus consumption should be separated by at least 2 hours.[11] C/I with Phenylpropanolamine, which is found in many OTC allergy, cold, and upper respiratory infection drugs. [9]

There are seven groups of herbs that have significant side effects that are referenced in the herb descriptions in this chapter. These include the anthraquinone containing laxatives, anticoagulant and antiplatelet herbs, thujone containing herbs and unsaturated pyrrolizidine alkaloids. Additionally, this section discusses the concerns associated with tannins, hormonally-active constituents, and herbs that affect blood sugar levels.

Anthraquinone (AQ) containing laxatives

Buckthorn Bark, Cascara Sagrada, Chinese Fo-Ti, Turkey Rhubarb and Yellow Dock.

Cautions: Laxative doses should be used for no more than

2 weeks. Long term use of laxatives may produce dependence and result in symptoms called "laxative abuse.[20]

American Herbal Products Association (AHPA) recommended labeling states "Do not use this product if you have abdominal pain or diarrhea. Consult a health care provider prior to use if you are pregnant or nursing. Discontinue use in the event of diarrhea or watery stools. Do not exceed recommended dose. Not for long-term use." [3]

The formulas described in this book use these herbs in a dose that is safe and effective.

Use is contraindicated in children under 2 years, in inflammatory intestinal disease, in obstruction of the bowel, in abdominal pain of unknown origin, and should be limited to less than 14 days duration. [20, 3, 6]

Anticoagulant and Antiplatelet properties of herbs

Herbs with anticoagulant properties with coumarin constituents or that effect platelet aggregation:

Angelica, anise, arnica, asafoetida, bogbean, boldo, capsicum, celery, chamomile, clove, danshen, dong quai, fenugreek, feverfew, garlic, ginger, ginkgo, ginseng (Panax), horse chestnut, horseradish, licorice, meadowsweet, prickly ash, onion, papain, passionflower, poplar, quassia, red clover, turmeric, wild carrot, wild lettuce, willow.

> *Caution:* Interactions with Anticoagulant and Antiplatelet Drugs

Herbs that have a mild or moderate effect on "thinning" the blood or decreasing platelet aggregation or blood clotting can increase the effect of medication, such as warfarin (coumadin) or aspirin, that thins the blood in heart and circulatory problems. This can increase the risk of bleeding in some people both from cuts on the skin and internal bleeding from a trauma or injury. Herbs can also increase the effect of other herbs with similar effects. Although multiple herbs are likely to cause problems in healthy individuals it possible individuals in fragile health could experience a significant anticoagulant effect.

The formulas described in this book use these herbs in a dose that is safe and effective.

Thujone

These herbs contain some thujone in their natural form:

Mugwort, oak moss, oriental arborvitae, sage, tansy, thuja (cedar), and tree moss.

> *Caution:* Thujone is a toxic oil . It is present in very small amounts in herbs but may be as high as 50% in some essential oils such as thuja oil which are not for internal use. Herbs that contain small amounts of thujone can be used in limited quantities in herbal formulas. These formula's have a duration of use that is appropriate for the small amount of thujone that is present. Avoid thujone containing herbs that will add to the dosage.

Mechanism of Action: The constituent, thujone is chemically related to camphor. As the amount of thujone ingested is increased, the toxic effect becomes pronounced, leading to increased salivation and redness of the mucous membranes and pelvic viscera. Thujone heightens and alters the effect of alcohol. Researchers think thujone has a mind-altering effect similar to tetrahydrocannabinol, the active constituent marijuana. Chronic thujone poisoning can lead to epileptic seizures, delirium and hallucinations.

The formulas described in this book use these herbs in a dose that is safe and effective.

Unsaturated Pyrrolizidine Alkaloids (UPA)

UPA's are present in Coltsfoot, Comfrey, Eupatorium and Ragwort.

> *Cautions:* These herbs have a cumulative toxicity and should not be used as single herbs. Their use in formulas should be in low dosage and for short periods of time alternating with formula's that are UPA free. There are 2 fundamental groups of PA s. The saturated PA's are nontoxic while the unsaturated PA's are toxic. The toxicity of UPAs takes a predictable course of action: liver damage known as veno-occlusive disease progressing to cirrhosis. A number of the UPA s have been shown to be mutagenic and/or carcinogenic. Any internal use should be limited to 4-6 weeks of use with a total of no more than 100 mcg. per year. UPA's are C/I in pregnancy and lactation. [19]

The formulas described in this book use these herbs in a dose that is safe and effective.

Tannins-

Tannins are phenolic compounds with astringent properties.
Tannins bind and precipitate proteins, which can effect the
absorption of certain pharmaceuticals. These are not problematic unless large doses of tannins are consumed. Tea and coffee
are high in tannins and due to the tendency for large consumption of these beverages may affect some drugs. *The Botanical
Safety Handbook* cites an association of increased esophogeal and
nasal cancer with the consumption of tannins. They further
mention that G/I disturbances are traditionally associated with
tannin containing plants.

Hormonally Active Herbs

Plants such as Saw Palmetto, Vitex, Black Cohosh and Ginseng
have steroidal components which mildly effect human hormone
activity. This class of plants can potentiate the effect of some
drugs and hormones and antagonize the effects of others. These
herbs can be of significant concern in estrogen sensitive breast or
prostate cancer. These have a theoretical interaction with pharmaceutical hormonal therapy. Hormone replacement therapy,
oral contraceptives, and conventional treatment for prostate disorders fall into this category. The concern is strictly theoretical
at this point.

Herbs Effecting Blood Sugar

Some herbs have been shown to effect the blood sugar level.
Some have a increase blood sugar, a hyperglycemic effect or
decrease it, a hypoglycemic effect. Diabetics and individuals with
reactive hypoglycemia should be aware of any effects of herbs
that they use. Awareness when introducing new substances is
the key, diabetics should pick up any changes when they monitor
their sugar. Hypoglycemic individuals can usually monitor their
symptoms. Diabetics may need to adjust insulin accordingly.
Keep in communication with your physician if this is the case.

LIST OF HERBS WITH CAUTIONS,
CONTRAINDICATIONS AND DRUG
INTERACTIONS

Arnica-*Arnica latifolia*

Caution: Toxic Arnica should not be used internally as a single herb product. It can be used safely in formulas when used as directed. Arnica is used in several proprietary medications that are recognized formulas with multiple herbs. [2]

Acute overdose is accompanied by vomiting and diarrhea, stimulation of heart rate, dizziness or tremor.[2] Some sources C/I internal use altogether especially as a single ingredient product. [1, 3]

Approved by German Commission E monographs for use in fever, colds, bronchitis.

American Herbal Products Association (AHPA) recommended labeling: "To be used only under the supervision of an expert qualified in the appropriate use of this substance." [3]

Minimal risk for external use— Allergic dermatitis may result in sensitive people or with long term use. C/I on open wounds or broken skin. [3, 6]

Contraindication: C/I in pregnancy. [3, 6]

Ashwaganda-*Withania somnifera*

Cautions: none found.

Contraindications: C/I in pregnancy. [3, 6]

Drug Interaction

Because of sedative action, may mildly potentiate the effect of antidepressant and anxiety drugs. [42]   May potentiate effects of amphetamines and barbituates. [3] Contains beta sitosterol, a hormonally active component, which theoretically could interfere with hormone therapy, including oral contraceptives. [7, 12]

Astragalus membranaceus

Cautions: None found.

Contraindications: none found.

Drug Interaction: Immunostimulants are contraindicated with immunosuppressants such as Cyclophosphamide for organ transplants. [8] May potentiate the effect of blood thinners such as Coumadin. [67]

Barberry-*Berberis vulgaris*

No health hazards or side effects associated with proper use. [67]

Cautions: Dosages of barberry root over 4 mg will cause vomiting, diarrhea, nosebleed and light stupor.[67]

Contraindications: C/I in pregnancy due to berberine content. [3]

Drug Interaction

There are mixed results reported when mixing berberine containing plants with Doxycline and Tetracycline-type antibiotics. More information is needed. [11, 13]

Basil-*Ocimum basilicum* (the following applies to therapeutic doses)

No health hazards have been associated with proper administration or therapeutic doses. [67]
Caution: Estragole, a component of basil concentrated in oil of basil, has shown carcinogenic potential in animals [49]
Oil of basil is not recommended for extended therapeutic use.
Contraindications: C/I during pregnancy and lactation. Not recommended for infants or toddlers. (Due to essential oil component estragole). [3, 6]
Drug Interaction
None found.

Bilberry- *Vaccinium myrtillus*

Caution: Appears safe in reasonable amounts. More data is needed.
Contraindications: none found.
Drug Interaction
May have hypoglycemic properties; therefore could enhance diabetic medications. [7, 68]

Bitter Orange- *Citrus aurantium* (the following apply to therapeutic doses)

Caution: There are reports of problems (colic, convulsions, death) in children with the consumption of large doses. Bitter orange is photosenstizing. [3, 18, 68]
Contraindications: Pregnancy, due to antifertility properties of citrantin. The presence of synephrine signifies potential C/I with hypertension. [18, 68]
Drug Interaction
Coumarins are listed indicating possible potentiation of Warfarin, aspirin and other anti-coagulants. Not to be used prior to surgery. [4, 8] Theoretical interactions exist with stimulants such as caffeine and CNS stimulant drugs such as phenylpropanolamine because of increased risk of hypertension or cardiovascular complications. Because of stomach acid production associated with bitter orange, may interfere with antacids, sucralfate, H2 antagonists, or proton pump inhibitors. [68]

Black Alder-*Alnus serrulatta*

No health hazards or side effects associated with proper use. [67]

Drug Interaction

Contains tannins; large doses may decrease absorption of codeine, ephedrine, pseudoephedrine, theophylline and aminophylline. [9, 11, 13]

Black Cohosh-*Cimicifuga racemosa*

Caution: Is effectively used for symptoms of menopause but does not provide protection from osteoporosis as hormone replacement therapy claims. Overdose (12 grams) may cause vomiting, dizziness, headache and lowered blood pressure. [3]

Contraindications: C/I in pregnancy due to a risk of spontaneous abortion. [3]

Drug Interaction

Can increase the effect of blood pressure lowering medication. Theoretical interaction with oral contraceptives due to estrogenic activity. [7, 25]

Black Haw-*Viburnum prunifolium*

Caution: No health hazards or side effects known with proper administration.

Has small amount of oxalic acid, caution if a history of kidney stones is present. [3]

Contraindications: none found.

Drug Interactions

Contains coumarins in small amounts, thus potentiation of anti-coagulant pharmaceuticals such as Warfarin is possible. [7 18]

Black Walnut-*Juglans nigra*

No health hazards known with proper use.

Caution: One source cautions against prolonged use, due to possible mutagenic qualities of juglone. [3]

Drug Interaction

Contains tannins, large doses may decrease absorption of codeine, ephedrine, pseudoephedrine, theophylline and aminophylline. [9, 11, 13]

Bladderwrack-*Fucus vesiculosis*

Contains iodine, which is essential for the production of thyroid hormone.

Caution: Iodine in excess of 150 mcg./day can induce or aggravate a hyperthyroidism. Due to the variability of the

iodine content this herb should not be used as a single herb in large doses.[67]
Contraindications: In overactive thyroid conditions, including partial thyroid removal or Hashimoto's thryoiditis.[3, 6] Not recommended for long-term therapeutic use.
Drug Interactions
Limit intake with anticoagulants due to high levels of Vitamin K. [27]

Bloodroot- *Sanguinaria canadensis*

No health hazards or side effects known with proper use. [67]
Caution: In large amounts causes nausea and vomiting. [2]
Contraindications: C/I pregnancy[1]
Drug Interactions
None found.

Blue Flag-*Iris versicolor*

Caution: Fresh root may cause mucosal irritation, nausea and vomiting. [3]
Contraindications: pregnancy. [3]
Drug Interactions
None found.

Buchu-*Barosma betulina*

No health hazards or side effects known with proper use. [67]
Caution: Kidney infections are serious conditions and should be treated with medical supervision.
Contraindications: C/I in pregnancy. [3, 6]
Felter states that "large doses may produce stomach or bladder irritation.[38] Color and odor of urine may be altered by this plant. [36]

Buckthorn Bark-*Rhamnus cathartica*

Caution: Laxative doses should be used for no more than 2 weeks. Long term use of laxatives may produce dependence and result in symptoms called "laxative abuse.[20]
Contains 2-7% of anthranoid derivatives. [20] See anthraquinone containing laxatives.
Contraindications: Contraindicated in acute abdominal pain, bowel obstruction, and appendicitis. C/I in children under 12 and pregnancy. [3]
Drug Interaction
Potassium loss is increased and should be supplemented if

using drugs that also stimulate potassium loss (diuretics) in order to prevent cardiac rhythm changes. Use with licorice may also stimulate potassium loss. C/I with cardiac glycosides (digitalis). [20]

Bugleweed-*Lycopus virginica*

Caution: Causes decreased thyroid hormone activity. Headache is a possible side effect, corrected by reduction of dose. [20]

Contraindications: C/I in hypothyroid or thyroid enlargement. [3, 6] C/I in pregnancy due to anti-gonadotropic and anti-thyrotropic actions. [3, 6, 20] C/I in lactation due to anti-prolactin activity. [6, 20]

Drug Interactions
Can interfere with thyroid hormone formation and function and decreases iodine absorption. [3, 6, 20]
Listed as a hypoglycemic [6] and therefore may interact with endocrine system pharmaceuticals such as antidiabetics, corticosteroids, and oral contraceptives. [7]

Bupleurum falcatum

Caution: Low toxicity. [4]
Contraindications: No C/I found.
Drug Interaction
Interferon therapy [10]

Burdock-*Arctium lappa*

Caution: None found.
Contraindications: C/I in pregnancy. [6]
Drug Interaction
Listed as a hypoglycemic in large doses [12] may enhance insulin and antidiabetic medications. [7]

Butterbur-*Petasites frigida*

Caution: Toxic Contains unsaturated pyrrolizidine alkaloids. These herbs should not be used as single herbs and their use in formulas should be in low dosage and for short periods of time. The toxicity of UPAs takes a predictable course of action: liver damage known as veno-occlusive disease progressing to cirrhosis. Any internal use

should be limited to 4-6 weeks of use with a total of no more than 100 mcg of UPA's per year. [19, 1] See Unsaturated Pyrrolizidine Alkaloids.
Contraindication: C/I in pregnancy and lactation. [6, 19]
Drug Interactions
None found.

Calamus -*Acorus calamus*

No health hazards or side effects known with proper use. [67]
Caution: Volatile oil is noted to cause dermatitis in some cases when coming into contact with skin. [28]
No other cautions with American variety, Indian calamus contains asarone which is not recommended. [3 28]
Contraindication: C/I in pregnancy. [6]
Drug Interactions
None found.

California Poppy-*Eschscholzia californica*

No health hazards or side effects with proper use. [67]
Caution: Recommended labeling in Australia reads "Warning: Do not exceed the stated dose." [3]
Contraindication: pregnancy. [3]
Drug Interactions
May cause additive effects with MAO-inhibitors, antidepressants, antipsychotics, anxiolytics, dopaminergics, analgesic and antiepileptic and ulcer-healing drugs. [3, 4, 7, 8, 22]
Concomitant use should be under supervision of healthcare professional.

Cardamom-*Elettaria cardamomum*

Caution: The oil is a cholegogue; it stimulates gall bladder to secrete bile. If gallstones or gall bladder disease is present, pain and colic may result.
Contraindication: Commission E advises use only under physician's supervision in case of gallstones. [1]
Drug Interactions
None found.

Cascara Sagrada-*Rhamnus purshiana*

Contains 6% of anthranoid derivatives. [20] See anthraquinone containing laxatives.
Caution: Laxative doses should be used for no more than 2 weeks. Long term use of laxatives may produce dependence and result in symptoms called "laxative abuse." [20]

**American Herbal Products Association (AHPA)
recommended labeling** states "Do not use this product if
you have abdominal pain or diarrhea. Consult a health care
provider prior to use if you are pregnant or nursing.
Discontinue use in the event of diarrhea or watery stools.
Do not exceed recommended dose. Not for long-term
use." [3]

Contraindication: in children under 2 years, in
inflammatory intestinal disease, in obstruction of the bowel,
in abdominal pain of unknown origin, and should be
limited to less than 14 days duration. [20, 3, 6]

Drug Interaction
Potassium loss is increased and should be supplemented if
using drugs that also stimulate potassium loss (diuretics) in
order to prevent cardiac rhythm changes. Use with licorice
may also stimulate potassium loss. C/I with cardiac
glycosides (digitalis), due to increased potassium loss with
potential increase of toxicity. [20]

Catnip-*Nepeta cataria*

No health hazards or side effects known with proper use. [67]
Caution: None found.
Contraindication: pregnancy. [3, 6]
Drug Interactions
None found.

Cat's Claw-*Uncaria tomentosa*

Low toxicity seems likely; and "no major toxicity problems
appear in the world literature." [45]
Caution: Common name of Una de Gato may be confused
with several other plants. Cat's Claw used for over 8 weeks
has produced decreased serum estradiol and progesterone. [67]
Contraindications: C/I in pregnancy (based on traditional
use as a contraceptive). [3, 44] One source C/I use in children
under 3 years old, hormone therapy, and patients
undergoing skin grafts, organ transplants or blood plasma
treatment in hemophiliacs. [3]
Drug Interactions
See contraindications.

Celandine-*Chelidonium major*

Caution: This herb may have a cumulative toxicity. It is not
to be used as a single remedy. It should only be used in low
dosage as a part of a formula and the duration of the use of

the formula should be limited. Celandine has been recently implicated in at least ten cases of hepatitis involving five different brand products manufactured in Germany. [67] AHPA clarifies that the fresh plant is associated with "severe irritation of the digestive system", but this side effect is not noted with dried plant. [3] Occasional poisonings have been reported in humans.
Contraindication: C/I in pregnancy [1,3] and children. [3]
Drug Interactions
None found.

Celery-*Apium graveolens* (the following C/I apply to therapeutic doses)

Caution: Allergic reactions noted, including anaphylactic shock. Furocoumarins indicate potential photosensitizing qualities, although these are not reported. [3,18,43,68]
Contraindication: kidney disorders. [3,68]
Drug Interactions
Sedative properties may mildly potentiate the effect or antidepressant and anxiety drugs. [7,68] May increase the effect of PUVA therapy, due to psoralen content (furocoumarin). Coumarins indicate possible potentiation of anti-coagulant pharmaceuticals such as Warfarin. [7,18,68]

Chamomile-*Matricaria recutita*

No health hazards or side effects known with proper use. [67]
Caution: Mild and rare contact allergy is noted. [22]
Contraindication: pregnancy. [6]
Drug Interactions
None found.

Chaparral -*Larrea tridentata*

Caution: This herb has a cumulative toxicity. It is not to be used as a single remedy. It should only be used in low dosage as a part of a formula and the duration of the use of the formula should be limited.
There are reports of serious poisonings, acute hepatitis, kidney and liver damage. Nordihydroguaiaretic acid (NDGA), a constituent of chaparral was removed by the FDA from the "Generally Regarded As Safe" (GRAS) list, due to toxicity. NDGA is toxic to the kidneys. [20]
AHPA recommended labeling: "Seek advice from a health care practitioner before use if you have a history of liver disease. Discontinue use if nausea, fever, fatigue, or jaundice occur (e.g., dark urine or yellow discoloration of the eyes)." [3] AHPA concluded that liver toxicity appears to

be an idiosyncratic reaction with pre-existing liver conditions. [3]
Contraindication: C/I in pregnancy and lactation.
Drug Interactions
Amino acid constituents indicate potential interaction with Monoamine Oxidase Inhibitors (MAOI). [43] May interfere with "tissue compatibility procedures in the blood transfusion laboratory." [20]

Chaste Tree Berry-*Vitex agnus-castus*

Caution: Suppresses lactation. Occasional occurrence of rashes. 1 Rare side effects include nausea or headaches. [46]
Contraindication: C/I in pregnancy and lactation. [1,3,6]
Drug Interaction
Suppresses Follicle Stimulating Hormone, which is similar to the effect of oral contraceptives and may interfere with sex hormone treatment. [3,7] Stimulates dopamine which potentially would interfere with dopamine-receptor antagonists. [1]

Cinnamon Essential Oil, *Cinnamon verum*

No health hazards or side effects with proper use. [67]
Caution: Medium potential for skin sensitization. Internal use of essential oils should be limited to 4 weeks, allow 2 weeks break between courses of treatment. [16]
Contraindication: C/I in pregnancy.
Drug Interaction
None found.

Cleavers-*Galium aparine*

No health hazards or side effects known with proper use. [67]

Codonopsis tangshen

No health hazards or side effects known with proper use. [67]
Drug Interaction
Immunostimulants in general are contraindicated with immunosuppressants such as Cyclophosphamide for organ transplants [8]

Cola Nut-*Cola nitida*   PDR and Natural database use Cola acuminata,

No health hazards or side effects known with proper use. [67]
The cola nut has Generally Recognized as Safe (GRAS) status in the US (11).
Caution: Stimulant containing caffeine may cause difficulty falling asleep, nervousness and stomach complaints.

Chronic use, especially in large doses, can cause habituation and psychological dependence. Physical withdrawal symptoms can occur with sudden discontinuation.
Contraindication: C/I in pregnancy and with gastric and duodenal ulcers. [1]

Drug Interaction
Possible C/I with antidepressants and SSRIs due to increased plasma concentration of xanthines. Also possible C/I with antihypertensives, due to antagonism.[4] Strengthening of the action of caffeine-containing drugs and beverages including Anacin, Bayer Select Headache, Excedrin, Midol Max Strength, NoDoz, and Vivarin. [1] Caffeine taken with ephedrine can increase thermogenesis and weight loss and cause agitation, tremors, and insomnia. May decrease absorption of tricyclic antidepressants and thus should be separated by at least 2 hours.[11] C/I with Phenylpropanolamine, which is found in many OTC allergy, cold, and upper respiratory infection drugs. [9]

Coleus forskohlii

No health hazards or side effects associated with proper use. [67]
Caution: Use caution with low blood pressure, gastric and peptic ulcers (appears to stimulate acid and pepsinogen secretion). [4, 17]

Drug Interaction
Caution should be used with allergy, hypertensive and asthmatic medications, due to possible potentiation. [4]

Comfrey-*Symphytum officinale*

Caution: This herb has a cumulative toxicity. It is not to be used as a single remedy. It should only be used in low dosage as a part of a formula and the duration of the use of the formula should be limited. Comfrey contains unsaturated pyrrolizidine alkaloids (UPA's) that are toxic to liver. Avoid internal use of over 100 mcg of UPA's per year. The root contains 10 times the amount of UPA as the leaves.

American Herbal Products Association (AHPA) recommended labeling: "For external use only, which should be limited to 4-6 weeks with a level of unsaturated pyrrolizidine alkaloids no greater than 100 mcg. Do not apply to broken or abraded skin. Do not use when nursing." AHPA goes on to say that the limitation may be overly cautious.[3]

Drug interactions
No known interactions. See Unsaturated Pyrrolizidine Alkaloids.

Chinese Coptis-*Coptis chinensis*

No health hazards or side effects with proper use.
Contraindication: C/I in pregnancy (uterine stimulant, emmenagogue) [3]

Corn Silk-*Zea mays*

No health hazards or side effects known with proper use. [67]
Caution: None found.
Contraindication: None found.
Drug Interaction
None found.

Corydalis-*Dicentra canadensis*

No health hazards or side effects known with proper use.
Caution: None found.
Contraindication: None found.
Drug Interaction
None found.

Damiana-*Turnera diffusa*

Caution: Overdose reactions: Tetanus-like convulsions and paroxysms following ingestion of 200 grams Damiana extract. [4]
Contraindication: C/I in pregnancy and lactation.
Drug Interaction
Contains 4% tannins, therefore in large doses may decrease absorption of iron, codeine, ephedrine, pseudoephedrine, theophylline and aminophylline. [8, 9, 11, 12]

Dandelion-*Taraxacum officinale*

Cautions: Use caution in cases of bile or intestinal blockage, acute gallbladder inflammation or gallbladder stones. [3, 6, 15, 24] Recommend consultation with medical professional for gall bladder ailments.
Contraindication: None found.
Drug Interaction
Possible potentiation with pharmaceutical diuretics. [13]

Devil's Claw—*Harpagophytum procumbens*

Caution: German Commission E recommending use in gallstones only after consultation with a physician. [1] Weiss, however, indicates the plant for gallbladder complaints. [2]

Contraindications: C/I in gallstones, duodenal and gastric ulcers. [1, 2, 3, 6, 24]

Two sources note a claim of oxytocin activity, indicating C/I during pregnancy. [7, 49]

Drug Interaction

A reported interaction with Warfarin indicates that caution should be used with anti-coagulant therapies, including Coumadin and Ticlopidine. [13] "Excessive doses" C/I with hypotensive therapies. [7]

Devil's Club-*Oplopanax horridum*

Cautions: None found

Contraindication: C/I in pregnancy and lactation. [67]

Drug Interaction

Considered hypoglycemic and therefore may enhance diabetic medications. [7]

Devil's Weed- *Tribule terrestre*

Caution: No reported cautions

Contraindication: Pregnancy and lactation.

Drug Interaction:

No reported drug interactions

Dong Quai-*Angelica sinensis*

Cautions: Use cautiously in diarrhea. [47, 51, 52]

Contraindications: C/I in pregnancy, excessive menses and hemorrhagic disease. [3]

The estrogenic effects of Dong Quai would suggest caution in estrogen sensitive diseases including breast, uterine and ovarian cancer, endometriosis and fibroids as we do not fully understand the effects of phytoestrogens in cancer.[68] Willard, states that side effects are rare. [29] Dong Quai is second only to licorice in frequency in Chinese formulas. [51]

Drug Interaction

C/I with anticoagulant or blood thinning pharmaceuticals such as Warfarin (coumadin) or aspirin because of enhanced potency causing bleeding. [13] See section on Anticoagulant herbs in this chapter.

Echinacea-*Echinacea purpura and angustifolia*

Is one of the most frequently taken herb in the U.S. with an excellent record of safety.

Cautions: Should not be used if allergies are present to composite family of plants.

Contraindications: A theoretical concern, not based on

adverse incidents, is expressed in Commission E monographs that caution be used for autoimmune conditions, organ transplants, AIDS, HIV and tuberculosis. [1]
Drug Interactions:
None known. [1, 4]

Elderberry-*Sambucus canadensis*

No health hazards or side effects known with proper use. [67]
Cautions: Ripe fruit must be used, due to cyanogenic glycosides in the unripe fruit, which can cause vomiting. [3]
Contraindication: None known.
Drug Interactions
None known.

Elecampane-*Inula helenium*

Caution: Irritating to mucous membranes. Overdose symptoms: Vomiting, diarrhea, spasms, and symptoms of paralysis caused by large doses. [1, 3] Contact dermatitis noted. [1, 6, 22]
Contraindication: C/I in pregnancy.
Drug Interaction:
None known.

Embelia ribes

Caution: Antifertility action noted in traditional use [14]
Contraindication: In pregnancy and with birth control pills.
Drug Interaction
Contains tannins, [12] therefore in large doses may decrease absorption of iron, [8] codeine, ephedrine, pseudoephedrine, theophylline and aminophylline. [9, 11, 13]

Ephedra or Ma Huang-*Ephedra sinica*

Cautions: Side effects include headache, insomnia, motor restlessness, irritability, headaches, nausea, vomiting, disturbances of urination, tachycardia. In higher dosage: increase in blood pressure, cardiac arrhythmia, development of dependency. [1]
American Herbal Products Association recommended labeling: "Seek advice from a health care practitioner prior to use if you are pregnant or nursing, or if you have high blood pressure, heart or thyroid disease, diabetes, difficulty in urination due to prostate enlargement, or if taking a MAO inhibitor or any other prescription drug. Reduce or discontinue use if nervousness, tremor, sleeplessness, loss of

appetite, or nausea occur."
Contraindication: C/I in pregnancy and lactation. Not
intended for use by persons under 18 years of age. Keep
out of the reach of children." [3]
Drug Interaction
Potentiation of effects with caffeine and caffeine-containing
drugs (e.g. Anacin R), adrenaline, ephedrine,
pseudoephedrine, phenylpropanolamine (e.g. Dimetapp, R
DayQuill R Allergy Relief, etc.), Corticosteroids and
cortisone-like drugs, steroids, phenelzine (Monoamine
Oxidase Inhibitor), epinephrine. [13]

Eyebright-*Euphrasia officinalis*

No health hazards or side effects known with proper use. [67]
Caution: None
Contraindications: C/I in pregnancy and lactation.
Drug Interactions
No Information

Fennel-*Foeniculum vulgare*

Caution: Rare skin and respiratory allergic reactions are
noted. [1]
Contraindication: C/I in pregnancy and young children. [1]
Drug Interaction
C/I with coumarin derivatives and other anti-coagulants.
27 Estrogenic activity noted thus may interfere with sex
hormone therapy, including oral contraceptives. [7 12]

Feverfew-*Tanacetum parthenium*

Caution: Reported side effects in 6-15% of users include
mouth ulceration or gastric disturbance and usually occur
within the first week of use. [3]
A post feverfew withdrawal including headaches, insomnia,
nervousness, fatigue and/or muscle stiffness have been
reported in as high as 10% of users who stop taking
feverfew abruptly. [8]
Contraindications: C/I in pregnancy and breastfeeding. [6, 3]
Drug Interaction
Inhibits arachadonic acid which is a precursor to
prostaglandins involved in clotting; therefore, C/I with
anti-coagulants. [2]

Figwort- *Scrophularia nodosa*

No health hazards or side effects known with proper use. [67]
Caution: none found.

Contraindications: Due to lack of pharmacological and toxicity data, Newall, et al recommend avoiding use during pregnancy and lactation. [43]

Drug Interaction

Figwort has similar chemical makeup as other cardiac glycosides and simultaneous use can increase the risk of cardiac glycoside toxicity. Cardiac glycoside-containing herbs include black hellebore, Canadian hemp roots, digitalis leaf, hedge mustard, lily of the valley roots, motherwort, oleander leaf, pheasant's eye plant, pleurisy root, squill bulb leaf scales, strophanthus seeds, and uzara. [68]

Chinese Fo-Ti-*Polygonatum multiflorum*

No health hazards known with proper use. [67]

Caution: Raw and cured have different pharmacological activity. Both contain anthraquinones, thus C/I with diarrhea. [3] The cured is preferred, as anthraquinones are greatly reduced. Raw root is considered cathartic [3] and more toxic. [18]

Garcinia cambogia

Insufficient data exists to assess the safety of this plant. It appears to be non-toxic and safe.

Caution: N/A

Contraindication: N/A

Drug Interaction: N/A

Garlic-*Allium sativum*

Caution: Commission E warns us that the "odor of garlic may pervade the breath and skin," [1] beware! Instances of allergic reaction, GI symptoms, heartburn, nausea and intestinal flora changes are noted. [1, 19]

Contraindication: Pre-existing gastrointestinal irritation. AHPA advises caution in use with children and lactation. [3]

Drug Interaction

Potentiate effect of warfarin, aspirin and other anti-coagulants. Not to be used prior to surgery. [4, 8]

Yellow Jasmine-*Gelsemium sempervirens*

Health risks following the proper administration and dosage are not recorded. [67]

Caution: Very toxic when used as single herb, recommended use only in formulas at safe dosage. Alkaloids are "extremely toxic." Fatalities are reported from as little as 4 ml of a fluid extract (1:1) or 3 leaves. Chewing leaves or sucking flower nectar has resulted in severe poisoning of children. Symptoms of toxicity include respiratory depression, weakness, double vision, dilated pupils, and ptosis (drooping of eyelids). [18]

Contraindication: C/I in pregnancy. [6]

Drug Interaction

Potentiates analgesic effects of aspirin and phenacetin. [18]

Gentian-*Gentiana lutea*

Caution: The AHPA editors note that gentian's "irritating qualities are maximized in tincture form and minimized as a tea." [3] King's tells us that large doses may "oppress the stomach, irritate the bowels, and even produces nausea and vomiting, as well as fullness of pulse and headache." [15]

Contraindication: C/I in gastric or duodenal ulcers, in gastric irritation or inflammation, stomach irritation or inflammation and stomach ulcers. [2, 3, 6, 15, 24] C/I in pregnancy. [43]

Drug Interaction

None Known [1]

Geranium- *Geranium maculatum*

Health risks following the proper administration and dosage are not recorded. [67]

Caution: In constipation due to high tannin content. [4]

Contraindication: C/I in pregnancy and lactation.

Drug Interaction: Contains 10-30% tannins, therefore moderate doses may decrease absorption of iron, codeine, ephedrine, pseudoephedrine, theophylline and aminophylline. [8, 9, 11]

Ginger-*Zingiber officinalis* (the following C/I apply to thera peutic doses)

Caution: Heartburn,

Contraindication: Gallstones (cholegogue effect) [6] Commission E gives a contraindication to ginger in morning sickness because it has some abortifacient properties. Other research provides evidence that ginger is effective and safe at 250 mg 4 times daily. [1 67]

Drug Interactions

C/I with antacids, due to possible antagonism of mucosal irritation. [4] Avoid use with blood thinning pharmaceuticals such as warfarin and aspirin. [4]

Ginkgo-*Ginkgo biloba*

Caution: headaches, gastric disturbances and allergic reactions are possible but rare. [21]

Contraindication: C/I with epileptic patients as it may lower seizure threshold. [1] C/I in pregnancy and lactation. [8]

Drug Interaction

C/I with pharmaceutical blood thinning agents such as warfarin, heparin, and other anti-coagulants and prior to surgery. [23] Caution should also be used in combination with milder blood thinners (i.e. aspirin) and with herbal blood thinners. [8, 23] Stated to diminish the effectiveness of anti-convulsants. [8]

Ginseng, American-*Panax ginseng*

Caution: Hormonal-like effects are recorded as are the "relatively rare side effects, ...only with high doses and/or use over very long periods of time." [3] These side effects include sleeplessness, nervousness, diarrhea (particularly in the morning) and menopausal bleeding.[3]

Ginseng abuse syndrome was reported in 1979 and is prolonged use of high dose Panax with caffeine producing insomnia, headache, nervousness and vomiting.

Enlargement of breasts in males has been reported.

Ginseng in face cremes has caused vaginal bleeding in post menopausal women. People with cardiovascular disease or diabetes should use with caution and preferably under professional guidance.

Contraindication: C/I ginseng in cases of very high blood pressure (systolic over 180 mm Hg) over use can result in "headache, insomnia, palpitations, and a rise in blood pressure." [24] Commission E lists numerous possible C/I, side effects, or drug interactions with Panax but states that few if any are confirmed.[13] C/I in pregnancy and lactation.

Drug Interactions

C/I with warfarin and other anti-coagulants. [8] Headache, tremors and manic-like symptoms reported when used concurrently with Phenelzine an MAO inhibitor. [6] Hypoglycemic effects of Panax may potentiate diabetic medication. [3]

Ginseng, Siberian-*Eleutherococcus senticosus*

Caution: No health hazards or side effects associated with proper use. [67]

Contraindication: Conflicting statements exist about its use in hypertension. The German Commission E C/I the use in hypertension, [1] while Huang attributes a blood pressure lowering effect to the use of the herb. [3] Others report that it should be avoided only in individuals with a blood pressure greater than 180/90 mm/HG. [3, 20]

Drug Interactions

May enhance the serum levels of patients on digitalis, increase the effect of insulin and hypoglycemic agents and potentiate the effects of blood thinners, warfarin and aspirin. One source indicates an increase effect with antibiotics, possibly due to increased T-lymphocyte activity. [6] Used in Russia in cancer care to increase the tolerance of the patients to the adverse effects of chemotherapy and radiation therapy. [20]

Glycerin

No health hazards or side effects known with proper use. [67]

Caution: Glycerin is metabolized to glucose or glycogen. Diabetes patients run the risk that use of a moderate quantity of glycerin may result in transitory sugar in the urine. This is not likely with the quantity in alcohol free herbal extracts. [48]

Drug Interaction

Potentially interferes with insulin in frequent, moderate quantities by slightly increasing blood sugar.

Goldenrod-*Solidago odora*

Caution: Consult a practitioner in chronic kidney disorders. [3, 6, 20]

Contraindication: C/I in pregnancy and lactation.

Drug Interaction: C/I with pharmaceutical diuretics, including loop, thiazide, and potassium-sparing diuretics due to possible potentiation of activity. [13]

Goldenseal Root-*Hydrastis canadensis*

Caution: Extended use may cause digestive disorders attributed to mucous membrane irritation and changes in the colon microflora.

Contraindication: Pregnancy, because of the alkaloids' uterine stimulation. Use in ear canal C/I if ear drum is ruptured. [6]

Drug Interaction

Hydrastis has an antagonistic effect decreasing the effect of Heparin as an anticoagulant. [11 67]

Gotu Kola-*Centella asiatica*

No health hazards or side effects known with proper use.
Caution: None known.
Contraindication: C/I in pregnancy [6]
Drug Interaction
None known.

Grape Seed

Caution: N/A
Contraindication: N/A
Drug Interaction
Potentiation of anti-coagulant pharmaceutical is possible,
due to tocopherol content. [68]

Gravel Root- *Eupatorium purpureum*

Caution: This herb may have a cumulative toxicity. It is not
to be used as a single remedy. It should only be used in low
dosage as a part of a formula and the duration of the use of
the formula should be limited. Unsaturated pyrrolizidine
alkaloid containing plant.
Contraindication: C/I in pregnancy, lactation, and not for
long term use. [3]
AHPA recommended labeling states "For external use only.
Do not apply to broken or abraded skin. Do not use when
nursing." [3] King's, however, states that it can be used for
long periods of time "without ill results". [15]
Drug Interactions
no information
*Read about Unsaturated Pyrrolizidine Alkaloids in this
chapter.*

Green Tea-*Camellia sinensis*

No health hazards known with proper use. [67]
Cautions: Nervous system stimulant, may irritate sensitive
stomachs due to tannin (addition of milk will bind tannin
and reduce symptoms). [3]
Contraindications: Caution with use in kidney disorders,
due to increased urinary output. Caution with use in
duodenal ulcers because of increased gastric acid secretion.
Caution with use in tachycardia and heart arrhythmias due
to increased heart rate. Caution with use in anxiety, is a

nervous system stimulant. [6] Pregnant women and children should limit intake to maximum of 250 mg a day (3 cups).

Drug Interactions

High in tannins and thus may decrease absorption of iron, codeine, ephedrine, pseudoephedrine, theophylline, aminophylline and atropine. [9, 11, 13] If taken with ephedrine can increase thermogenesis and weight loss plus cause agitation, tremors, and insomnia. [6] Excessive amounts combined with MAOI pharmaceuticals could cause a hypertensive crisis. [6] May decrease absorption of tricyclic antidepressants and thus consumption should be separated by at least 2 hours.[11] C/I with Phenylpropanolamine, which is found in many OTC allergy, cold, and upper respiratory infection drugs. [9]

Grindelia robusta

No health hazards known with proper use. [67]

Caution: High doses reported to cause irritation of the stomach and kidney. [3]

Contraindication: Pregnancy and lactation.

Drug Interaction

none reported

Gymnema sylvestre

No health hazards known with proper use.

Caution: none found.

Contraindication: may be a mild gastric irritant. [4]

Drug Interaction

Caution with diabetics as it lowers blood sugar, may potentiate diabetic medication and lower sugar to low. [7, 13]

Hairy Goat Weed-*Epimedium grandiflorum*

Dosage used in formula is safe.

Cautions: Extended use of Japanese epimedium may result in dizziness, vomiting, dry mouth, thirst, and nosebleed. [3] Large doses of Japanese epimedium may cause respiratory arrest and exaggeration of tendon reflexes to the point of spasm. [3]

Contraindication: Pregnancy and lactation. Insufficient information availible.

Drug Interaction:

No interactions are known to occur, and there is no known

reason to expect a clinically significant interaction with epimedium.

Helonias -*Chamaelirium luteum*

No health hazards or side effects known with proper use. [67]
Caution: Saponin content may cause gastric upset.
Contraindication: pregnancy. [3]
Drug Interaction
No information

Hops-*Humulus lupulus*

No health hazards or side effects known with proper use. [67]
Caution: as a sedative in depression. [22]
Contraindication: pregnancy and lactation. [43]
Drug Interaction
Because of sedative activity, use may potentiate antidepressant drugs. [7]

Horsetail-*Equisetum arvense*

No health hazards or side effects recorded with proper use. [67]
Caution: none.
Contraindication: In patients with edema with cardiac or renal dysfunction. Not recommended for children. [3]
Drug Interaction
May increase toxicity of digitalis if excessive potassium loss from the diuretic effect. [6]

Hyssop- *Hyssopus officinalis*

No health hazards recorded with proper use. [67]
Caution: Isolated cases of muscle spasm after taking 10-30 drops of the volatile oil after several days (2-3 drops of oil for children). [18]
Contraindication: pregnancy. [3,6]
Drug interaction
No information

Jamaican Dogwood-Piscidia erythrina

No health hazards or side effects recorded with proper use. [67]
Caution: Sedative effect may aggravate depression and insomnia with restlessness.[4]
Contraindication: C/I in pregnancy and cardiac insufficiency. [22]
Drug Interaction: none known

Jambul Seed-*Syzygium jambolana*

No health hazards or side effects recorded with proper use. [67]
Caution: Indications for use are to lower blood sugar in
diabetics. Monitoring blood sugar is essential.
Drug Interactions
Hypoglycemic herbs may potentiate diabetic medications. [7]

Jujube Dates-*Ziziphus jujube*

No health hazards or side effects recorded with proper use. [67]

Juniper Berry-*Juniperis communis*

No health hazards or side effects recorded with proper use. [67]
Caution: Use for short term only, long term use may cause
kidney irritation and damage. [67]
Contraindication: Pregnancy and kidney infection. Do not
use for more than 4-6 weeks in succession. [1, 3, 6]
Drug Interactions
Potentiation with pharmaceutical diuretics, including loop,
thiazide, and potassium-sparing diuretics. [13]

Kava Kava-*Piper methysticum*

Caution: Motor reflexes and judgement while driving may
be reduced when using Kava. Not to be used for more than
3 months unless under medical advice. High doses can
increase liver enzymes (GGT) with normalization after
discontinuation. Prolonged use can result in yellow skin,
nails and hair discoloration, which resolves upon
discontinuation of kava. [1, 3, 6, 20]
Contraindication: Not recommended for use under age 18.
C/I in endogenous depression, reported to increase the
danger of suicide. C/I in pregnancy and lactation. [8]
Drug Interaction
Do not mix with alcohol, potentiates the effects of alcohol.
Potentiation of effect of CNS depressants (barbituates) and
psychoactive drugs. Because of sedative activity may reduce the
effectiveness of antidepressants. [18] Kava can antagonize the
effect of levadopa in Parkinson's and should be avoided. [1, 3, 6]

Kelp-*Nereocystis luetkeana*

No health hazards or side effects recorded with proper use. [67]
Contains iodine, which is essential for the production of
thyroid hormone.
Caution: Iodine in excess of 150 mcg./day can induce or

aggravate a hyperthyroidism. Due to the variability of the iodine content this herb should not be used as a single herb in large doses.[67]

Contraindications: In overactive thyroid conditions, including partial thyroid removal or Hashimoto's thryoiditis.[3] [6] Not recommended for long-term therapeutic use.

Drug Interaction:
Due to high levels of Vitamin K, limit intake with anticoagulants. [27]

Lavendar -*Lavandula officinalis*

No health hazards or side effects recorded with proper use. [67]
Cautions: N/A
Contraindications: C/I in pregnancy[3, 6, 53]
Drug Interaction
"An interaction exists with pentobarbital: the sleeping time is increased." [58] Because of the antidepressant effects, likely to potentiate other barbituates and sedative drugs. [7, 27]

Lemon Balm-*Melissa officinalis*

No health hazards or side effects recorded with proper use. [67]
Cautions: N/A
Contraindications: N/A
Drug Interactions
Its sedative actions may potentiate other sedative drugs such as barbituates. [7, 27]

Licorice-*Glycyrrhiza glabra*

Deglycyrrhized licorice does not cause the kidney imbalance and potassium loss.
Cautions: In sensitive individuals, prolonged use longer than 6 weeks may result in pseudoaldosteronism; elevated sodium and water retention; low potassium; edema in the legs and heart problems including arrhythmias. [6, 3, 60-62, 20] Avoid prolonged use unless under qualified supervision.[3]
Contraindications: C/I with high blood pressure, C/I in potassium deficiencies or heart disease, congestive heart failure, or edema. C/I with pregnancy, diabetes, kidney insufficiency and liver disorders. [3, 6, 20, 60-62]
Drug Interaction
C/I with digoxin and corticosteroid treatment, loop and thiazide diuretics, spironolactone or amiloride. [3, 6, 7, 8, 9, 13] Shown to have a supportive effect against ulcers in long-term aspirin treatment. [13]

Life Root-*Senecio aurus*

Caution: Contains hepatotoxic Unsaturated Pyrrolizidine Alkaloids (UPA's, senecine, senecifoline) [6]
Contraindication: C/I in pregnancy, due to UPA content, emmenagogue activity, and teratogenic effects; C/I in lactation, due to excretion of UPAs into milk. [6]
Read Unsaturated Pyrrolizidine Alkaloids in this chapter.

Linden Flowers-*Tilia spp.*

No health hazards or side effects recorded with proper use. [67]
Cautions: N/A
Contraindications and Drug interactions: N/A

Lobelia inflata

No health hazards recorded with proper use. [67]
Caution: Overdose may cause nausea and vomiting; diarrhea, abdominal pain, cardiac arrhythmias, headache, respiratory difficulty. [3, 18] Like nicotine, which is in the same family, lobelia is first a CNS stimulant and then a depressant.[18, 29] Overdose may result in convulsion and collapse. [18, 36]
Contraindication: C/I in pregnancy. [36, 24]

Lomatium dissectum

Caution: Can cause skin rashes when used internally. [3]
Brinker states that Lomatium contains photosensitizers and thus can cause photodermatitis .
Contraindication: C/I in pregnancy. [3] C/I during excessive exposure to sunlight, or during ultraviolet light exposure (therapeutic or cosmetic surgery). [6]
Drug interactions: N/A

Lungwort Lichen-*Sticta pulmonaria*

No health hazards or side effects recorded with proper use. [67]
Caution: N/A
Contraindication: N/A
Drug interactions: N/A

Maca-*Lepidium meyenii*

Regarded as safe in amounts used in food. [70]
Cautions: No adverse reactions reported. [68]
Contraindication: No adverse reactions reported. [68]
Drug interactions
No interactions reported or expected to occur. [68]

Maitake Mushroom-*Grifola frondosa*

Cautions: N/A
Contraindications: N/A
Drug interactions
Immunostimulants are contraindicated with
immunosuppressants such as Cyclophosphamide for organ
transplants. [8] Said to be hypoglycemic, therefore may
potentiate insulin therapy. [68]

Marshmallow-*Althea officinalis*

No health hazards or side effects recorded with proper use. [67]
Caution: Reported to have "hypoglycemic activity", [18] thus
caution should be used in people with low blood sugar.
Contraindications: Mucilages in general are C/I in
"bronchial and catarrhal conditions." [4]
Drug Interaction
May delay absorption of other drugs taken simultaneously.
[1, 20] Listed as a hypoglycemic [18] and potentiate diabetic
medications. [7]

Mayapple Root-*Podophyllum peltatum*

Caution: This herb may have a cumulative toxicity. It is not
to be used as a single remedy. It should only be used in low
dosage as a part of a formula and the duration of the use of
the formula should be limited.
Overdose Symptoms: May induce vomiting and cathartic
diarrhea. Accidental poisonings of podophyllum have
produced death. May produce gastro-intestinal irritation
and inflammation. [15]
Contraindication: C/I in Pregnancy. [6, 20] C/I in gallstones
and intestinal obstruction. [6]
Drug Interaction
Leptandra, hyosycamus or belladonna modifies the cathartic
effects. [15]
Only aged or roasted root should be used.

Meadowsweet-*Filipendula ulmaria*

No health hazards or side effects recorded with proper use. [67]
Caution: Contains salicylates in the flower, [12] thus avoid
intake if salicylate sensitivity exists. [1, 22]
Contraindication: N/A
Drug Interaction
C/I with salicylate-containing pharmaceuticals, such as
Pepto-Bismol (Bismuth subsalicylate).[13]

Milk Thistle-*Silybum marianum*

No health hazards or side effects recorded with proper use. [67]
Cautions: Mild laxative effect reported. [1, 18] No toxicity has
been found, even in large doses. [18]
Contraindication: N/A
Drug Interaction
Protective against hepatotoxins. [6, 18, 2] Often used to protect
against deleterious effects of hepatotoxic drugs such as
acetaminophen and chemotherapy. [0]

Mistletoe-*Viscum flavescens*

Cautions: Not to be used as single herb but only in a
formula or under direction of a qualified health
professional. The herb/leaf is nontoxic but overdose by the
fruit causes vomiting and diarrhea and can include muscular
spasms to the point of convulsions, nausea and respiratory
difficulty.[35] Do not exceed recommended dose. [3]
Contraindications: C/I in protein hypersensitivity (contains
toxic lectins) and chronic-progressive infections such as
tuberculosis and AIDS. [3]
Drug Interactions: N/A

Motherwort- *Leonurus cardiaca*

No health hazards or side effects recorded with proper use. [67]
Cautions: overdose over 3.0 g may cause diarrhea, uterine
bleeding, and stomach irritation. [3]
Contraindications: C/I in pregnancy (emmenagogue,
uterine stimulant). [3]
Drug Interaction
Because of sedative activity use may potentiate
antidepressant drugs. [43]

Mugwort-*Artemesia vulgaris*

No health hazards or side effects recorded with proper use. [67]
Cautions: Wormwood products in US required to be free of
thujone, an oil that is a neurotoxin.
Contraindications: C/I in pregnancy. [3, 6] Not appropriate
for use if duodenal ulcers present. [4]
Drug Interaction: N/A

Muira Pauma-*Ptychopetulum olacoides*

No health hazards or side effects recorded with proper use. [67]
Caution: N/A
Contradiction: C/I in pregnancy and lactation.
Drug Interaction
Hormonal components identified [12, 54] indicating potential

interaction with sex hormone treatment. [7]

Contains tannins, [12] therefore in large frequent doses may decrease absorption of iron, codeine, ephedrine, pseudoephedrine, theophylline and aminophylline. [8, 9, 11, 13]

Mullein - *Verbascum olympicum*

No health hazards or side effects recorded with proper use. [67]

Myrrh- *Commiphora molmol*

No health hazards or side effects recorded with proper use. [67]
Caution: The AHPA editors note irritation to kidneys and diarrhea resulting from doses of over 2.0-4.0 grams. [3]
Contraindication: C/I in pregnancy [3, 6] and in "excessive uterine bleeding." [3]

Neem Leaves - *Azadirachta alba*

No health hazards or side effects recorded with proper use. [67]
Caution: Leaf fraction stated to delay blood clotting time [14]
Contraindication: C/I with anti-coagulant therapy as may potentiate or with coagulant therapy with surgery as it will antagonize.

Nettle (Stinging) - *Urtica dioica*

No health hazards or side effects recorded with proper use. [67]
Caution: Mild stomach irritation rarely occurs with intake.
Contraindication: Patients who are allergic to stinging nettles. Brinker C/Is in pregnancy 6 but other sources do not. [1, 3]
Drug Interaction: Listed as a hypoglycemic [6] and therefore may interact diabetic medication. [7]

Night Blooming Cereus - *Cereus grandiflorus*

No health hazards or side effects recorded with proper use. [67]
Cautions: Use in formula only not as single herb unless with guidance with qualified professional. Intake of fresh juice causes itching on skin.
Contraindications: Brinker cautions in hypertension or over-active heart conditions, due to cardioactive properties. [6] Potential side effects of the tincture in large doses include: gastric irritation, mental confusion, hallucination, slight delirium, quickened pulse, constrictive headache.   The importance of proper dose is emphasized. [15]
Drug Interaction
No information.

Oat Seed (Wild Milky) -*Avena sativa*

No health hazards or side effects recorded with proper use. [67]
Cautions: None found.

Olive Leaf-*Olea europaea*

Caution: No reported cautions.
Contraindication: pregnancy and lactation.
Drug Interaction:
May potentiate blood pressure lowering effects. [71]

Oregano Essential Oil-*Origanum vulgare*

Caution: Internal use of essential oils should be limited to a maximum of 4 weeks. In chronic cases allow 2 weeks break between courses for 1 week of treatment. [16]
Contraindication: Do not use during pregnancy.
Drug Interaction
No information.

Oregon Grape-*Berberis aquifolium* (Mahonia aquifolium)

No health hazards or side effects recorded with proper use. [67]
Caution: No information.
Contraindication: C/I in pregnancy due to berberine content [3] C/I in bile duct obstruction, acute live disease, infected gall bladder and liver cancer. [4]
Drug Interaction
There are mixed results reported when mixing berberine containing plants with Doxycline and Tetracycline-type antibiotics. More information is needed. [11, 13]

Osha-*Ligusticum porteri*

Caution: No information.
Contraindication: C/I in pregnancy. [3]
Drug Interaction: Contains phytosterols [37] and thus use may interfere with sex hormone treatment, including oral contraceptives. [7]

Passionflower-*Passiflora incarnata*

No health hazards or side effects recorded with proper use. [67]
Caution: May cause depressant effect to skeletal and smooth muscle, and decrease blood pressure. [36]
Contraindication: C/I in pregnancy. [6]
Drug Interaction
Because of sedative activity use may potentiate antidepressant drugs. Maltol, a sedative component of

Passiflora, is known to increase sleeping time when combined with hexobarbital. [6]

Pau D'Arco-*Tabebua impetiginosa*

Caution: N/A
Contraindication: N/A
Drug Interaction
N/A

Peppermint-*Mentha piperita*

No health hazards recorded with proper use. [67]
Caution: Commission E recommends consultation with a practitioner before using with gallstones. [1]
Contraindication: Gallstone carriers often experience colicky pain with use. C/I in gallstones and hiatal hernia (upper sphincter of stomach) which causes a relaxation of the sphincter aggravating the symptoms of stomach pain. [6 12, 19]
DeSmet states that no data on peppermint or spearmint oil was recovered from the literature suggesting peppermint is safe during pregnancy or lactation. [19]

Peppermint Oil- *Mentha piperita*

Caution: Some GI irritation is reported. Internal use of essential oils should be limited to a maximum of 4 weeks. In chronic cases allow 2 weeks break between courses for 1 week of treatment. [31] "The no effect level for peppermint oil for humans was calculated at 10 mg/kg per day." Rare allergic reactions are reported. Excessive intake of oil has resulted in 2 cases of muscle fibrillation (twitching), in both cases reduction of intake resulted in a reversal of the condition. [19]
Contraindications: Do not use essential oils internally during pregnancy.
Drug Interaction
N/A

Black Catnip*Phyllanthus amarus*-

No health hazards or side effects recorded with proper use. [67]
Caution: Very bitter herb.
Contraindication: N/A
Drug Interaction
N/A

Pipsissewa- *Chimaphila umbellata*

No health hazards or side effects recorded with proper use. [67]

Caution: Long term use is limited because of hydroxyquinone glycoside, chimaphilin (a major constituent of Pipsissewa), is shown to be a moderate contact sensitizer causing occasional contact dermatitis.[2955]

Moore states that when used for "short-or long-term skin eruptions, the first two or three cups a day may temporarily aggravate but then considerably shorten the duration of the symptoms." [26]

Contraindication: N/A
Drug Interaction
N/A

Plantain-*Plantago lanceolata*

No health hazards or side effects recorded with proper use. [67]
Caution: N/A
Contraindication: N/A
Drug Interaction
N/A

Pleurisy Root-*Asclepias tuberosa*

No health hazards or side effects recorded with proper use. [67]
Caution: May cause nausea, vomiting and diarrhea. [3,43]
Contraindication: C/I in pregnancy [3,6,43] and in lactation. [43]
Drug Interaction: Caution may potentiate cardiac drug therapy, due to presence of cardiac glycosides. [43]

Poke Root-*Phytolacca americana*

Caution/Toxic: This herb is not to be used as a single remedy. It should only be used in low dosage as a part of a formula and the duration of the use of the formula should be limited.

AHPA labeling recommendations are "To be used only under the supervision of an expert qualified in the appropriate use of this substance." [3] Dosage guidelines must be adhered to. Overdose commonly involves nausea, protracted vomiting, sometimes with blood, profuse sweating, severe abdominal cramps and pain, diarrhea, headache, dizziness and tachycardia. All recently described patients recovered within 24-48 hours, often with the aid of supportive care. [15,20]
Contraindication: C/I in pregnancy and lactation. [43]

Prickly Ash-*Xanthoxylum clava-herculis*

Caution: Use caution with stomach or intestinal ulcers or

intestinal inflammation due to mucosal irritation.
Contraindication: In pregnancy and lactation, due to
emmenagogue effect and irritating qualities.[1,2]
Drug Interaction
Possible interaction with antacids (antagonism, increased
mucosal irritation) With general medication, there is
potential increased absorption form mucosal surfaces and
increased metabolism of drug. [3]

Propolis Resin

Caution: If bee allergy or multiple pollen allergies should
start with small testing dosage.
Contraindication: None found.
Drug Interaction
None found.

Pygeum-*Pygeum africanum*

Caution: None found.
Contraindication: None found.
Drug Interaction
Hormonal activity decreases testosterone and cholesterol in
prostate while raising adrenal hormones. [59] Potential
interference with sex hormone therapy.[7]

Quassia-*Picaraena excelsa*

No health hazards or side effects recorded with proper use. [67]
Caution: Occasional mild dizziness has been reported with
single herb use. [18]
Contraindication: In pregnancy.
Drug Interaction
None found.

Rauwolfia vomitoria and spp.

Caution: This herb has a potential for Toxicity: It should
only be used as a single herb by herbal specialists only.
Otherwise it should only be used in low dosage as a part of
a formula and the duration of the use of the formula should
be limited. Its indication in hypertension is to lower blood
pressure and slow the heart rate via decreased catacolamine.
It acts as a characteristic central depressant and sedative.
Use with caution in depression. Weiss pointedly remarks
that Rauwolfia's action has a specific toxic effect with long-
term large dose use, which may "develop into genuine
melancholia ...with a tranquilizing effect like Valium". All
in all, Weiss concludes that Rauwolfia is one of the most

gentle and effective agents for hypertension. He points out it is best to start with small doses and titrate up. If sedation effects become "too powerful" reduce the dose again. [2] Side effects are minimal but possible at the small to medium dose and also include nasal congestion, fatigue and erectile dysfunction. [2]

Contraindication: C/I in pregnancy, lactation, depression, ulceration and pheochromocytoma. [6 67]

Drug Interaction: With digitalis and other heart medications it severely lowers the heart rate. Greatly increase the impairment with alcohol. May potentiate the effect of medications for anxiety and neuroleptic conditions.

Red Clover-*Trifolium pratense*

No health hazards or side effects recorded with proper use. [67]
Caution: contains a number of estrogen like components.
Contraindication: C/I in pregnancy. [3]
Drug Interaction
Avoid use for 7-14 days prior to surgery. Coumarin-containing plant and thus C/I with anti-coagulant or coagulant therapy. [6] There are a number of hormonally active components [12] indicating a potential interaction with sex hormone treatment, including oral contraceptives. [7] Read Anticoagulant and Antiplatelet properties of herbs in this chapter.

Red Root-*Ceonothus americanus*

No health hazards or side effects recorded with proper use. [67]
Caution: Astringent due to high tannin content.
Contraindication: C/I in pregnancy. [3]
Drug Interaction
Contains tannins, therefore in large doses may decrease absorption of iron, codeine, ephedrine, pseudoephedrine, theophylline and aminophylline. [8, 9, 11, 13]

Red Raspberry Leaf-*Rubus idaeus*

No health hazards or side effects recorded with proper use. [67]
Cautions: None found. Often recommended in the last month of pregnancy to prepare for childbirth.
Contraindication: N/A
Drug Interactions: N/A

Reishi Mushroom-*Ganoderma lucidum*

Caution: Rare side effects, dryness of mucous membranes,

stomach upset. Nosebleed and bloody stools noted after heavy and continuous use for 3-6 months due to blood thinning effect. [3]

Contraindication: N/A

Drug Interactions: Simultaneous use of herbs that have anticoagulant or antiplatelet activity can theoretically increase the risk of bleeding in some people. Simultaneous use with herbs that lower blood pressure might produce hypotension. [68]

Rosemary-*Rosmarinus officinalis* (the following C/I apply to therapeutic doses)

No health hazards or side effects recorded with proper use. [67]

Caution: Overdose using very large quantities for purpose of miscarriage can lead to coma spasm, vomiting and death.

Contraindication: C/I in pregnancy due to uterine stimulation and abortifacient properties. [3, 6]

Drug Interactions

No information.

Sage-*Salvia officinalis* (the following C/I apply to therapeutic doses)

No health hazards or side effects recorded with proper use. [67]

Caution: Not for long-term use. Do not exceed recommended dose. [3, 20, 43]

Sage Essential Oil is toxic and is not used internally, it contains 35-50 % thujone (a toxic ketone). [43]

Contraindication: C/I in pregnancy, used traditionally to reduce lactation 3 which would signify a C/I for desired lactation.

Drug Interactions

May interfere with hypoglycemic therapy, anti-convulsant therapy and may potentiate sedative drugs. [43]

Contains tannins, therefore in large doses may decrease absorption of iron, codeine, ephedrine, pseudoephedrine, theophylline and aminophylline. [9, 11, 13]

Sarsaparilla-*Smilax officinalis, spp.*

Cautions: can cause gastrointestinal irritation due to saponins).

Avoid confusion with Indian or false sarsaparilla (Hemidesmus indicus). [67]

Contraindications: C/I in Pregnancy. [67]

Drug Interaction

Sarsaparilla can increase digitalis absorption potentiating its effect. Has mild hormonal properties and thus may interfere with sex hormone therapy.[7]

Saw Palmetto-*Serenoa repens*

No health hazards or side effects recorded with proper use. [67]
Caution: Commission E reports rare and mild stomach problems as a side effect and recommends regular physician visits when treating enlarged prostate. [1]
Contraindication: C/I in pregnancy and lactation. Long-term and large dose toxicology studies on rats resulted in no negative effects and had no influence on fertility. [4]
Drug Interaction
Patients with hormone sensitive cancers should discuss usage with physician. Hormonal properties, and thus may interfere with sex hormone therapy, including oral contraceptives.[7]

Schizandra chinensis

No health hazards or side effects recorded with proper use. [67]
Caution: Rare side effects of appetite suppression stomach upset and hives. [1]
Contraindication: N/A
Drug Interaction
N/A

Sheep Sorrel-*Rumex acetosella*

No health hazards or side effects recorded with proper use. [67]
Caution: Only a very large amount of leaves eaten can create an oxalate poisoning. Use cautiously if a history of kidney stones is present, due to oxalates. [3]
Contraindication: N/A
Drug Interaction
Contains tannins, therefore in large doses may decrease absorption of iron, codeine, ephedrine, pseudoephedrine, theophylline and aminophylline. [9, 11, 13]

Skullcap-*Scutellaria lateriflora*

No health hazards or side effects recorded with proper use. [67]
Caution: Overdoses of the tincture cause giddiness, stupor, confusion of mind, twitching of the limbs, intermission of the pulse and other symptoms indicative of epilepsy, for which in diluted strength and small doses it has been

successfully given." [32]
Contraindication: Sedative effect could aggravate depression.
Drug Interaction
Because of sedative activity, [4] use may potentiate anxiety drugs or antagonize antidepressant drugs. [7]

Chinese Skullcap-*Scutellaria baicalensis*

Caution: N/A
Contraindication: N/A
Drug interactions: N/A

Slippery Elm-*Ulmus rubra*

No health hazards or side effects recorded with proper use. [67]
Caution: Mucilages in general are C/I in "bronchial and catarrhal conditions." [4]
Contraindication: N/A
Drug interactions: N/A

Spearmint-*Mentha spicata*

No health hazards recorded with proper use. [67]
Caution: Commission E recommends consultation with a practitioner before using with gallstones. [1]
Contraindication: Gallstone carriers often experience colicky pain with use. C/I in gallstones and hiatal hernia (upper sphincter of stomach) which causes a relaxation of the sphincter aggravating the symptoms of stomach pain. [6,12,19]
DeSmet states that no data on peppermint or spearmint oil was recovered from the literature suggesting spearmint is safe during pregnancy or lactation. [19]
Drug interactions: N/A

Spilanthes acmella

Caution: N/A
Contraindication: N/A
Drug interactions: N/A

Squawvine-*Mitchella repens*

Caution: Long history of use, no cautions reported at therapeutic dosages. [72]
Contraindication: Pregnancy (abortifacient) and lactation (insufficient information)
Drug Interaction:
No reported interactions.

St. John's Wort-*Hypericum perforatum*

Caution: Fair-skinned [and immune-compromised] individuals should avoid excessive exposure to the sun while taking, due to the slight risk of photosensitization. [1, 3]

Contraindication: Brinker C/I in pregnancy 6 although other sources do not share this concern. [1, 3, 4]

Drug Interaction

As compared with pharmaceutical antidepressants, Hypericum is found to be as effective with far fewer and less serious side effects. [64] May interact with tricyclic antidepressants, selective seratonin reuptake inhibitors (SSRIs), and other kinds of anti-depressant medications. Use together only under a physician's guidance.[8, 13] Concerns were once raised about potential interaction with MAOI therapy, due to some preliminary research indicating MAOI activity. [3] However, subsequent research shows little to no evidence of MAOI activity and the C/I is not considered relevant.1 C/I with photosensitizing drugs like piroxicam or tetracycline hydrochloride. [8] Recent research has shown an increase in induction of CYP3A4 of the cytochrome P450 pathway. This indicates that Hypericum could interfere with even more pharmaceuticals than previously thought. 65 Bergner lists potentially serious drug interactions with an AIDS drug (indinavir) and the post heart transplant anti-rejection drug (cyclosporin). [66]

Stillingia-*Stillingia sylvatica*

Cautions: This herb is not used as a single remedy but is used in a small to moderate dosage in formula's. Fresh root contains a caustic latex and may be irritating to mucosa.[3] Ellingwood claimed that large doses would increase cardiac activity; cause excessive bronchial secretion, vomiting and bilious purging; cause a peculiar GI burning sensation; and exhaustion. [33]

Contraindication: C/I during lactation.

Drug Interaction

Contains tannins, therefore in large doses may decrease absorption of iron, codeine, ephedrine, pseudoephedrine, theophylline and aminophylline. [9, 11, 13]

Suma-*Pfaffia paniculata*

No health hazards recorded with proper use. [3]

Cautions: Inhalation of powdered root is known to cause

"occupational asthma." [68]
Contraindication: N/A
Drug Interaction
Immunostimulants are contraindicated with immunosuppressants such as Cyclophosphamide for organ transplants. Hormonal properties, and thus may interfere with sex hormone therapy, including oral contraceptives.[7, 8, 69]

Thuja-*Thuja occidentalis*

Caution: Toxic due to thujone content unless eliminated during processing. This herb is not used internally as a single herb although it may safely be used in small dosage in a formula. Not for long term use; do not exceed recommended dose...Should be taken internally only occasionally. [3]

Overdose symptoms from use of large dose as an abortifacient are vomiting, queasiness, painful diarrhea, and mucous membrane hemorrhaging. [67]

Contraindication: C/I in pregnancy (abortifacient) and in lactation. [3, 39]

Drug Interactions: N/A

Thyme-*Thymus vulgaris*

No health hazards or side effects recorded with proper use. [67]

Caution: Low potential for sensitization. [67]

Contraindication: C/I in pregnancy. [6] King's lists as an emmenagogue. [15]

Drug Interactions: N/A

Thyme Essential Oil-*Thymus vulgaris*

Caution: Internal use of essential oils should be limited to a maximum of 4 weeks. In chronic cases allow 2 weeks break between courses for 1 week of treatment. [16]

Contraindication: C/I in pregnancy.

Drug Interactions: N/A

Turkey Rhubarb-*Rheum palmatum*

Caution: Anthroquinone containing laxatives. Spasmodic stomach and abdominal symptoms can occur as a side effect to its purgative action on the bowel. Use caution if history of kidney stones is present. Do not use in excess of 8-10 days. [3] Significant loss of electrolytes via diarrhea can occur causing symptoms of low potassium. Not recommended as an individual herb but to be used in a formula for a short time. Recommended AHPA labeling: "Do not use this product if

you have abdominal pain or diarrhea. Consult a health care provider prior to use if you are pregnant or nursing. Discontinue use in the event of diarrhea or watery stools. Do not exceed recommended dose. Not for long-term use." [3]
Contraindication: C/I in intestinal inflammatory conditions, obstruction of the intestines, and abdominal pain of unknown origin. Not for children under 12. [3]
Drug Interactions:
Contains anthraquinones and anthraquinone glycosides.[19] Read anthroquinone containing laxatives in this chapter.

Turmeric-*Curcuma longa*

No health hazards or side effects recorded with proper use. [67]
Cautions: none.
Contraindication: C/I with bile duct obstruction, gallstones, stomach ulcers or hyperacidity. [1,3,6] Commission E recommends consultation with a physician for use in gallstones. 1 C/I in pregnancy and lactation. [3]
Drug Interactions
May potentiate the effect of coumadin and aspirin as blood thinning agents causing bleeding problems. [4] Please refer to anticoagulant section of this chapter.

Usnea-*Usnea barbata*

No health hazards or side effects recorded with proper use. [67]
Cautions: N/A The LD50 is reported to be 22.53 g/kg which is a very safe herb. [59]
Contraindications: N/A
Drug Interactions
N/A

Uva Ursi-*Arctostaphylos uva ursi*

Cautions: Classified as a GI irritant due to large tannin content. [3] Large doses may lead to nausea and vomiting. [22] Liver damage has occurred with long term use especially in children. See a practitioner for guidance on long-term use.
Contraindication: C/I pregnancy, lactation and children under 12. C/I in kidney disorders, digestive irritation, with acidic urine or with remedies which produce acidic urine (i.e. cranberry juice). [3]
Drug Interaction
Contains 15-20% tannins, therefore in large doses may decrease absorption of iron, codeine, ephedrine, pseudoephedrine, theophylline and aminophylline. [9,11,13]

Valerian-*Valeriana officinalis*

Cautions: Valepotriates in Valerian are toxic, but they are so unstable as to degrade quickly in to less toxic metabolites and are poorly absorbed. [3, 21] Despite the valepotriates, acute toxicity is considered to be very low. Following long term use headaches, restless ness and insomnia may appear. More research is needed. [21]

Contraindications: C/I in pregnancy and lactation.

Drug Interaction

May potentiate barbituates. [8] Possible enhanced sedative effects when combined with Alpha-blockers. [4] Because of sedative activity [22] use may potentiate antianxiety, analgesic and antiepileptic medications but may antagonize antidepressant drugs.[7]

Wild Cherry-*Prunus serotina*

No health hazards or side effects recorded with proper use. [67]

Cautions: "Not for long-term use; do not exceed recommended dose." [3] King's states that Wild Cherry is "best adapted to chronic troubles." [15]

Contraindication: C/I in pregnancy. [6]

Drug Interaction

Sedative action [15, 33] a possible potentiation of hypnotics, anxiolytics, and antagonism to antidepressant drugs. Duke lists P-coumaric acid [12] which indicates possible interaction with anti-coagulants. [7]

Wild Indigo-*Baptisia tinctoria*

No health hazards or side effects recorded with proper use. [67]

Caution: Overdoses (like 30 gm.) are toxic and can cause vomiting and diarrhea. [3]

Quinolizidine alkaloids can produce toxicity when used long term, and cause gastrointestinal symptoms with high doses. [6]

Contraindication: C/I in pregnancy. As a single remedy, not for long-term use except under the supervision of a qualified practitioner.

Drug Interaction

C/I with coumarin pharmaceuticals and other anti-coagulants, due to coumarin constituents. [27]

Wild Yam-*Dioscorea villosa*

No health hazards or side effects recorded with proper use. [67]

Caution: Said to produce vomiting in "large doses" of the

tincture.[15] 2-10 ml of tincture is given as a dose by Willard, with 2-4 ml of fluid extract. [29]

Contraindication: C/I in pregnancy and lactation. Stimulates the excretion of bile so would be contraindicated in obstruction of the bile ducts.

Drug Interaction: diosgenin in wild Yam has a potentiation of estrogen medications. It also decreases the anti-inflammatory effect of indomethacin by increasing the excretion.[67]

Willow-*Salix species*

No health hazards or side effects recorded with proper use. [67]

Caution: Avoid intake if salicylate sensitivity exists.[1,22]

Contraindication: C/I in pregnancy and lactation

Drug Interaction

Contains salicylates and tannins [3] thus, C/I with salicylate-containing pharmaceuticals, such as aspirin and Pepto-Bismol (Bismuth subsalicylate).[13] Contains tannins, therefore in large doses may decrease absorption of iron, codeine, ephedrine, pseudoephedrine, theophylline and aminophylline. [8,9,11,13]

Witch Hazel-*Hamamelis virgiana*

No health hazards or side effects recorded with proper use. [67]

Caution: Reported side effects are rare and include stomach irritation and contact dermatitis (topical application).[3,4]

Contraindication: none found.

Drug Interaction

Contains tannins, [12] therefore in large doses may decrease absorption of iron, [8] codeine, ephedrine, pseudoephedrine, theophylline and aminophylline. [9,11,13]

Wormwood-*Artemesia annua and A. absynthium*

Cautions: Wormwood naturally contains thujone, which is required to be taken out in all U.S. products. The essential oil should not be used internally.

Contraindications: C/I in pregnancy, and in stomach or intestinal ulcers (irritating to GI tract) [3,6]

Drug Interaction

Contains coumarins [12] and thus C/I with anti-coagulants. [7] Contains tannins, up to 12%[12] therefore in large doses may decrease absorption of iron, codeine, ephedrine, pseudoephedrine, theophylline and aminophylline. [8,9,11,13] Thujone containing herbs are C/I with seizure medication as it lowers the seizure threshold.

Yellow Dock-*Rumex crispus*

No health hazards or side effects recorded with proper use. [67]
Cautions: Despite some anthraquinones present, there is a mild laxative effect at most. Due to oxalates present, use caution if there is a history of kidney stones.[3]
Contraindications: C/I pregnancy and lactation.
Drug Interaction
N/A

Yerba Santa-*Eriodictyon californicum*

No health hazards or side effects recorded with proper use. [67]
Cautions: N/A
Contraindications: N/A
Drug Interaction
N/A

Yohimbe- *Corynanthe yohimbe*

Cautions: Yohimbine increases blood pressure, heart rate, and motor activity; is a central nervous system stimulant; and may cause anxiety. Caution should be used in cases of depression, anxiety, or other psychiatric disorders. Not recommended for excessive or long-term use. [22, 3]
Contraindications: Include heart disease, high blood pressure, chest pain, glaucoma, pregnancy, children, chronic inflammation of the sexual organs or prostate, liver and kidney disease. [22, 3]
Drug Interaction
A number of theoretical drug interactions exist: with large amounts of caffeine-containing herbs and ephedra (increased risk of hypertensive crisis), monoamine oxidase inhibiting pharmaceuticals, alpha 2-adrenergic blocking pharmaceuticals, antihypertensives, beta-blockers, Clonidine, Guanabenz, naloxone, phenothiazines, sympathomimetics, and tricyclic antidepressants. [68, 3, 13]

Yucca spp.

No health hazards or side effects recorded with proper use. [43]
Cautions: Side effects include G/I disturbances and mucous membrane irritation. [68]
Contraindications: N/A
Drug Interaction
N/A

MASTER REFERENCE LIST

1. Blumenthal M. *et al.* Ed. *The Complete German Commission E Monographs.* Austin: American Botanical Council; 1998.

2. Weiss RF. *Herbal Medicine.* Beaconsfield: Beaconsfield Pub Ltd; 1988.

3. McGuffin M, *et al.* Ed. *AHPA's Botanical Safety Handbook.* Boca Raton: CRC Press; 1997.

4. Bone K and Mills S. *Principles and Practice of Phytotherapy.* Edinburgh: Churchill Livingstone; 2000.

5. Bone K. Autoimmune Disease: A Phytotherapeutic Perspective. *Townsend Let.* 1999: Aug/Sept; 94-98.

6. Brinker F. *Herb Contraindications and Drug Interactions.* Sandy: Eclectic Inst; 1997.

7. Newall C and Phillipson JD. "Interactions of Herbs with Other Medicines." Online. Internet. [4/26/00]. Available WWW: http://www.ex.ac.uk/phytonet/phytojournal/

8. Miller L. Herbal Medicinals: Selected Clinical Consideration Focusing on Known or Potential Drug-Herb Interactions. *Arch Intern Med.* 1998; 158: 2200-11.

9. Brown D. Common Drugs and Their Potential Interactions with Herbs or Nutrients. *HNR.* 1999; 6(2): 124-41.

10. Brown D. Common Drugs and Their Potential Interactions with Herbs or Nutrients. *HNR.* 1999; 6(3): 209-22.

11. Brown D. Common Drugs and Their Potential Interactions with Herbs or Nutrients. *HNR.* 1999; 6(4): 282-94.

12. Duke J. Dr. Duke's Phytochemical and Ethnobotanical Databases. 29 September 1998. Online. Internet. [9/29/98]. Available WWW: http://www.ars-grin.gov/cgi-bin/duke/activity.pl

13. Healthnotes. "Drug Interactions Summary." 1999. Online. Internet. [5/9/00]. Available WWW: http://www.enutrition.com/healthnotes/

14. Kapoor LD. *Handbook for Ayurvedic Medicinal Plants.* Boca Raton: CRC Press; 1990.

15. Felter HW and Lloyd JU. *King's American Dispensatory.* Portland: Eclectic Med. Pub; 1983 (orig 1898).

16. Tisserand RB. *The Art of Aromatherapy.* NY: Destiny Books; 1977.

17. Snow JM. Coleus forskohlii Willd. (Lamiaceae). PJBM. 1995 Autumn; 1(2): 39-42.

18. Leung A and Foster S. *Encylclopedia of Common Natural Ingredients.* NY: Wiley; 1996.

19. DeSmet PAGM. *Adverse Effects of Herbal Drugs. Vol 1.* Berlin: Springer-Verlag; 1993.

20. DeSmet PAGM. *Adverse Effects of Herbal Drugs. Vol 2.* Berlin: Springer-Verlag; 1993.

21. DeSmet PAGM. *Adverse Effects of Herbal Drugs. Vol 3.* Berlin: Springer-Verlag; 1993.

22. Bradley P. Ed. *British Herbal Compendium Vol 1.* Dorset: British Herbal Med Assoc.; 1992.

23. Bergner P. "Herb-drug Interactions." Medical Herbalism. 1997. Online. Internet. [5/20/99]. Available WWW: http://medherb.com/92DRGHRB.HTM

24. Bradley P. Ed. *British Herbal Compendium Vol 1.* Dorset: British Herbal Med Assoc.; 1992.

25. Hudson T. *A Woman's Guide to Herbal Care.* Brevard: Herbal Res Pub; 1998.

26. Moore M. *Medicinal Plants of the Mountain West.* Santa Fe: Museum of NM Press; 1979.

27. Meletus CD and Jacobs T. *Interactions between Drugs and Natural Medicines.* Sandy: Eclectic Med Pub; 1999.

28. Motley TJ. The Ethnobotany of Sweet Flag, Acorus calamus (Araceae). *Economic Botany.* 1995; 48(4): 397-412.

29. Willard T. *Wild Rose Scientific Herbal.* Alberta: Wild Rose College of Nat Healing.; 1991.

30. Hoffman D. *The Holistic Herbal.* Ca: Element Books, 1988.

31. Tisserand RB. *The Art of Aromatherapy.* NY: Destiny Books; 1977.

32. Grieves M. *A Modern Herbal.* Vol 2. NY: Dover; 1971 (orig. 1931).

33. Ellingwood F. *American Materia Medica, Therapeutics and Pharmacognosy.* Portland: Eclectic Med Pub, 1985.

34. Lyle TJ. *Physio-Medical Therapeutics, Materia Medica and Pharmacy.* London: National Assoc of Med Herbalists, 1932 (orig. 1897).

35. Brinker F. "Viscum flavescens, V. album." From *Eclectic Dispensatory of Botanical Therapeutics,* vol. II. Sandy: Eclectic Med Pub; 1993.

36. Brooks S. ed. Botanical Toxicology. *Protocol J. Bot Med.* 1995; 1(1): 147-158.

37. Boon H and Smith M. *The Botanical Pharmacy.* Quebec: Quarry health Books, 1999.

38. Felter HW. *The Eclectic Materia Medica, Pharmacology, and Therapeutics.* Portland: Eclectic Med Pub, 1985.

39. Bartram T. *Encyclopedia of Herbal Medicine.* Dorset: Grace Pub, 1995.

40. Huang KC. *The Pharmacology of Chinese Herbs.* Boca Raton: CRC Press;1993.

41. Auf'mkolk M, *et al.* Inhibition by certain plant extracts of the binding and adenylate cyclase stimulatory effect of bovine thyrotropin in human thyroid membranes. *Endocrinology.* 1984 Aug; 115(2): 527-34.

42. Lindner S. Withania somnifera. *Aust J of Med Herbalism.* 1996; 8(3): 78-82.

43. Newall C, *et al. Herbal Medicines:A Guide for Health-Care Professionals.* London: Pharmaceutical Press, 1996.

44. Duke J and Vasques R. *Amazonian Ethnobotanical Dictionary.* Boca Raton: CRC Press; 1994.

45. Anonymous. Cat's Claw. *The Lawrence Review of Natural Products.* 1996 Apr; 1-3.

46. Snow J. *Vitex agnus-castus* L. (Verbenaceae). *Prot J Bot Med.* 1996; 1(4): 20-23.

47. Bensky D and Gamble A. *Chinese Herbal Medicine Materia Medica.* Seattle:Eastland Press, 1986.

48. Reynolds J ed. *Martindale: The Extra Pharmacopeoeia.* London: Pharmaceutical Press; 1993.

49. Wren RC. *Potter's New Cyclopaedia of Botanical Drugs and Preparations.* Great Britain: CW Daniel, 1988.

50. Anonymous. Dong Quai. *The Lawrence Review of Natural Products.* 1990 April.

51. Pederson M. *Nutritional Herbology.* Indiana: Whitman, 1995.

52. Zhu DPQ. Dong Quai. *Am J of Chinese Med.* 1987; XV(3-4), 117-125.

53. McQuade-Crawford A. *Herbal Remedies for Women.* Rocklin: Prima Pub, 1997.

54. Anonymous. "Muira Pauma." Online. Internet. [9/1/00]. Available WWW: http://www.rain-tree.com/muirapuama.htm

55. Hausen BM and Schiedermair I. The sensitizing capacity of chimaphilin, a naturally-occurring quinone. *Contact Dermatitis.* 1988; 19(3): 180-3.

56. Baldo BA, *et al.* Allergens from plantain (*Plantago lanceolata*). Studies with pollen and plant extracts. *Int Arch Allergy Appl Immunol.* 1982; 68(4): 295-304.

57. Morgan MS, *et al.* English plantain and psyllium: lack of cross-allergenicity by crossed immunoelectrophoresis. *Ann Allergy Asthma Immunol.* 1995 Octr; 75(4): 351-9.

58. Guillemain J, *et al.* Neurodepressive effects of the essential oil of Lavandula angustifolia Mill. *Ann Pharm Fr.* 1989; 47(6): 337-43.

59. Dobrescu D, *et al.* Contributions to the complex study of some lichens-Usnea genus. Pharmacolgical studies on *Usnea barbata* and *Usnea hirta* species. *Rom J Physiol.* 1993 Jan-Jun; 30(1-2): 101-7.

60. Bernardi, et. al. Effects of a prolonged ingestion of graded doses of licorice by healthy volunteers. *Life Sciences.* 1994; 55(11): 863-72.

61. Farese, Jr. et. al. Licorice-induced hypermineralocorticoidism. New Eng J Med. 1991; 325(17): 1223-27.

62. Takeda, et. al. Prolonged Pseudoaldosteronism Induced by Glycyrrhizin. *Endocrinol Japon.* 1979; 26(5): 541-7.

63. Stanford JL, *et al.* Rauwolfia use and breast cancer: a case-control study. *J Natl Cancer Inst.* 1986 May; 76 (5): 817-22.

64. Josey ES and Tackett RL. St. John's Wort: a new alternative for depression? *Int J Clin Pharmacol Ther.* 1999 Mar; 37(3): 111-9.

65. Moore L, *et al.* St. John's Wort induces hepatic drug metabolism through activation of the pregnane X receptor. Published online before print June 13, 2000, 10.1073/pnas.130155097; *Proc Nat Acad Sci USA.* 2000 June 20; 97(13): 7500-7502.

66. Bergner P. "Hypericum, Drug Interactions, and Liver Effects." 2000. Online. Internet. [10/25/00]. Available WWW: http://medherb.com/hypericum-drug-herb.html

67. Gruenwald J, et. al. PDR for Herbal Medicines. 2nd ed. Montvale, NJ: Medical Economics Company, Inc., 1998.

68. Natural Medicines Comprehensive Database, naturaldatabase.com, Stockton, Ca. 2001

69. Taylor L. "Suma." 1996. Online. Internet. [9/1/2000]. Available WWW: http://rain-tree.com/suma.htm

70. The Review of Natural Products by Facts and Comparisons. St. Louis, MO: Wolters Kluwer Co., 1999.

71. Cherif S, *et al.*,A clinical trial of a titrated Olea extract in the treatment of essential arterial hypertension. J Pharm Belg 1996 Mar-Apr;51(2):69-71.

72. Native American Indian Resources website. URL http://indy4.fdl.cc.mn.us/~isk/food/parttrib.html.

CHAPTER 10

FREQUENTLY ASKED QUESTIONS ON THE USE OF HERBAL EXTRACTS

1. How is dosage determined?

Dosages of liquid extracts are determined through two factors:

a. Consideration is given for the concentration of the extract

b. Consideration is given for the specific use of the extract

A third factor may mitigate the recommended dose and that is the weight and constitution of the individual using the herb. If an individual is heavier or has a more robust constitution the higher range of the suggested use may be consumed. Contrary if a person weighs less or has a more fragile constitution the lower range of the suggested use should be consumed. Please keep in mind that not all brands of extracts carry the same concentration. The recommended dosages suggested in this book are therapeutic dosages and are intended to deliver the therapeutic response. (Please see Chapter 3 in this book)

2. How long should I take an herbal extract?

The nature of the condition should determine the length of use of the herbal extract. If the condition is acute or is of a superficial nature, the extract may be used for a shorter period of time such as 1-3 weeks. If the condition is chronic or deeper than it is appropriate to use the extract for 3-4 months or longer. There are always exceptions and it is wise to always follow the recommendations provided on the label. Regardless of how long the extract is used please consider the following rule of thumb: If an extract is to be used for more than one week then take six days on and one day off. If an extract is used for more than six weeks then take six weeks on and one week off with a day off each week. If an extract is to be used for more than six months then take six months on and one month off with a day off each week. The periodic time off from using the herbal extract allows for the full benefit of the herb to be fully integrated into the constitution.

3. How do I recognize the quality and concentration of herbal extracts in the market?

Without standards set by regulatory authorities governing

quality and concentration, the quality and concentration of herbal products are really determined by the integrity (or lack of it) of the manufacturing companies. Here are the procedures that an herbal retailer or consumer should follow and questions that should be asked when establishing which brand to choose and use:

Establishing Quality of the Product:

❑ Does the manufacturer grow or purchase only certified organic and ecologically, wild-crafted and GMO free herbs?

❑ Are the herbs harvested at the peak of their therapeutic activity?

❑ Are test results available to show the bio-active integrity of the originating plant material?

❑ Is the bio-activity of the plant material tested before the product is harvested or purchased?

❑ Are microbial tests and heavy metal detection tests completed on all raw material purchased?

❑ Is the extraction methodology unique for each herb?

❑ Is the product manufactured under strict GMP (Good Manufacturing Practices) compliance guidelines following approved SOP's (Standard Operating Procedures)?

Establishing Concentration of the Product:

❑ What is the procedure used to insure that the products have a consistent level of bio-activity?

❑ Is every batch tested to insure concentration consistency ?

❑ Are the products concentrated utilizing "Full Spectrum Standardization"?

❑ What assurances are given so that the product meets or exceeds the stated label information?

Establishing Full Label Disclosure:

❑ Does the label disclose whether the herbs are certified organic or ecologically wildcrafted?

❑ Does the label disclose the latin binomial and part of the plant used in the product?

❑ Does the label disclose the amount of extract and/or the amount of known active ingredients?

❑ Does the label disclose all added solvents, excipients, fillers, binders, etc?

❑ Does the label disclose a legible lot number and best buy date?

❑ Does the label represent the required "Supplement Facts" Box accurately?

4. Why is there alcohol in herbal extracts?

Pure grain alcohol is used to prepare herbal extracts because it functions very well as a solvent and as a preservative. The properties of alcohol enable it to effectively mobilize the constituents that are active in plants from with the plants cell wall and bring them into solution. This is simply a process of pre-digesting the plant. In this way when the extract is ingested there is 100 % absorption and 100 % bioavailability. This is so important especially if one's digestive functions are impaired or one needs a response from the herbal preparation quickly. Liquid herbal extracts work quickly. Because they do not need to move through the first pass of the liver for digestion, they enter the bloodstream immediately and effect their receptor sites within the body within minutes after consumption. Pure grain alcohol also acts as a wonderful preservative. A liquid herbal extract will remain stable for over 5 years while crude herb capsules and tablets tend to degrade very quickly. Effectiveness of herbal tablets and capsules containing dry crude herbs is minimal.

5. How much alcohol am I consuming per dose when I take a liquid extract?

Very little indeed!! If an average dose of an herbal extract is 30-40 drops and the herbal preparation contains 50 % alcohol, then one is consuming 15-20 drops of alcohol with the herbal extractive matter miscible within it. This is simply much less alcohol ingested than if one were to eat a ripened piece of fruit (by virtue of the sugars in fruit that are converted to alcohol when the fruit is consumed). However if one has a background of alcohol sensitivity or cannot consume products with alcohol, then it is recommended that the alcohol-free liquid extracts or the alcohol-free liquid extracts in vegetable capsules (Liquid Phyto-Caps™) be used.

6. Are alcohol-free herbal extracts as concentrated as the alcohol extracts?

Not for all companies! In fact only the most reputable companies capable of extracting first with USP grain alcohol then distilling off the alcohol and testing the finished product with HPLC instruments can claim that the alcohol free products are as concentrated as the alcohol extracts. Many companies extract the herbs for their alcohol free products with vegetable glycerin. Unfortunately, vegetable glycerin is not a good solvent and cannot effectively extract the same constituents the grain alcohol can extract.

7. Can I combine several extracts or formulas and take them together?

Because herbal preparations have specific constituents that target specific receptor sites within the body, it is important that they be taken thoughtfully. Unless specifically indicated, it is best to take one herbal preparation apart from another by allowing at least twenty minutes to pass. Many herbs do combine well together and in fact are enhanced when combined together. Herbal compounds that are scientifically formulated enable the formula to produce a result that is specific and desirable. It takes much knowledge to properly combine herbal preparations together. When unsure whether two or more single herbs or preparations may be combined together, please refer to the information contained within this book, ask an herbal professional, or space each preparation by at least twenty minutes.

8. Can I use herbal extracts safely during pregnancy?

Although there are many herbs that are safe to use during pregnancy, it is recommended on all the information in this book that the herbs should not be used during pregnancy. We do this because we believe that if you are pregnant and wish to use herbs to maintain a strong and healthy pregnancy that you consult a naturopathic doctor, licensed herbalist or licensed holistic health practitioner qualified to guide you in the safe use of herbs during pregnancy.

9. Are there any herb/drug interactions that I should be concerned about when using herbs?

There certainly may be interactions between prescription drugs and herbs. We suggest that if you are currently using a prescription drug that you consult your medical doctor or a naturopathic physician before taking herbs. Throughout history and in cultures all over the world, herbs have been used safely as medicine. Herbal medicines have produced relatively few incidences of harm when used intelligently and as recommended. Also herbal medicines have a long history of producing effective results without the harmful side effects that prescriptive drugs produce. Please consult the information contained within Chapter 9.

10. What is the best way to take liquid herbal extracts?

There are several ways to consume liquid herbal extracts safely and effectively. What follows below is a summary of some of the ways to ingest liquids with the first being the very finest:

a. Add drops to a small amount of warm water.

b. Place drops directly into the mouth or under the tongue.

c. Add drops to a small amount of herbal tea such as peppermint or fennel.

d. Add drops to a small amount of diluted juice such as grape or apple juice.

e. Add drops to a vegetarian "00" capsule and swallow quickly before capsule dissolves with a small amount of warm water.

11. Can children use herbal extracts safely?

Yes! In fact liquids are the preferred method for children to consume medicinal remedies. Herbal extracts for children that have been clinically tested by naturopathic physicians have been shown to be remarkably effective. They are formulated to address specific aliments that children commonly experience and they taste great! They should not be sweetened with sugar like popular children's remedies may be, but rather they should be formulated with gentle and pleasant tasting herbs that children truly love. To learn more about herbs for children please read "A Parent's Guide to Children's Herbal Care" by Dr. Mary Bove.

12. What are Herbal Solutions for Healthy Living?

Herbal Solutions for Healthy Living is a unique line of herbal products formulated, developed, and manufactured for the herb market. These formulations utilize a patented Liquid Phyto-Cap™ technology, and address many of the lifestyle concerns experienced by many individuals who purchase herbal supplements today.

13. What are Liquid Phyto-Caps™?

Liquid Phyto-Caps™ represent a patented extraction technology that delivers a concentrated full spectrum alcohol-free liquid extract in a 100% vegetarian capsule. Because these products are concentrated and in full liquid solution, Liquid Phyto-Caps™ can offer you the superior bioavailability and faster absorption of a liquid delivery system, in the convenience of a vegetarian capsule.

14. Are Liquid Phyto-Caps™ concentrated enough?

Yes! In fact each capsule delivers 2-10 times the amount of dry herb equivalent derived from capsules containing powdered herb. This means that for every Liquid Phyto-Cap™ you derive 2-10 times more value when compared to herbal powders in capsules. And better yet they are already in an assimilable form so you will absorb more from each capsule when compared to herbal powders in capsules. Please note beneath the Supplement Facts Box on each label that the crude herb equivalent amount is specified.

15. Are Liquid Phyto-Caps™ Standardized?

Currently there are 34 items offered in this product line. There are 10 single herb products that are fully standardized utilizing Full Spectrum Standardization. There are 24 blended herbal formulas as well. In many of these formulas the primary active herbs are standardized utilizing the same Full Spectrum Standardization.

16. What does Full Spectrum Standardization mean?

Full Spectrum Standardization represents an extraction, concentration and analytical process utilizing only certified organic/ecologically wild-crafted herbs that are processed without the use of harsh non-ingestible solvents,* high heat, high vacuum, or other chemical processes that isolate the active constituents while discarding other constituents naturally occurring in the plant (considered by some companies to have no value). This process captures the wholeness of the herb while concentrating it in a way that maintains the natural balance of each plant's constituents.

17. Are certified organic herbs used to prepare Liquid

Phyto-Caps™?

Yes! In fact many of the herbs are grown utilizing organic methods on farms certified through Oregon Tilth. When an herb is not possible to cultivate, conscientious wild-crafters are employed to harvest those herbs in an ecologically responsible manner in each herbs natural protected habitat.

18. Are Liquid Phyto-Caps™ 100% Vegetarian?

Yes! Every product is encapsulated using a vegetable cellulose capsule. This technology is patented and represents an alcohol-free, non-oil base liquid extract in a vegetarian capsule. All other soft-gel capsules are made with animal gelatin and are made with an oil base that can be difficult for many individuals to digest.

* Commercial manufacturers of herbal products often use these solvents such as hexane, acetone, methanol, etc. to extract and purify their herbs. These solvents cause greater toxic wastes and air pollution to be generated as a consequence of herbal extraction than is necessary.

Index

B

C

D

H

I

N

O

S

T

U

V